T0384846

BLACK COUPLES THERAPY

Most research and couples therapy modalities tend to be normed on white European American couples and fail to include research on Black couples. This volume fills a void in the theory, research, and practice of couples therapy where clinicians have historically not been specifically trained to provide culturally responsive care when addressing the unique experiences and needs of Black couples. It aims to provide students, researchers, and allied mental health professionals with greater awareness, knowledge, and competency in working with Black couples. It assists therapists in developing a working alliance with Black couples and places an emphasis on cultivating environments that are instrumental to decreasing relationship distress and disconnection. *Black Couples Therapy* provides a comprehensive overview of the research and theory behind race and collective identity as well as romantic coupling, illustrated by examples of practice.

DR. YAMONTE COOPER is a scholar, author, professor of counseling, adjunct professor of clinical psychology, clinical director of the West Coast Sex Therapy Center, Licensed Professional Clinical Counselor (LPCC), and Certified Sex Therapist Supervisor (CST-S). As a Fulbright scholar, Dr. Cooper has exchanged best practices globally in career counseling and development.

DR. ERICA HOLMES is a licensed clinical psychologist, educator, author, speaker, and consultant. As executive director of Champion Counseling Center, associate program chair and director of the Trauma Specialization at Antioch University, and founder of HOMMs Consulting, she has provided psychotherapy, training, consultation, and research services to individuals and organizations for over twenty years.

BLACK COUPLES THERAPY

Clinical Theory and Practice

EDITED BY

YAMONTE COOPER

El Camino College

ERICA HOLMES

Antioch University

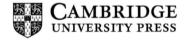

CAMBRIDGE
UNIVERSITY PRESS

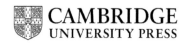

Shaftesbury Road, Cambridge CB2 8EA, United Kingdom

One Liberty Plaza, 20th Floor, New York, NY 10006, USA

477 Williamstown Road, Port Melbourne, VIC 3207, Australia

314–321, 3rd Floor, Plot 3, Splendor Forum, Jasola District Centre, New Delhi – 110025, India

103 Penang Road, #05-06/07, Visioncrest Commercial, Singapore 238467

Cambridge University Press is part of Cambridge University Press & Assessment, a department of the University of Cambridge.

We share the University's mission to contribute to society through the pursuit of education, learning and research at the highest international levels of excellence.

www.cambridge.org
Information on this title: www.cambridge.org/9781009205627

DOI: 10.1017/9781009205665

First published 2023

A catalogue record for this publication is available from the British Library.

Library of Congress Cataloging-in-Publication Data
NAMES: Cooper, Yamonte, 1974– editor. | Holmes, Erica, 1970– editor.
TITLE: Black couples therapy : clinical theory and practice / edited by Yamonte Cooper (El Camino College, Los Angeles), Erica Holmes (Antioch University, Los Angeles).
DESCRIPTION: Cambridge, United Kingdom ; New York, NY : Cambridge University Press, 2023. | Includes bibliographical references and index.
IDENTIFIERS: LCCN 2022045256 (print) | LCCN 2022045257 (ebook) | ISBN 9781009205627 (hardback) | ISBN 9781009205658 (paperback) | ISBN 9781009205665 (epub)
SUBJECTS: LCSH: Couples therapy–United States. | African American couples. | African American couples–Mental health services. | African Americans–Mental health services.
CLASSIFICATION: LCC RC488.5 .B567 2023 (print) | LCC RC488.5 (ebook) | DDC 616.89/1562–DC23/eng/20221021
LC record available at https://lccn.loc.gov/2022045256
LC ebook record available at https://lccn.loc.gov/2022045257

ISBN 978-1-009-20562-7 Hardback
ISBN 978-1-009-20565-8 Paperback

Contents

Figures

Tables

Contributors

JESHANA AVENT-JOHNSON, The Intimacy Seminars and Psychological Services, USA

BEVERLEY BOOTHE, Life Enrichment Counseling Center Inc., USA

MOE A. BROWN, Transcendent Therapy and Consulting LLC, USA

CYNTHIA CHESTNUT, Capella University, USA

SATIRA STREETER CORBITT, Ascensions Psychological Services Inc., USA

DANIELLE Y. DRAKE, California Institute of Integral Studies, USA

LAURA DUPITON, Eastern University, USA

ADIA GOODEN, Adia Gooden, LLC, USA

DAKTARI SHARI R. HICKS, Optimum Specialists, USA

BRIAN R. HUMPHREY, PsychSynergy Behavioral Health, USA

TENIKA L. JACKSON, Antioch University, USA

RONECIA LARK, California State University Dominguez Hills, USA

JONATHAN MATHIAS LASSITER, Rowan University, USA

HEATHER C. LOFTON, Northwestern University, USA

KATHERINE MCKAY, Private Practice, USA

DARYL M. ROWE, Pepperdine University, USA

SANDRA LYONS ROWE, Retired, USA

ALICE SHEPARD, The City University of New York, USA

JESSICA M. SMEDLEY, Smedley Psychological Services LLC, USA

LEKEISHA A. SUMNER, U.S. Department of Veterans Affairs, USA

Foreword

Historically, the psychotherapy field has devoted scant attention to the therapeutic needs of clients of color. Adamantly and feverishly adhering to claims of color-blindness and the insistence that all couples and families are essentially the same has contributed to a massive dearth of knowledge and understanding among therapists regarding providing culturally and racially sensitive therapy to clients of color. Claims of *not seeing color* while simultaneously denying the impact of racial oppression on the everyday lives of People of Color have dangerously supported and continue to perpetuate approaches to therapy that are guided by a centrality of whiteness (Hardy, 2022).

The 2020 murder of private citizen George Floyd and the ensuing racial unrest that followed were stark reminders of our society's ongoing struggles with race, whiteness, and our affectionate heartwarming claims of color blindness. One of the many byproducts of the 2020 worldwide racial uprising was the poignant reminder that issues of race needed to be confronted and appropriately addressed throughout all domains of society, and this certainly would include the field of psychotherapy – a profession where historically virtually all the stewards and gatekeepers have been disproportionately white and male. In the psychotherapy field, the Gurus, "Masters," "Fellows," and Distinguished Professors have been disproportionately white and male, often espousing doctrines offered as "objective truths" proclaimed to be widely applicable to all, while remaining deeply oblivious to the inherent racially based biases and centrality of whiteness embedded within them. Needless to say, a significant and radical expansion of *what has been*, requires interrogation and a change in course. As McGoldrick and Hardy (2019) asserted, a revisioning of therapy with greater attention devoted to the impact of race, class, gender, sexual orientation, and a host of other significant contextual variables is sorely needed. The *one size fits all* "cookie cutter" approach that we have historically subscribed to throughout the field, is not only outdated but potentially harmful as well. We need the birthing of a new set of ideas, ways of being, thinking and approaches designed to meet the needs of today's complex and racially diverse world. This book, *Black Couples Therapy: Clinical Theory and Practice*, edited by Yamonte Cooper and Erica Holmes, is a major step in this direction.

Cooper and Holmes have not only assembled an impressive group of diverse theoreticians and clinicians to contribute to this groundbreaking clinical anthology, but they also have been thoughtful and comprehensive regarding the range of salient topics that are covered. This book, unlike many of its companion couples therapy publications, recognizes the complexity and diversity of the coupling experience. In so doing, they and the contributing authors overtly acknowledge that NOT all couples are white, heterosexual, and cisgender. The book challenges the prevailing and popular notion that "couples therapy" is "couples therapy" and essentially all couples are the same. Seasoned practitioners and those with considerably less experience will find this book to be a timely, relevant, and insightful resource. Clinicians of all backgrounds and level of experience will appreciate the ways in which the editors as well as the contributing authors delicately and skillfully address issues in much the same ways in which these issues often emerge in therapy.

As the book title asserts, the editors strike a very fine balance between exposing the reader to important clinical theory that provides a conceptual framework for therapeutic intervention, and specific strategies for working with specific clinical populations that reflect the rich diversity of Black couples. This book is a must read for today's couples' therapists, especially those who are committed to providing culturally attuned, racially sensitive couples therapy.

Kenneth V. Hardy, PhD
Eikenberg Institute for Relationships
New York, USA

REFERENCES

Hardy, K. V. (2022). *The enduring, invisible, and ubiquitous centrality of Whiteness*. Norton.
McGoldrick, M., & Hardy, K. V. (2019). *The re-visioning of family therapy* (3rd ed.). Guilford Press.

Acknowledgments

To my friend and loving spouse RW, I appreciate your unyielding support. Thank you, Emory & Virginia, Edna, and the rest of my family, for your love and support. Thank you, Erica, with the deepest gratitude for joining me on this project. Yamonte Cooper, Ed.D.

Thank you to my husband, ADG, for your unconstrained love and support. Thank you to my son, Jace, and bonus daughter, Kendelle, for so generously sharing me with the world. Thank you to all of my kinfolks. I am because you are. I would like to thank Yamonte Cooper for inviting me to be a part of this extraordinary body of work. Most importantly I want to thank God for everything. Erica Holmes, PsyD.

We thank each contributing author for your time and talent. A special acknowledgement to Katherine McKay may you continue to be remembered through your work. We thank the entire publishing team at Cambridge University Press.

Introduction

Black relationships in the United States have endured over the past four centuries and been instrumental in the survival of Black[1] people as a source of companionship and love. Simultaneously, Black relationships have been undermined by 400 years of structural anti-Black racism that includes slavery, white terrorism, and institutional decimation comprising hyperincarceration. In addition, the domestic slave trade caused the dissolution of marriages in over 30 percent of enslaved Black couples (Hunter, 2017). However, despite these overt attacks on Black love, Black people continued to show their commitment to coupling. The importance of Black relationships was demonstrated with the practice of jumping the broom, which was symbolic of the union among Black couples, during a time when it was illegal for enslaved Black Americans to legally marry (Parry, 2020). Although marriage rates have decreased for Black people, when queried, they continue to place a high value on and desire marriage (Phillip et al., 2012).

Romantic partnerships have long been highly valued among Black Americans. Black Americans are more likely to endorse marriage among couples than white Americans (Saad, 2006). Opinion pieces on Black love and relationships proliferate in the popular media, which indicates a huge interest in Black love and relationships. This volume represents a departure from these anecdotal impositions and provides theory, research, and practice, placing emphasis on the fact that couples therapy is a very specific area of research, specialization, and practice. Traditionally, the topic of therapy with Black couples has been incorporated into books that address family therapy. This volume fills a void in the theory, research, and practice of couples therapy where clinicians have historically not been specifically trained to provide culturally responsive care in addressing the unique experiences and needs of Black couples. Further, most research and

---

[1] Black is capitalized in this book to recognize the struggle of Black Americans in the United States. Black and African American are used interchangeably.

couples therapy modalities tend to be normed on European American couples and do not include research on Black couples. This includes the omission of social conditions that impact Black couples and their relational dynamics such as the legacy of slavery and anti-Black racism. This text provides a new and refreshing entry into the field of couples therapy using theory, research, and clinical experience to modify common couples therapy modalities and integrate cultural context, which can increase applicability, relevance, and efficacy with Black couples.

The impetus for this volume was the recognition that there was a significant gap in the literature on couples therapy with Black couples. This gap was noticeable in our graduate training and left us with very few resources to reference in our clinical work. As Black therapists working with Black couples, we became accustomed to modifying current Eurocentric couples therapy modalities. This was necessary for them to be viable in application and practice with Black couples. Therefore, this text will assist clinicians and graduate students in providing culturally responsive care to Black couples. Each chapter is written by a clinician who provides expertise on various topics and populations of Black couples.

I.1   Overview of Chapters

This volume encompasses five sections and 16 chapters. Each section is composed of chapters with similar themes and focal areas. Each chapter was written to stand independently; therefore, they do not need to be read in sequential order. This allows the reader to select chapters most relevant to their work or curiosity. Each chapter is structured to provide a socio-cultural understanding of the factors that influence African American coupling, the impact of anti-Black racism and manifestation in the couple dynamic, along with intervention strategies. A list of questions is provided at the end of each chapter to encourage the reader to reflect on the main themes and their application. The following are chapter overviews.

I.1.1   Part I Racism and Identity

Chapter 1, written by Cynthia Chestnut, details research findings on patterns of African American couples' positive and negative stereotyping of each other and others in the general African American community. This chapter highlights the impact of internalized messages, both positive and negative, on the relational self. Chapter 1 sets the tone for the remainder of the book, in that it underscores the impact of socialization within a context of anti-Black racism that affects the ways that the couple perceives themselves and their partners.

In Chapter 2, authors Heather C. Lofton and Adia Gooden, examine the impact of the Strong Black Woman (SBW) schema on Black women's ability to seek and engage in healthy romantic interpersonal relationships. Embodied by unyielding strength and unlimited capacity when navigating daily roles, interpersonal interactions, and life tasks, the SBW schema affects trust and vulnerability and thus intimacy. This chapter reviews the history and development of the SBW schema and how this schema manifests in the lived experiences of Black women in romantic relationships. The chapter concludes with specific recommendations for working with women who adopt the SBW schema to help foster healthy romantic relationships.

Chapter 3, authored by Jonathan M. Lassiter, completes Part I by discussing ways in which religion, spirituality, and romance intersect in the lives of Black American same-gender-loving (SGL) individuals. Ways in which religion and spirituality influence the development, maintenance, dynamics, and quality of Black American SGL men's romantic and sexual relationships are explored. The chapter concludes with strategies based on Afrocentric psychology to assess and intervene when working with clients along with recommendations for future clinical research in this area.

I.1.2 Part II Fundamentals for Healthy Coupling

In Chapter 4, Daryl M. Rowe and Sandra Lyons Rowe detail an approach to cultivating and sustaining healthy marital relationships that is grounded in the emerging field of African-centered psychology. This approach privileges the lived experiences of African Americans and summarizes a marriage empowerment program, Conversations in Marriage© (CIM), which uses African proverbs to promote situational learning. The authors discuss the essential need to explicitly incorporate cultural issues when working with African American couples, provide an overview of the cycle of healthy relationships, highlight the legacy of healthy families of African ancestry, stress the importance of a participatory approach, and describe introducing and incorporating African proverbs to stimulate engagement. Each element is discussed from a perspective that centers marriage within a framework of community, growth, empowerment, and sustainability.

Chapter 5, written by Erica Holmes, Ronecia Lark, and Jessica M. Smedley urges the reader to consider the importance of premarital counseling and education for engaged African American couples. The authors begin by discussing the psychological, social, and economic benefits of marriage, while highlighting the decline of African American marriages in the United States. The authors then analyze how the legacy of anti-Black racism and discrimination/oppression have shaped the African American family structure, impacted marriage rates, and marriage success. The chapter concludes with an outline of a proposed premarital workbook for African American heterosexual couples that specifically addresses their unique history and challenges experienced in marriages.

I.1.3   Part III Adapting Major Therapeutic Approaches for Work with African American Couples

In Chapter 6, Yamonte Cooper examines Emotionally Focused Therapy (EFT) with Black couples. The author stresses the importance of the integration of clinical considerations (e.g., racial realities of anti-Blackness) when using EFT with Black couples to provide an appropriate adaptation that is a culturally responsive couples therapy. The author argues that adult attachment must be conceptualized from a network approach (e.g., multiple relationships/collectivism) instead of only a dyadic perspective. The author further examines important factors such as acculturation, anti-Black racism, internalized stereotypes, SBW schema, and John Henryism in providing culturally responsive care and clinical interventions that strengthen EFT treatment approaches with Black couples.

Chapter 7 by Satira Streeter Corbitt explores the historical trauma and challenges faced by Black couples and the resulting impact of Dr. Joy DeGruy's explanatory theory of Post-Traumatic Slave Syndrome (PTSS). The central theory of the Gottman Method for couples therapy is reviewed along with special considerations when working with Black couples. Case conceptualizations of three African American couples impacted by PTSS and treated using Gottman method interventions is presented to illustrate integration of the theory and practice.

Chapter 8, written by Moe A. Brown, uses a Narrative Therapy lens to addresses the challenges that often arise for Black transgender men and their romantic partners when seeking support in therapy. The author defines key terminology related to gender identity and discusses other facets of identity, like biological sex, gender identity, gender expression, gender presentation, and sexual orientation. Its application to clinical practice with Black transgender men and their romantic partners is also presented. Further, the chapter provides a summary of primary Narrative Therapy concepts and uses a case example to illustrate Narrative Therapy with Black transgender men and their romantic partners.

In Chapter 9, Beverley Boothe discusses ways in which Harville Hendrix's Imago Relationship Therapy can be adapted to support African American couples experiencing relationship conflict. The author introduces the main tenets of Imago Relationship Therapy and discusses ways that it can enable the African American couple to look at their childhood story, increase awareness of their connections, identify their triggers, and decide to move from an unconscious to a conscious way of relating. The author concludes with a clinical vignette to illustrate its application.

Chapter 10, by Alice Shepard and Katherine McKay, explores Eye Movement Desensitization Reprocessing Therapy (EMDR) as a critical approach needed to address trauma's neurological, emotional, and relational impact. It provides a culturally relevant model of applying EMDR to create a healing space for building self-efficacy, worth, trust, and intimacy within Black romantic partnerships.

I.1.4 Part IV Sex and Intimacy

Chapter 11 by Danielle Y. Drake and Daktari Shari R. Hicks explores sociopolitical factors, including gender roles and power dynamics that affect sexual intimacy among heterosexual Black couples. Culturally specific factors that can promote resilience are highlighted with a view toward increasing the understanding of Black heterosexual relationships as emotionally supportive spaces, with an emphasis of intentional intimacy as acts of social justice. Creative interventions for use in clinical practice are offered to assist in expanding sexual intimacy with Black couples.

In Chapter 12, Jeshana Avent-Johnson explores intimacy, sex, and desire as important elements to personal and relational well-being. Johnson asserts that there is a unique challenge that can hamper the development of these elements given the historical backdrop of oppression that contributes to significant stressors in the lives of these couples. Helping Black couples to understand how they make meaning of sex, intimacy, and interactions with their partner, while maintaining a clear sense of self in context of their physical and emotional closeness, has been positively associated with sexual desire, intimacy, and couple satisfaction. Hence, this chapter explores the role of differentiation, the impact it has on a Black couple's intimate life, and how clinicians can help facilitate the process of increasing the couple's levels of differentiation, thus, breathing life into the relationship.

Chapter 13 by Laura Dupiton and Cynthia Chestnut explores infidelity in Black committed relationships. The authors discuss emotional and

psychological wounds caused by systemic oppression, internalized stereotypes, and other factors that often cause Black men and women to wear a
mask and not show up as their authentic selves. The sociological phenomenon called *covering* is discussed to conceptualize ways Black men and
women, in relationship, have learned to protect themselves from further
emotional bruising. The authors conclude with a case study using
Narrative Therapy to address *covering* while attending to the language
used to shape a couple's reality.

I.1.5   Part V Special Topics

In Chapter 14, Tenika L. Jackson emphasizes the necessity for clinicians to
assist their Black lesbian clients who experience infertility with the biological, psychological, social, and emotional aspects of the process. The author
seeks to help therapists acquire an understanding of the process and unique
challenges of conceiving a child within a lesbian relationship. The impact
of factors such as social stigma, societal expectations based on gender
expression, and generalized labels such as infertile are explored. Further,
the chapter discusses the process of intrauterine insemination, in vitro
fertilization, and adoption within the lesbian community and specifically
the Black lesbian community. Clinicians will learn how the journey to
conceive a child impacts the Black lesbian relationship and what helping
professionals need to do to effectively help their clients weather the storm.

Chapter 15 by Brian R. Humphrey explores the seldom discussed topic
of infertility in men: more specifically Black men. Race and ethnicity can
impact how male factor infertility is understood, communicated, and
managed. The aim of this chapter is to synthesize available research
regarding biopsychosocial variables of male factor infertility with African
American men while offering support considerations.

Chapter 16 authored by Lekeisha Sumner centers on African American
couples facing medical illness and its impact. This chapter highlights
research and theory relevant to couples coping with medical illness within
sociohistorical and culturally relevant conceptual frameworks in clinical
practice. The chapter concludes by offering considerations for clinical
practice.

This volume will serve as a resource for clinicians and graduate students
working with Black couples and can challenge any preconceived notions or
biases that clinicians may have about Black couples. The information
contained in this volume will assist therapists in developing a working

alliance with Black couples. The therapeutic relationship with Black couples can cultivate an environment that is instrumental in decreasing relationship distress and disconnection. Therefore, clinicians will be able to provide culturally responsive care and clinical interventions that inform treatment approaches.

REFERENCES

Hunter, T. W. (2017). *Bound in wedlock: Slave and free black marriage in the nineteenth century.* Harvard University Press.

Parry, T. D. (2020). *Jumping the broom: The surprising multicultural origins of a black wedding ritual.* UNC Press Books.

Phillips, T., Wilmoth, J., & Marks. L. (2012). Challenges and conflicts. strengths and supports: A study of enduring African American marriages. *Journal of Black Studies, 43*(8), 936–952.

Saad, L. (2006, July 14). *Blacks committed to the idea of marriage.* Gallup. https://news.gallup.com/poll/23767/Blacks-Committed-Idea-Marriage.aspx

PART I

Race, Racism, and Identity

CHAPTER I

Internalized Stereotypes and the Impact on Black Couples

Cynthia Chestnut

African Americans' self-perceptions have changed since the time of slavery, but the residual effects of slavery continue to exert a negative influence on African Americans' views of themselves through internalized negative stereotypes (Allen et al., 1992; Baldwin & Hopkins, 1990; Kelly & Floyd, 2001; Parham & Helms, 1985; Sellers, 1993; Taylor & Zhang, 1990). Internalized negative stereotypes among African Americans are believed to contribute to the income disparity between African Americans and white Americans, to disproportionate incarceration rates among African American males, and to elevated rates of drug addiction among African Americans (Adams & Dressler, 1988; Boyd-Franklin, 1989; Boyd-Franklin & Franklin, 1998; Clark et al., 1999; Hardy, 2001; West, 1993). However, income disparity is not of any doing of African Americans but the deliberate systematic socioeconomic deprivation of African Americans from slavery to Jim Crow. Mass incarceration/criminalization is not a change in behavior among African American men but a change in policy. Drug addiction is equal among African Americans and whites and in some instances more so whites. These ideas lend themselves to cultural pathology/inferiority and can blame Black people for the socially engineered conditions that they live and die in (Alexander & West, 2012; Blumstein, 1982; Charles & Luoh, 2010; Y. Cooper, personal communication, August 29, 2021; Darity, 2005; Darity et al., 2001). Researchers have also attributed declining marital rates, lack of marital commitment, and obstacles to couple relationship adjustment among African Americans to internalized negative stereotypes that have persisted as residual effects of slavery (Kelly & Floyd, 2001; Taylor & Zhang, 1990).

African Americans have the lowest rate of marriage of any U.S. ethnicity. In 2000, the marriage rate among African Americans was 48 percent, compared to Hispanics (68 percent), Asian Pacific Islanders (80 percent), and white/non-Hispanic couples (83 percent; U.S. Census Bureau, 2000).

Compared to white women, African American women are 25 percent less likely to have ever been married and about half as likely to be currently married (U.S. CensusBureau, 2008). African Americans report greater unhappiness in their marriages than do whites, and they are less likely to remarry after divorce (Cutrona et al., 2003; Franklin, 1980; Jewell, 1983).

Lower rates of marriage among African Americans have been attributed to high rates of mortality, drug addiction, and incarceration that limit the number of available African American men (Eichler, 2004; Lawson & Thompson, 1994). The lower levels of marital satisfaction observed among African American couples have been attributed in part to female partners' negative perceptions of male partners arising from African American women's higher levels of educational and occupational attainment (Aborampah, 1989; Broman, 1993), to financial stress associated with occupational discrimination (Turner & Noh, 1983), and to polygyny among African American males resulting in part from high rates of male mortality and incarceration (Eichler, 2004; Lawson & Thompson, 1994; Pinderhughes, 1989).

Many clinicians working with African American couples have reported that internalized negative stereotypes may be a root cause of the conditions that lower marriage rates and marital satisfaction among African American couples. Clinicians have found that in many African American couples who are experiencing marital difficulties, both partners have been socialized into believing negative stereotypes about themselves and each other (Boyd-Franklin, 1989; Franklin, 1980; Jewell, 1983; Kelly & Floyd, 2001; Pinderhughes, 1989). Such couples blame each other for their displaced rage and disillusionment. Their rage and disillusionment are thought to be effects of intergenerational pain, unresolved anger from racism and discrimination, and internalization of a poor sense of self due to negative cultural connotations of skin color (Franklin, 1980; Jewell, 1983; Pinderhughes, 1989). Many African Americans have struggled with racial identity and with distinguishing their anger from what has been projected onto them. The internalization of anger in response to racism has become a characteristic residing within African American identity. African Americans may project this internal conflict onto their relationships with friends and co-workers, as well as onto their intimate partners, while feeling confused regarding the origin of their anger and its projection (Boyd-Franklin, 1989).

Despite indications that internalized negative stereotypes lower rates of marriage and marital satisfaction among African American heterosexual couples, few researchers have investigated this topic (Kelly & Floyd, 2001;

Taylor, 1990). A number of studies have been conducted to examine the significance of marriage in American culture at large (Cutrona et al., 2003; Lynch & Blinder, 1983; Olson, 1999; Steinberg et al., 2001). Much has also been written on professionals' views of factors affecting relationship adjustment in heterosexual couples (e.g., Locke & Wallace, 1959; Spanier, 1976; White, 1989; Zeifman & Hazan, 1997). However, there have been few investigations of the commonplace relationship dilemmas resulting from internalized negative stereotypes among ethnic minority couples, including African Americans (Jewell, 1983; Kelly & Floyd, 2001; Taylor & Zhang, 1990).

This study was conducted to examine the impact of internalized negative stereotypes that are conveyed, projected, and experienced by African American romantic partners on the relationship factors of cohesion, consensus, satisfaction, affection, and overall couple adjustment. The impact of these dynamics on treatment considerations with couples of various demographic statuses was also explored. The following section is an overview of the theoretical and empirical literature that formed the background of this research (Chestnut, 2009).

1.1   Literature and Hypotheses

This brief review of the literature is a discussion of the empirical and theoretical background of this research. The first section is a description of the background of couple adjustment and social exchange theory. The second section indicates the background of current scholarly understandings of symbolic interactionism and its relationship to African Americans' experiences and self-perceptions. In the third section, the relationships between couple adjustment and social exchange theory and symbolic interactionism are discussed in relation to the need for this study. The fourth section is a list of the hypotheses derived from the review of the literature.

1.1.1   Couple Adjustment and Social Exchange Theory

The central premise associated with social exchange theory is the characterization of relationships as extended markets in which individuals act out self-interest with the goal of maximizing profits (Spanier, 1976). In couple relationships, individuals voluntarily enter and remain in a relationship because they experience a profit, in the sense that the rewards of the relationship outweigh its costs. Couple adjustment theory has its roots in the social exchange framework, which Spanier (1976) used to explore the role of marital quality and other, related factors as mediators of marital stability. The social exchange framework is focused on variables that mediate the formation, maintenance, breakdown, and dynamics of exchanges within the couple relationship. Spanier adopted this framework to emphasize the role of reciprocity and exchange in marriage, applying his concept of marital adjustment to better understand reciprocity in role consensus, satisfaction, affection, and cohesion.

In couple adjustment theory, reciprocity is believed to stabilize marital relationships by helping to establish a network of interdependent duties and expectations (Spanier, 1976). Each person in the relationship must provide the rewards that the other person wants in order to receive, in exchange, the rewards that he or she values. Over time, this stable pattern of role expectations and obligations is expected to alleviate the sense of indebtedness and obligation one partner has to the other, thereby establishing reciprocity as a norm.

Couple adjustment is viewed as "a process of movement along a continuum that can be evaluated in terms of proximity to good or poor adjustment" (Spanier, 2001, p. 23). Couple adjustment includes several different dimensions, including couple cohesiveness, couple consensus, expressions of affection, and couple satisfaction (Spanier, 1976). Couple cohesiveness is the degree to which a couple shares common interests and activities. Couple consensus is the degree of agreement between partners on important matters. Expressions of affection indicate the quality of emotional communication between partners, whereas couple satisfaction indicates a couple's desire to continue their relationship, with satisfied couples being more likely to maintain their commitment.

1.1.2   Symbolic Interactionism Theory

Symbolic interactionism theory is focused on the connection between symbols, or shared meanings, and interactions, which include verbal or nonverbal actions and communications. The theory indicates that human beings work in concert to create and maintain symbols, which in turn shape human behavior (LaRossa & Reitzes, 1993). Symbols provide the context for social interactions, which, in turn, enable participants to develop a concept of self by assessing and assigning value to their activities (LaRossa & Reitzes, 1993). Individuals assess their performance in a role according to a perceived social consensus about the expectations for that role, and they feel more competent and satisfied when their performance is high according to those consensus expectations (White & Klein, 2002). Individuals are more likely to experience dissatisfaction and strain in their role, however, when they encounter a lack of broad consensus on the social expectations for that role, and particularly when they encounter contradictory expectations (White & Klein, 2002).

Social interactionism has a particular significance for African Americans for two reasons. First, being an African American is, itself, a social role, and African Americans are likely to identify with that role rather than regard themselves as performers who are distinguishable from the role of being a member of the African American ethnicity (Nobles, 1973, 1991). Thus, Nobles argued that for African Americans, there is no distinction between self-identity and ethnic identity. The second reason social interactionism is particularly significant for African Americans is that the ethnic identity with which self-identity is so intimately bound has traditionally had a negative meaning in U.S. culture (Du Bois, 1964).

As a consequence, African Americans often struggle to maintain a positive perception of themselves and their ethnicity in the face of cultural forces that continually impose negative connotations on African American identities (Allen & Bagozzi, 2001; Broman et al., 1988). The moment-to-moment confrontation with cultural disparagements of African American identities has negative effects on African Americans' physiological health and psychological well-being, and socioeconomic disparities that are consequences of negative cultural perceptions of African Americans are likely to reinforce the internalization of negative stereotypes (Allen & Bagozzi, 2001; Allen et al., 1992; Broman et al., 1988).

The internalization of negative stereotypes affects identity development, self-actualization, self-esteem, and psychological functioning among African Americans (Cross, 1995; Taylor, 1990). For example, Gatewood (1988) and Okazawa-Rey et al. (1986) discussed discrimination within African American communities based on skin tones and hair texture. Intragroup discrimination based on internalized negative stereotypes may be manifested in derogatory language, including "big-lips, liver-lips, burred-heads, fuzzy-heads, kinky-haired, nappy-headed, big-legs, high-ass, apes, and monkeys," and by the perception among African Americans themselves that dark skin is ugly (Udry et al., 1971, p. 723). Boyd-Franklin (1989) and Pinderhughes (1989) argued that African Americans have also internalized negative stereotypes of themselves as lazy, unintelligent, weak, and giving up easily.

1.1.3   The Relationship between Couple Adjustment
and Symbolic Interactionism

Couple adjustment theory based on a framework of reciprocity and social exchange indicates that partners in a marriage will experience their relationship as profiting from them when its benefits appear to outweigh its costs (Spanier, 1976). The benefits of a marriage can include access to a desirable sexual partner and mate, companionship, and resource-sharing, and costs can include conflict with the partner, inequitable resource-sharing, and lower self-esteem associated with having a partner of low social status. The relationship between the conclusions drawn from symbolic interactionism theory in the preceding section and couple adjustment based on social exchange is that internalized negative stereotypes are likely to reduce the partner's perceived value and exacerbate experiences of relationship costs among African American couples (Franklin, 1980; Jewell, 1983; Taylor & Zhang, 1990).

Internalized negative stereotypes reduce African American couple adjustment in the same ways they lower African Americans' self-perceptions. For example, Franklin (1980) and Jewell (1983) argued that Black men tend to perceive Black women as emasculating and aggressive, whereas Black women tend to perceive Black men as passive and submissive. These complementary, internalized stereotypes support negative perceptions about Black men's refusing to commit to long-term relationships with Black women, and Black women's lack of awareness and sensitivity to how they emasculate and act aggressively toward Black men.

In relationships, biases about the self or the partner may be projected onto the partner, challenging the sustainability of the relationship (Franklin, 1980; Jewell, 1983). Couples reporting marital distress are more likely to manifest internalize negative stereotypes than couples who are not experiencing distress, and couples who reported more internalized racism have tended to report less marital satisfaction (Taylor & Zhang, 1990). Kelly and Floyd's (2001) study demonstrated that the combination of internalized negative stereotypes and high Afrocentricity (i.e., self-identity as African American and strong endorsement of goals for ethnic advancement in opposition to oppression) for men were associated with decreased perceptions of partner dependability and decreased dyadic adjustment for both partners with low consensus and couple satisfaction. High Afrocentricity also resulted in low couple adjustment for both African American partners' indication variables such as consensus, cohesion, affectionate expression, and couple satisfaction were positively related. Allen and Hatchett (1986) reported that religiosity was associated with the internalization of negative stereotypical beliefs about Blacks.

Although age, education, number of years married, employment, money, prestige of occupation, and children have been examined in some studies on African Americans, Kelly and Floyd (2001) suggested that more research should be conducted to investigate the relationships between demographical variables and internalized negative stereotyping. However, there have been few studies of couple dynamics that have included African Americans as subjects (McRoy & Fisher, 1982; Reis & Patrick, 1996, Reis & Shaver, 1988; Simpson, 1987, 1990; Whiting & Crane, 2003; Zeifman & Hazan, 1997).

1.1.4 Hypotheses

The findings in the research studies reviewed indicated the following hypotheses: (a) African Americans held negative stereotypes about other African Americans; (b) income was negatively related to internalized stereotypes about African Americans; (c) education was negatively related to internalized stereotypes about African Americans; (d) Afrocentricity was negatively related to internalized stereotypes about African Americans; and (e) religiosity was negatively related to internalized stereotypes about African Americans.

1.2 Methods and Results

A quantitative research design with a cross-sectional time frame was utilized in this study. This design was intended to develop a portrait of African Americans' perceptions of positive and negative stereotypes and the quality of their couple adjustment in their heterosexual relationship at time of study. The following research questions were answered in this study:

RQ1. Will negative stereotypes about African Americans be related to couple cohesion, couple consensus, couple affectionate expression, couple satisfaction, and overall couple adjustment?

RQ2. Will there be a relationship between demographic variables and African American couples' negative stereotyping of each other, and couple adjustment?

1.2.1   Participants

The study was conducted using a convenience (nonprobability) sample of African Americans in a heterosexual couple relationship. All participants identified as African American, were at least second-generation U.S. citizens, were at least 18 years of age, and were in a heterosexual relationship with another identifying African American. A power analysis determined that eighty participants be recruited with 50 percent African American males and 50 percent females meeting the inclusion/exclusion criteria (Nunnally, 1978). A mass email was sent to Drexel University students, staff, faculty of the College of Nursing and Health Professions, the Department of Student Life, and individual student organizations of interest of Drexel University. Mass emails were sent to Smartmarriages. com Listserv, Pennsylvania Association of Liaisons and Officers of Multicultural Affairs (PALOMA), and the Pan African Network. Flyers were distributed throughout Drexel University's surrounding community. As a result, 160 agreed to take the survey. Out of the 160 participants, 142 African American heterosexuals in a couple relationship completed the entire survey, including 41 males and 101 females. A total of eighteen participants started the survey but did not complete it in its entirety.

1.2.2   Survey

The survey included three parts, the first of which was the Stereotype Scale. Kelly and Floyd (2001) adapted the scale from Allen et al. (1989). The Stereotype Scale was modified by the researcher to include five new items to measure opinions about African Americans' endorsing stereotypes regarding skin color and media influences. These items were (a) think that portrayals of Blacks in media (TV, movies) are pretty accurate, (b) prefer lighter skinned women, (c) want to be like sports and entertainment celebrities, (d) prefer lighter skinned men, and (e) want to look like the women they see in media (TV, movies, ads). Higher scores indicated that African Americans endorse more negative and fewer positive adjectives on the Stereotype Scale.

The second part of the survey was the demographic survey. Demographic variables were developed to provide a description of the African American couples who will participate in this study. The demographic survey (questions 93–110) was developed by the author to examine African Americans' gender, age, financial status and employment, marital or couple status, length of the relationship, education, commitment to a long-term relationship, substance abuse history, and mental health diagnosis, as well as their religious organization attendance, children, and imprisonment.

The third part of the survey was the Dyadic Adjustment Scale (DAS), questions 61–92, which was derived from previous marital adjustment measures (Locke, 1947; Locke & Williamson, 1958; Terman, 1938). This part of the survey was used to measure couple adjustment, the dependent variable in this study. During the scale development phase, items included in the DAS were evaluated by three judges for content validity to determine whether they were relevant measures of dyadic adjustment for contemporary relationships, consistent with nominal definitions suggested by Spanier and Cole (1976) for adjustment and its components (satisfaction, cohesion, affection, and consensus) in carefully worded fixed choice responses (Spanier, 2001). A factor analysis (Spanier & Cole, 1976) was conducted on the initial 40 items to test the adequacy of the working definition of dyadic adjustment, to determine which items should remain on the final scale, and to assess how each item on the scale related to the other.

Construct validity (variables accurately measure the construct of interest) about the DAS was determined by how it is characterized in other studies measuring content validity (to determine the relevancy of the measure; Spanier & Cole, 1976), criterion-related validity (to make accurate predictions; (Spanier, 1976), and concurrent and predictive validity (predict subsequent performance or behavior) (Markowski & Greenwood, 1984; Meredith et al., 1986). Convergent validity (overlap between different tests that measure the same construct) was established when Spanier (1976) correlated the DAS with Locke and Wallace's (1959) Marital Adjustment Scale. The correlations among married respondents were 0.86 and the divorced respondents were 0.88 in Spanier's (1976) study.

The instruments chosen to measure the variables are the Stereotype Scale, which is a Likert ordinal scale ranking each response, and the DAS, which is a Likert ordinal scale ranking the scores of the respondents. Two of the items are measured nominally and the concepts are multidimensional. The stereotype concepts are measured within two dimensions, positive and negative, for each of the three subcategories: African Americans in general, African American men, and African American women. The couple adjustment concepts are measured within four dimensions, including couple cohesion, couple consensus, affectionate expression, and couple satisfaction. The demographic variables are largely nominal.

1.2.3   Data Analysis

Data were entered into SPSS 15.0 (SPSS Inc., 2005) for Windows. Descriptive statistics were conducted on each of the variables. Multivariate analyses of variance (MANOVAs) were used to examine the influence of Stereotypes, Affective Expression, Dyadic Cohesion, Dyadic Satisfaction, and Dyadic Consensus. Stereotypes are defined as negative stereotypes of Black females, which are discussed as Negative Black Female in this study; negative stereotypes of Black males, which are discussed as Negative Black Male; and positive stereotypes of Blacks in general, Black males, and Black females are discussed as Positive Black. The Dyadic Adjustment abbreviations are Affective Expression Dyadic Cohesion (AEDH), Dyadic Cohesion (DH), Affectionate Expression (AE), Dyadic Satisfaction (DS), Dyadic Consensus 1 (DC1), and Dyadic Consensus 2 (DC2). The ANOVA examined only the demographic variables that had a significant effect from the MANOVA. Multiple regressions were conducted and Negative Black Female, Negative Black Male, or Positive Black Stereotypes predict DAS, Demographics and DAS variables predict total DAS. Three linear regressions (Negative Black Female, Positive Black, and Negative Black Male) were conducted to predict total DAS by male and female. Eight independent sample *t*–test were conducted to assess differences on Negative Black Female, Positive Black, Negative Black Male, and total DAS. Independent *t*–tests were conducted on Positive Black by group and linear regressions were conducted to assess committed relationship predicting Positive Black Stereotypes by males and females.

1.3   Results

Pearson *r* correlations were conducted to assess if relationships exist among the original total DAS in this study, Negative Black Female, Positive Black, and Negative Black Male (Table 1.1).

The results are presented in Table 1.1 where significant positive correlation coefficients were revealed between the total DAS and Positive Black, DAS and between Negative Black Female and Positive Black with Negative Black Male. Positive significant correlation coefficients indicate that as one variable increases the corresponding variable will also increase. Negative correlation coefficients were revealed between Negative Black Female with Positive Black. Negative significant correlation coefficients

Table 1.1. *Correlation matrix among original DAS subscales and stereotypes*

	Total DAS	Negative Black Female	Positive Black				
Negative Black Female	0.020	−0.127	0.011	0.011	**−0.022**		
Positive Black	0.119	0.045	0.179*	0.063	**0.156**	**−0.376****	
Negative Black Male	0.052	−0.163	0.048	−0.013	**−0.012**	**0.268****	**0.209***

Note. * $p < 0.05$, ** $p < 0.01$.

Table 1.2. *Correlations between Stereotype Scales and revised DAS scores*

DAS		Stereotypes		
		Negative Black Female	Positive Black	Negative Black Male
AEDH	Pearson correlation	−0.055	0.060	0.044
	Sig. (2-tailed)	0.513	0.482	0.599
	N	142	142	142
DS	Pearson correlation	−0.024	0.028	−0.099
	Sig. (2-tailed)	0.773	0.738	0.240
	N	142	142	142
DC1	Pearson correlation	0.056	0.145	0.033
	Sig. (2-tailed)	0.509	0.085	0.699
	N	142	142	142
DC2	Pearson correlation	−0.018	0.114	0.047
	Sig. (2-tailed)	0.833	0.176	0.577
	N	142	142	142
Total DAS	Pearson correlation	−0.009	**0.193***	0.002
	Sig. (2-tailed)	0.917	**0.021**	0.981
	N	142	142	142

indicate that an inverse relationship exists suggesting as one variable increases the corresponding variable will decrease.

Correlations were conducted between the three Stereotype subscales and the five DAS subscales presented in Table 1.2.

One of the correlations was statistically significant at the 2-tailed significance 0.021 level between Positive Black and total DAS, suggesting that African Americans indicated a positive relationship between DAS and Positive Black stereotypes. All other correlations were positively correlated and not significant.

Table 1.3. *Multiple regression on demographic variables predicting total DAS*

	B	SE	Beta	t	Sig.
(Constant)	3.119	0.735		4.243	0.000
Gender	−0.031	0.077	−0.043	−0.398	0.691
Age	−0.003	0.004	−0.089	−0.636	0.526
Marital status	−0.193	0.103	−0.280	−1.872	0.065
Length of relationship	0.000	0.005	0.010	0.067	0.946
Committed relationship	0.333	0.121	0.327	2.761	**0.007**
Employed	−0.007	0.089	−0.009	−0.080	0.936
Income	0.000	0.000	−0.096	−0.768	0.445
Education	−0.019	0.073	−0.028	−0.256	0.798
Substance abuse	−0.049	0.185	−0.038	−0.266	0.791
Partner substance abuse	−0.076	0.206	−0.059	−0.371	0.712
Prison	0.418	0.238	0.216	1.753	0.083
Partner prison	−0.408	0.338	−0.173	−1.207	0.231
Religious institution	0.117	0.110	0.158	1.062	0.291
Partner religious institution	−0.095	0.112	−0.137	−0.848	0.399
Same religious institution	0.061	0.103	0.091	0.594	0.554
Children	−0.039	0.102	−0.051	−0.381	0.704

A multiple regression was conducted to assess if gender (male vs. female), age, marital status (married vs. not), length of relationship, committed relationship (yes vs. no), employed (yes vs. no), income, education (college graduate vs. nongraduate), substance abuse (yes vs. no), partner substance abuse (yes vs. no), prison (yes vs. no), partner prison (yes vs. no), attend religious services (yes vs. no), partner attends religious services (yes vs. no), partner and you attend the same religious services (yes vs. no), and children (yes vs. no) predicts total DAS (Table 1.3).

The results of the regression were not significant F (16, 81) = 1.30, p = 0.217 and the independent variables accounted for (R^2) 20.5 percent of the variance in total DAS. The results of the regression are summarized in Table 1.3. "Committed relationship" has a high relationship to the total DAS. Prison and marital status have significant relationship to total DAS; however, prison skewed low.

A multiple regression was conducted to assess if gender (male vs. female), age, marital status (married vs. not), committed relationship (yes vs. no), employed (yes vs. no), education (college graduate vs. nongraduate), substance abuse (yes vs. no), partner substance abuse (yes vs. no), prison (yes vs. no), partner prison (yes vs. no), attend religious services (yes vs. no), partner attends religious services (yes vs. no), partner and you

Table 1.4. *Regression of Stereotype Scale of Positive Black factors on covariates*

| | Coefficients[a] | | | | |
| | Unstandardized Coefficients | | Standardized Coefficients | | |
Model	B	Std. Error	Beta	T	Sig.
(Constant)	2.611	0.810		3.223	0.002
What is your gender?	0.136	0.103	0.123	1.312	0.192
What is your age?	0.003	0.004	0.061	0.617	0.539
Married Y/N	−0.057	0.127	−0.052	−0.451	0.653
Do you feel you are in a committed relationship?	−0.055	0.170	−0.032	−0.326	0.745
Are you employed?	0.016	0.117	0.013	0.137	0.891
What is your education status?	−0.025	0.041	−0.055	−0.602	0.549
Do you have a substance abuse history?	−0.582	0.242	−0.253	−2.403	**0.018**
Do your partner have a substance abuse history?	0.102	0.192	0.057	0.529	0.598
Have you ever been in prison?	0.632	0.307	0.209	2.056	**0.042**
Have your partner ever been in prison?	−0.411	0.285	−0.152	−1.443	0.152
Do you attend a religious institution?	0.221	0.141	0.192	1.561	0.121
Do your partner attend a religious institution?	−0.110	0.151	−0.103	−0.730	0.467
Do you and your partner attend the same religious institution?	−0.113	0.141	−0.110	−0.800	0.425
How many children do you have that are 18 years and under?	−0.024	0.037	−0.060	−0.650	0.517

[a] Dependent variable: Positive Black

attend the same religious services (yes vs. no), and children (yes vs. no) predicts Positive Black Stereotypes (Table 1.4).

The results of the regression were not significant. The results of the regression are summarized in Table 1.4. Substance abuse history and Prison have a high relationship to the Positive Black Stereotypes. Therefore, substance abuse and prison have significant prediction to Positive Black Stereotypes, although they both skewed low.

A multiple regression was conducted to assess if gender (male vs. female), age, marital status (married vs. not), committed relationship (yes vs. no), employed (yes vs. no), education (college graduate vs. nongraduate), substance abuse (yes vs. no), partner substance abuse (yes vs. no),

Table 1.5. *Regression of Stereotype Scale of Negative Black Female factors on covariates*

	Coefficients[a]				
	Unstandardized Coefficients		Standardized Coefficients		
Model	B	Std. Error	Beta	T	Sig.
(Constant)	2.567	0.790		3.250	0.001
What is your gender?	0.166	0.101	0.139	1.642	0.103
What is your age?	0.010	0.004	0.220	2.467	**0.015**
Married Y/N	0.042	0.124	0.036	0.343	0.732
Do you feel you are in a committed relationship?	−0.200	0.165	−0.108	−1.212	0.228
Are you employed?	−0.110	0.115	−0.082	−0.962	0.338
What is your education status?	0.092	0.040	0.191	2.309	**0.023**
Do you have a substance abuse history?	0.243	0.236	0.098	1.027	0.306
Do your partner have a substance abuse history?	−0.313	0.187	−0.162	−1.670	0.097
Have you ever been in prison?	−0.064	0.300	−0.020	−0.215	0.830
Have your partner ever been in prison?	0.369	0.278	0.127	1.328	0.187
Do you attend a religious institution?	−0.218	0.138	−0.176	−1.578	0.117
Do your partner attend a religious institution?	0.056	0.147	0.049	0.380	0.704
Do you and your partner attend the same religious institution?	0.250	0.137	0.227	1.819	0.071
How many children do you have that are 18 years and under?	0.054	0.036	0.127	1.520	0.131

[a] Dependent variable: Negative Black Female

prison (yes vs. no), partner prison (yes vs. no), attend religious services (yes vs. no), partner attends religious services (yes vs. no), partner and you attend the same religious services (yes vs. no), and children (yes vs. no) predicts Negative Black Female Stereotypes (Table 1.5).

The results of the regression were not significant. The results of the regression are summarized in Table 1.5. Age and education have a high relationship to the Positive Black Stereotypes. Therefore, age and education have significant prediction to Negative Black Stereotypes.

An ANOVA on Negative Black Female and Negative Black Male was conducted to examine the mean differences by gender (Table 1.6).

Table 1.6. *ANOVA on Negative Black Female and Negative Black Male by gender*

Dependent Variable	F	Sig.	Eta	Power	Female M	Female SD	Male M	Male SD
Negative Black Female	11.95 (3.35)	0.001	0.08	0.93	0.04	0.40	−0.21	0.42
Negative Black Male	11.96 (1.94)	0.001	0.08	0.93	4.18	0.50	3.84	0.59

Note. Numbers in parentheses present the mean squared error.

Table 1.7. *ANOVA on Negative Black Female by level of education*

Dependent Variable	F	Sig.	Eta	Power	Completed High School M	Completed High School SD	Completed College M	Completed College SD
Negative Black Female	3.64 (1.00)	0.01	0.10	0.87	3.62	0.83	4.10	0.49

Note. Numbers in parentheses present the mean squared error.

Males have a negative relationship to Negative Black Female Stereotypes and females had a positive relationship to Negative Black Female Stereotypes. Females also had a positive relationship to Negative Black Male Stereotypes and a higher mean than males. Therefore, the ANOVA on Negative Black Male by gender was significant F (1, 141) = 11.96, $p <$ 0.001, suggesting that females had a larger mean (M = 4.18, SD = 0.50) than males (M = 3.84, SD = 0.59). The ANOVA on Negative Black Female by gender was significant F (1, 141) = 11.95, $p <$ 0.001, suggesting that females had a larger mean (M = 0.04, SD = 0.40) than males (M = −0.21, SD = 0.42). See Table 1.6 for further details.

An ANOVA of Negative Black Female Stereotypes was conducted on education to further assess the Negative Black Female factors (Table 1.7)

The ANOVA on Negative Black Female by level of education was significant F (4, 138) = 3.64, $p <$ 0.01, suggesting that respondents who had completed college had a larger mean (M = 4.10, SD = 0.49) than respondents who had completed high school (M = 3.62, SD = 0.83). See Table 1.7 for further details.

A multiple regression was conducted to assess if gender (male vs. female), age, marital status (married vs. not), committed relationship (yes vs. no), employed (yes vs. no), education (college graduate vs. nongraduate), substance abuse (yes vs. no), partner substance abuse (yes vs. no), prison (yes vs. no), partner prison (yes vs. no), attend religious services (yes vs. no), partner attends religious services (yes vs. no), partner and you attend the same religious services (yes vs. no), and children (yes vs. no) predicts Negative Black Male Stereotypes (Table 1.8).

Table 1.8. *Regression of Stereotype Scale on Negative Black Male factors on covariates*

| | Coefficients[a] | | | | |
| | Unstandardized Coefficients | | Standardized Coefficients | | |
Model	B	Std. Error	Beta	t	Sig.
(Constant)	−0.813	0.641		−1.268	0.207
What is your gender?	0.248	0.082	0.272	3.029	**0.003**
What is your age?	0.007	0.003	0.206	2.182	**0.031**
Married Y/N	−0.006	0.100	−0.007	−0.059	0.953
Do you feel you are in a committed relationship?	0.211	0.134	0.148	1.573	0.118
Are you employed?	−0.095	0.093	−0.092	−1.025	0.308
What is your education status?	0.011	0.032	0.030	0.346	0.730
Do you have a substance abuse history?	−0.006	0.192	−0.003	−0.031	0.975
Do your partner have a substance abuse history?	0.029	0.152	0.020	0.194	0.847
Have you ever been in prison?	−0.069	0.243	−0.028	−0.285	0.776
Have your partner ever been in prison?	−0.092	0.225	−0.041	−0.407	0.685
Do you attend a religious institution?	0.017	0.112	0.018	0.155	0.877
Do your partner attend a religious institution?	−0.074	0.119	−0.085	−0.624	0.534
Do you and your partner attend the same religious institution?	0.169	0.112	0.200	1.516	0.132
How many children do you have that are 18 years and under?	0.018	0.029	0.054	0.613	0.541

[a] Dependent variable: Negative Black Male

The results of the regression were not significant. The results of the regression are summarized in Table 1.8. Gender and age have a high relationship to the Negative Black Male Stereotypes. Therefore, gender and age have significant prediction to Negative Black Stereotypes.

An ANOVA was conducted to further examine the relations to Negative Black Male Stereotypes to the demographic covariates (Table 1.9).

Negative Black Male Stereotypes had a positive relationship to the demographic covariates, meaning they have a positive prediction to the covariates.

A regression analysis was conducted to examine predictions of the total DAS (Table 1.10).

Positive Black Stereotypes had a high prediction to the total DAS. The other variables have a low prediction to the total DAS.

Table 1.9. *ANOVA of Stereotype Scale on Negative Black Male factors by covariates*

ANOVA[b]					
Model	Sum of Squares	Df	Mean Square	F	Sig.
Regression	4.220	14	0.301	1.886	**0.034**[a]
Residual	19.816	124	0.160		
Total	24.037	138			

Table 1.10. *Regression of DAS on Stereotype Scale factors and significant covariates*

	Coefficients[a]				
	Unstandardized Coefficients		Standardized Coefficients		
Model	B	Std. Error	Beta	T	Sig.
1 (Constant)	−1.184	0.472		−2.511	0.013
Negative Black Female	0.110	0.077	0.145	1.427	0.156
Positive Black	0.216	0.078	0.265	2.753	**0.007**
Negative Black Male	−0.118	0.095	−0.119	−1.231	0.220
Do you feel you are in a committed relationship?	0.135	0.123	0.096	1.101	0.273

[a] Dependent variable: Total_DAS

Table 1.11. *T–tests by gender (male vs. female)*

	T	df	Sig.	Male		Female	
				M	SD	M	SD
Negative Black Female	−3.459	140	0.001	3.84	0.58	4.18	0.50
Positive Black	−0.673	140	0.502	2.09	0.51	2.15	0.51
Negative Black Male	−3.456	140	0.001	−0.21	0.41	0.04	0.39
Total DAS	−0.139	140	0.889	2.81	0.32	2.82	0.33

1.3.1   *Differences between Male/Female Scores*

Independent sample *t*-tests were conducted to assess if differences exist on Negative Black Female, Positive Black, Negative Black Male, and Total DAS by gender (male vs. female) (Table 1.11).

The results suggest that on Negative Black Female and Negative Black Male, females had a significantly larger mean as compared to males. Males had a lower means than females with DS, but it was not significant. Negative Black Female Stereotypes and Negative Black Males Stereotypes were significant, meaning differences did exist by gender. The results are summarized in Table 1.11.

1.3.2   *Summary of Results*

The significant findings in this study were as follows: (a) older age is correlated with Negative Black Female Stereotypes and Negative Black Male Stereotypes, (b) females had higher Negative Black Female Stereotypes and Negative Black Male Stereotypes compared to males, and (c) committed relationships and Positive Black Stereotypes related highly to African Americans Couple Adjustment. This current study also investigated if Positive Stereotypes, committed relationships, and couple adjustment were more significant between African American men or African American women, and the results show no differences between the genders.

1.4   Conclusions

1.4.1   *Relationship of Stereotype Scale to Dyadic Adjustment Scale*

Cronbach alpha scores changed when reliability was run and the alpha scores were significant with the three Stereotype components and the overall DAS were highly significant with DC fully contributing to that outcome. Correlations also supported the total DAS and Positive Black Stereotypes, which had significant positive correlations. The Stereotype Scale did not show any significant prediction in correlation analysis to support negative stereotypes predicting a negative relationship to DAS couple adjustment. African Americans did not respond significantly to items that suggest a negative relationship with DS and AE. These subscales (DAS) did not highly support the hypotheses. However, the DC subscale appeared to highly factor in the total DAS with African Americans and the DH subscale had significant correlation.

1.4.2 Relationship of Demographic Covariates to Couple Adjustment

A multiple regression was conducted to assess if gender (male vs. female), age, marital status (married vs. not), length of relationship, committed relationship (yes vs. no), employed (yes vs. no), income, education (college graduate vs. nongraduate), substance abuse (yes vs. no), partner substance abuse (yes vs. no), prison (yes vs. no), partner prison (yes vs. no), attend religious services (yes vs. no), partner attends religious services (yes vs. no), partner and you attend the same religious services (yes vs. no), and children (yes vs. no) predicts total DAS. Most of the results of the regression were not significant to the total DAS and the Demographics (independent variables). "Committed relationship" had the highest relationship to the total DAS. Prison and marital status have significant prediction to total DAS; however, prison skewed low by the number of participants responding to that item. Many participants identified as married in this study therefore perceived as a committed relationship. This indicates a value of high significance between committed relationships and couple adjustment among African Americans.

1.4.3 Relationship of Demographic Covariates to Stereotypes

Addressing the first question with the hypothesis, "African American couples have negative patterns of stereotyping and perceptions of couple adjustment," results indicated that patterns do exist. This study indicated that females had higher Negative Black Female and Negative Black Male stereotypes compared to men. This is a new insight to the patterns of endorsing negative stereotypes by African Americans. Previous research has found that males had greater endorsements of negative stereotypes than females (Kelly & Floyd, 2001). Nevertheless, gender and a pattern of negative stereotypes were results in this study as in a previous study (Kelly & Floyd, 2001). More research is needed to examine this change in consistency to explore how this is a change and what the indicators are.

Another significant phenomenon revealed in this research was that older Blacks endorsed more Negative Black Female and Negative Black Male stereotypes than Black males. Perhaps older Black females do not view these endorsements as stereotyping and relate to it as self-esteem; therefore, their view of their endorsements is indicative of a projection of poor self-esteem. This may suggest that the negative stereotypes endorsed refer to younger Black males and Black females who have not self-actualized as W. E. B. Du Bois describes the double consciousness theory

Du Bois (1964) explained this as the view of self through the eyes of hostile elements. The consequence is such that a person struggles to maintain a positive sense of self despite powerful forces pushing in the opposite direction. Perhaps older African American females view Black women in a struggle to hold on to a positive sense of self. As Allen and Bagozzi (2001) suggested, it takes tenacity for African Americans to hold on to a positive sense of self and the group despite the destructive aspects of the dominating culture historical intergenerational influence through the destructive experiences and oppression. The cohort of older African Americans were also identified in previous studies as endorsing negative stereotypes compared to younger African Americans. (Allen & Bagozzi, 2001; Allen et al., 1989; Allen & Hatchett, 1986; Allen et al., 1992). The findings of the current study partially support the first question that African American couples have negative patterns of stereotyping and perceptions of couple adjustment.

It also partially supports the second hypotheses from the second question: "There will be a relationship between demographic variables and African American couples' negative stereotyping and African Americans overall couple adjustment." The only demographic variable that had a significant relationship with African Americans' stereotyping and couple adjustment is commitment; however, this is a positive stereotype. Therefore, the hypotheses referring to negative stereotyping is not fully valid if positive stereotyping is considered acceptable. Pinderhughes (2002, 2008) suggested that stereotypes are valued as negative whether they sound positive or negative, and that they are considered a societal projection. The overall couple adjustment and Positive Black characteristics such as hard working, community oriented, intelligent, competent, and being proud of themselves are factors that contribute to African American's relationship. Perhaps African Americans view these positive stereotypes as qualities that contribute to character development, thus indicating these positive characteristics as admirable and to exchange these qualities or embrace these qualities while in a relationship influences commitment.

1.4.4   Limitations of the Study

The scales and subscales used in this study may be limitations in investigating stereotypes and their effects on African American couples adjusting in their relationships. However, the instruments used were able to provide partial support through the analysis used to investigate the research questions in this current study. A known limitation may be that this was a cross-sectional study, a design that is not appropriate for addressing issues of causality. Longitudinal and experimental designs may be necessary to examine causal relationships that may exist among the variables examined in this study.

Another limitation may be that this sample cannot be generalized to all African American marriages or couple relationships. Participants included 101 females and 41 males and may not represent African American responses at large. Also, approximately eighteen of those initially registered in the study did not participate. Thus, it is unclear as to how nonparticipants might differ from the couples in the study. This study was skewed toward higher education with thirty-one participants indicating they attended college and eighty-four indicating they completed college. The study is limited to self-report questionnaires. Limitations such as trust, self-esteem, mindfulness, romantic attachment, and racial identity were not examined as variables; therefore, these components were not weighed in the responses and may be factors in examining internalized racism with couple adjustment. This study did not survey couples. Only individuals in a couple relationship were surveyed, which may be another limitation to consider. This area of study has not been thoroughly addressed in the literature, and further examination is recommended using qualitative research, which may facilitate a closer and more dynamic description.

1.4.5   Clinical Implications

Negative stereotypes were not found to be significant predictor of African Americans' couple adjustment in this study. However, the existence of negative stereotypes in African American couple relationships was found to be significant. This suggested that negative stereotypes do exist in the components of couple adjustment, but commitment, positive stereotypes, and the couple's overall adjustment are significant factors to consider when treating couples.

Clinicians working with African American couples will need to consider the findings in this study while treating couples working to attain affection, satisfaction, closeness, and consensus in their relationships. Clinicians can help clients identify themes like sadness, shame, guilt, and pain experienced in their intimate relationships (Pinderhughes, 2008). They could use these findings as a narrative to bring healing and help them work toward desired goals of intimacy. Pinderhughes (2008) indicated that the undoing of negative consequences is imperative for mental health wellness. Further examination of studies developing inquiries of the identity development of African Americans in couple relationships may enable more insight and increase awareness of characteristics negatively affecting couple adjustment. Resilience may be a variable to explore in experimental designs investigating this phenomenon to gain insight in some of the outcomes of this study.

Clinicians need to query African American couples to help them understand the language they utilize in constructing their own narrative. Clinicians can help couples hear their narratives by echoing or mirroring back to them the concepts they convey in the language offered to describe their narrative. Also, clinicians can help the partners by having them extend these listening practices to each other. This intracultural approach between the partners may need to be discussed within the contexts of describing dominant constructs that influences their narratives for the sake of justice to be revealed and to ensure as much as possible the interplay of dominant cultural narratives that coexist in their stories. McCarthy and Byrne (2008) suggested that without this consideration the moral quest to help couples understand each other and themselves in the narrative will ultimately fail. Marginalized conditions such as poverty, gender, and ethnic origin may cause partners to feel excluded or silenced, and they may project the emotional and mental effects of these injuries or injustices to their partners.

The term "Stereotypes" may not be used between partners, but language such as lack of self-esteem, lack of confidence, and lack of self-respect, or the opposite such as too much self-esteem, too much confidence, and too much self-respect (when it appears one sided) may have a dominant place in their narratives. Clinicians would need to be mindful and careful to not force clients to fit within their proposed ideology of "culture" but to learn the language of the couple and have them convey the narrative of their culture and how their values and norms play out in their relationship. This suggests that clinicians assist with decoding language by adapting it to convey an expressive intention in a context that is fluid and suggest fair consideration for change.

Discussion Questions

1. How does *social exchange* theory help us to understand internalized negative stereotype's impact on mate selection for Black couples?
2. What significance does *social interactionism* have for African Americans? Why is this important when thinking about relationship development and satisfaction?
3. Name a few ways that negative and positive stereotypes impact African American couples' relationships.
4. Where would you begin your work with a Black couple who held negative stereotypes about Black men and women?

REFERENCES

Aborampah, O. (1989). Black male–female relationships. *Journal of Black Studies, 19*, 320–342.

Adams, J. P., & Dressler, W. W. (1988). Perceptions of injustice in a black community: Dimensions and variations. *Human Relations, 41*, 753–767.

Alexander, M., & West, C. (2012). *The new Jim Crow: Mass incarceration in the age of colorblindness.* New Press.

Allen, R. L., & Bagozzi, R. P. (2001). Consequences of the Black sense of self. *Journal of Black Psychology, 27*, 3–28.

Allen, R. L., Dawson, M. C., & Brown, R. E. (1989). A schema-based approach to modeling an African American racial belief system. *American Political Science Review, 83*, 421–441.

Allen, R. L., & Hatchett, S. (1986). The media and social reality effects: self and system orientations of Blacks. *Communication Research, 13*, 97–123.

Allen, R. L., Thornton, M. C., & Watkins, S. C. (1992). An African American racial belief system and social structural relationships: A test of invariance. *National Journal of Sociology, 6*(2), 157–186.

Baldwin, J. A., & Hopkins, R. (1990). African Americans and European American cultural differences assessed by the worldview. *Paradigm: An Empirical Analysis, 14*, 38–52.

Blumstein, A. (1982). On the racial disproportionality of United States' prison populations. *The Journal of Criminal Law and Criminology, 73*(3), 1259–1281.

Boyd-Franklin, N. (1989). *Black families in therapy: A multisystems approach.* Guilford Press.

Boyd-Franklin, N., & Franklin, A. J. (1998). African American couples in therapy. In M. McGoldrick & K. V. Hardy (Eds.), *Re-visioning family therapy: Race, culture, and gender in clinical practice* (pp. 268–281). Guilford Press.

Broman, C. L. (1993). Race differences in marital well-being. *Journal of Marriage and the Family, 55*, 724–732.

Broman, C. L., Neighbors, H. W., & Jackson, J. S. (1988). Racial group identification among black adults. *Social Forces, 67*, 146–158.

Charles, K. K., & Luoh, M. C. (2010). Male incarceration, the marriage market, and female outcomes. *Review of Economics and Statistics, 92*(3), 614–627. https://doi.org/10.1162/rest_a_00022

Chestnut, C. (2009). *The study of internalized stereotypes among African American couples* [Unpublished doctoral dissertation]. Drexel University.

Clark, R., Anderson, N. B., Clark, V., & Williams, D. R. (1999). Racism as a stressor for African Americans: A biopsychosocial model. *American Psychologist, 54*(10), 805–816.

Cross, W. E., Jr. (1995). The psychology of Nigrescence: Revisiting the Cross model. In J. G. Ponterotto, J. M. Casa, L. A. Suzuki, & C. M. Alexander (Eds.), *Handbook of Multicultural Counseling* (pp. 93–122). Sage.

Cutrona, C. E., Russell, D. W., Abraham, W. T., Gardner, K. A., Melby, J. N., Bryant, C., & Conger, R. D. (2003). Neighborhood context and financial strain as predictors of marital interaction and marital quality in African American couples. *Personal Relationships, 10*, 389–409.

Darity, W. (2005). Stratification economics: The role of intergroup inequality. *Journal of Economics and Finance, 29*(2), 144–153. https://doi.org/10.1007/bf02761550

Darity, W., Dietrich, J., & Guilkey, D. K. (2001). Persistent advantage or disadvantage?: Evidence in support of the intergenerational drag hypothesis. *American Journal of Economics and Sociology, 60*(2), 435–470. https://doi.org/10.1111/1536-7150.00070

Du Bois, W. E. B. (1964). *The souls of Black folk.* Fawcett. (Original work published 1903)

Eichler, T. P. (2004). *Race and incarceration in Delaware: A preliminary consideration.* Delaware Center for Justice; Metropolitan Wilmington Urban League. http://www.prisonpolicy.org/scans/RaceIncarceration.pdf

Franklin, C. W. (1980). White racism as the cause of Black male-female conflict: A critique. *The Western Journal of Black Studies, 4*, 42–49.

Gatewood, W. B., Jr. (1988). Aristocrats of color: south and north, the black elite, 1880–1920. *Journal of Southern History, 54*, 3–20.

Hardy, K. V. (2001). The African American experience and the healing of relationships. https://dulwichcentre.com.au/articles-about-narrative-therapy/african-american-experience/

Jewell, K. S. (1983). Black male/female conflict: Internalization of negative definition transmitted through imagery. *The Western Journal of Black Studies, 7*, 43–48.

Kelly, S., & Floyd, F. J. (2001). The effects of negative racial stereotypes and Afrocentricity on couple relationships. *Journal of Family Psychology, 156,* 110–123.

LaRossa, R., & Reitzes, D. C. (1993). Symbolic interactionism and family studies. In P. Boss, W. Doherty, R. LaRossa, W. Schumm, & S. Steinmetz (Eds.), *Sourcebook of family themes and methods: A contextual approach* (pp. 135–163). Plenum.

Lawson, E., & Thompson, A. (1994). Historical and Social correlates of African American divorce: Review of the literature and implication for research. *The Western Journal of Black Studies, 18*(2), 91–103.

Locke, H. J. (1947). Predicting marital adjustment by comparison of a divorced and happily married group. *American Sociological Review, 12,* 187–191.

Locke, H. J., & Wallace, K. M. (1959). Short marital adjustment and prediction test: their reliability and validity. *Marriage and Family Living, 21,* 251–255.

Locke, H. J., & Williamson, R. C. (1958). Marital adjustment: A factor analysis study. *American Sociological Review, 23,* 562–569.

Lynch, C., & Blinder, M. (1983). The romantic relationship: Why and how people fall in love, the way couples connect, and why they break apart. *Family Therapy, 10,* 91–104.

Markowski, E. M., & Greenwood, P. D. (1984). Marital adjustment as a correlate of social interest. *Individual Psychology Journal of Adlerian Theory, Research and Practice, 40,* 300–308.

McCarthy, I. C., & Byrne, N. O. (2008). A fifth-province approach to intercultural issues in an Irish context: Marginal illumination. In M. McGoldrick & K. V. Hardy (Eds.), *Re-visioning family therapy: Race, culture, and gender in clinical practice* (pp. 327–343). Guilford Press.

McRoy, S., & Fisher, V. L. (1982). Marital adjustment of graduate student couples. *Family Relations, 31,* 37–41.

Meredith, W. H., Abbott, D. A., & Adams, S. L. (1986). Family violence: Its relation to marital and parental satisfaction and family strengths. *Journal of Family Violence, 1,* 299–305.

Nobles, W. W. (1973). Psychological research and the black self-concept: A critical review. *Journal of Social Issues, 29,* 11–31.

(1991). Extended self: Rethinking the so-called Negro self-respect. In R. L. Jones (Ed.), *Black psychology* (3rd ed., pp. 295–304). Cobb and Henry Publishers.

Nunnally, J. (1978). *Psychometric theory* (2nd ed.). McGraw-Hill.

Okazawa-Rey, M., Robinson, T., & Ward, J. V. (1986). Black women and the politics of skin color and hair. *Women's Studies Quarterly, 14,* 13–14.

Olson, D. H. (1999). Overview of manual: In *David Olson's prepare/enrich counselor's manual,* Version 2000 (pp. 1–21). Life Innovations.

Parham, T. A., & Helms J. E. (1985). The relationship of racial, identity attitudes to self actualization of black students and objective states. *Journal of Counseling Psychology, 32,* 431–440.

Pinderhughes, E. (1989). *Understanding race, ethnicity & power: The key to efficacy in clinical practice.* The Free Press.

(2002). African American marriage in the 20th century. *Family Process, 41,* 269–282.

(2008). Black genealogy revisited: Restorying an African American family. In M. McGoldrick & K. V. Hardy (Eds.), *Revisioning family therapy: race, culture and gender in clinical practice* (pp. 114–134). Guilford Press.

Reis, H. T., & Patrick, B. C. (1996). Attachment and intimacy: Component processes. In E. T. Higgins & A. W. Kruglanski (Eds.), *Social psychology: Handbook of basic principles* (pp. 523–563). Guilford Press.

Reis, H. T., & Shaver, P. (1988). Intimacy as an interpersonal process. In S. Duck (Ed.), *Handbook of personal relationships* (pp. 367–389). Wiley.

Sellers, R. M. (1993). A call to arms for researchers studying racial identity. *Journal of Black Psychology, 19*(3), 327–332.

Simpson, J. A. (1987). The dissolution of romantic relationships: Factors involved in relationship stability and emotional distress. *Journal of Personality and Social Psychology, 53,* 683–692.

(1990). Attachment theory in modern evolutionary perspective. In *Handbook of attachment: Theory, research and clinical application* (pp. 115–140). Guilford Press.

Spanier, G. B. (1976). Measuring dyadic adjustment: New scales for assessing the quality of marriage and similar dyads. *Journal of Marriage and the Family, 38,* 15–28.

(2001). *Dyadic Adjustment Scale user's manual.* Multi-Health Systems.

Spanier, G. B., & Cole, C. L. (1976). Toward clarification and investigation of marital adjustment. *International Journal of the Sociology of the Family, 6,* 121–146.

SPSS, Inc. (2005). *SPSS base 15.0 user guide.* SPSS.

Steinberg, R. J., Hojjat, M., & Barnes, M. L. (2001). Empirical aspects of a theory of love as a story. *European Journal of Personality, 15*(3), 1–20.

Taylor, J. (1990). Relationship between internalized racism and marital satisfaction. *The Journal of Black Psychology, 16,* 45–53.

Taylor, J., & Zhang, X. (1990). Cultural identity in maritally distressed and nondistressed black couples. *The Western Journal of Black Studies, 14,* 205–213.

Terman, L. (1938). *Psychological factors in marital happiness.* McGraw-Hill.

Turner, R. J., & Noh, S. (1983). Class and psychological vulnerability among women: The significance of social support and personal control. *Journal of Health and Social Behavior, 24*(1), 2–15.

Udry, J. R., Bauman, K. E., & Chase, C. (1971). Skin color, status, and mate selection. *American Journal of Sociology, 76,* 722–733.

U.S. Census Bureau. (2000). *Statistical abstract of the United States* (114th ed.). U.S. Government Printing Office.

(2008). *Current Population Survey 2008 annual social and economic (ASEC) supplement.* https://www2.census.gov/programs-surveys/cps/techdocs/cpsmar08.pdf

West, C. (1993). *Race matters*. Vintage Books, Random House.

White, B. B. (1989). Gender differences in marital communication patterns. *Family Process, 28*, 89–106.

White, J. M., & Kline, D. M. (2002). *Family theories* (2nd ed.). Sage.

Whiting, J. B., & Crane, D. R. (2003). Distress and divorce: Establishing cutoff scores for the marital stress inventory. *Contemporary Family Therapy, 2*, 195–205.

Zeifman, D., & Hazan, C. (1997). Attachment: The bond in pair-bonds. In J. A. Simpson & D. Kenrick (Eds.), *Evolutionary social psychology* (pp. 237–263). Erlbaum.

CHAPTER 2

The Role of the Strong Black Woman Schema in Black Love and Relationships

Heather C. Lofton & Adia Gooden

2.1 Introduction

The Strong Black Woman (SBW) schema reflects how many Black women see themselves, how the world sees Black women, and how Black women are expected to engage in the world. The image of a strong Black woman is embodied by the exertion of unyielding strength and unlimited capacity when navigating daily roles, interpersonal interactions, and life tasks, all of which involve intense emotional and physical labor (Parks, 2010). In mainstream media, Black women are represented by messages of emotional restraint, power, and stamina; for example, "Black women don't cry in public" and "Black women have no choice but to be resilient." Although many Black women have benefitted from adopting the SBW schema, it also comes with a cost.

Specifically, personifying the SBW schema can make it difficult for Black women to seek and engage in healthy romantic relationships. In the modern context, Black romantic relationships are an opportunity for love and care and for Black people to have a space to retreat from the racism and sexism they experience in the world. However, Black women's connection to the SBW schema has both positive and negative impacts on both their public and their personal lives. In this chapter, we review the history and development of the SBW schema and how this schema manifests in the lived experiences of Black women in romantic relationships. Understanding this context provides better comprehension of the challenges Black women may face when dating and developing healthy intimate partner attachments, and can also offer helpful clinical insights when working with Black women clients in therapy.

2.2 Development and Manifestations of the Strong Black Woman Schema

The characteristics (e.g., always showing an invulnerable image to the world), narratives (e.g., that Black women must be strong to support their families and communities), qualities (e.g., selflessness, self-sacrificing, strong work ethic), and constraints (e.g., difficulty asking for what she needs, difficulty caring for herself) associated with the SBW schema have been ingrained in the lives of Black women since slavery. Examining Black womanhood during slavery reveals the complexities of the SBW construct's creation. It is evident in literature focused on romantic relationship among Black southern slaves, that platonic, familial, and romantic relationship building were not human rights granted to Black men and women (Robinson, 2007). To act on a basic human need for love and connection, enslaved men and women would risk their lives, secretly forming bonds and unions to solidify their love (Robinson, 2007). The risks involved in Black partnership during slavery informed a responsibility for Black men and women to protect and preserve Black union and loyalty as an expression of love. In many ways, the SBW schema reflects survival tactics Black women used during slavery when they and their loved ones were separated, threatened, and traumatized. These survival strategies resembled emotional suppression, ignoring internal stress responses, and operating with unrealistic psychological and physical capacity and self-expectation (Jones et al., 2022). The ability to suppress pervasive pain and suffering helped Black slaves and therefore came to signify a strength and power to survive. Ultimately, the skill of suppression became a core aspect of the SBW schema and was communicated over generations as fundamental to living. The power of this schema has been passed down through generations of Black women as grandmothers, mothers, aunts, sisters, and girlfriends communicated that this unyielding strength was necessary for survival (Nelson et al., 2016).

2.2.1 SBW Schema Development

2.2.1.1 Ethno-gendered Socialization

Focusing on the transmission of the SBW schema, researchers Brown and Tylka (2011) review the developmental process of socialization as one that supports resilience against discrimination. Ethno-gendered socialization refers to the way individuals were exposed to and taught values, perspectives, and overall survival techniques to navigate the intersections of race and gender (Brown & Tylka, 2011; Thomas & King, 2007). The SBW schema is often transmitted through ethno-gendered socialized messages and has both strengths and challenges; this socialization has enabled Black women to function with self-sufficiency and independence under difficult life circumstances and has also made it challenging for Black women to be vulnerable when receiving love from partners.

Black women have learned that acknowledging and responding to their feelings is either a sign of weakness and/or unacceptable. While this emotional suppression coping strategy may be helpful in some situations, several studies examining the SBW schema expose the associated risks of high levels of stress (Abrams et al., 2014; West et al., 2016). For young Black women, playing out the SBW schema often first happens in academic settings (Wang & Huguley, 2012). As young Black women start navigating academic institutions without their familial protective structures, being strong and stoic serve as the shields protecting Black women from vulnerabilities of oppression (Brown et al., 2009; Friend et al., 2011).

Further solidifying the salience of SBW narrative transmission, researchers Bailey-Fakhoury and Frierson (2014) conducted a specific examination of upper middle-class Black female students' experiences in predominantly white institutions. This study focused on a concept of "motherwork strategies" or survival tips and tools guided by the lived experiences of their mother figures. Black mothers teach their daughters how to survive a system that is not designed for their success. Young Black women are encouraged by their mothers to engage in preemptive behaviors, which are focused on ways to avoid or disarm an oppressive experience. Within these "motherwork strategies" lie scripts with culturally specific tenets of the SBW schema. The researchers noted that the middle-class Black mothers still communicated the importance of survival through their protective messages to their daughters, despite their socioeconomic status (Bailey-Fakhoury & Frierson, 2014). Strengthening the message, the SBW schema has helped Black women prevail in harmful spaces, demonstrating the ability to endure daily systemic stressors, overcome community constraints, and maintain emotional control, all while proclaiming no need for self-recuperation (Black & Peacock, 2011). However, Black women are also becoming more acquainted with the present-day risks of employing this unrelenting strength, which often prevents them from taking care of themselves and allowing others to care for them.

Barr and colleagues (2013) discuss the notion that young Black girls' marital beliefs are socialized based on the context of their upbringing. From a young age, families and communities communicate to Black girls that they should learn to be independent and take care of themselves and that they should also try to find a Black man who will take care of them one day (Wallace, 2007). These somewhat contradicting messages may be confusing for Black girls and women to navigate and leave them feeling a tension between the security of self-sufficiency and the vulnerability of expressing their desire for partnership. Black women are encouraged to find a Black male partner who can provide, yet societal constraints and generations of different SBW narratives have positioned Black women as providers (Hurt et al., 2014). Additionally, Wallace (2007) argues that the gendered socialization of Black boys and girls contributes to challenges that Black men and women have in romantic relationships with each other. Black boys learn that to be real men they must be dominant and aggressive while Black girls are taught to be independent and self-sufficient. These gendered ways of being are likely to clash in the context of a romantic relationship between a Black man and a Black woman if both partners adhere to their gendered socialization.

In addition to the messages Black girls receive, it is sadly not uncommon for Black girls to experience trauma from sexual assault, physical abuse, and witnessing violence in their family and communities. It is well known that adverse childhood experiences lead to negative mental and physical health outcomes in adulthood, and research has demonstrated that Black women who experience trauma are more likely to adopt the SBW schema (Harrington et al., 2010). Further, the experience of discrimination, harsh parenting, familial instability, and economic hardship contributes to cynical views of romantic relationships and marriage among Black male and female young adults (Kogan et al., 2013; Simons et al., 2012). Thus, it is conceivable that Black women who had harsh and traumatic experiences in their childhood not only may have challenges engaging in romantic relationships because of the SBW schema but may also be skeptical of the possibility that they will experience love, trust, and support in romantic partnerships.

2.2.2 *Contemporary Manifestations of the SBW*

Although there have been adaptations in what is believed to be essential to survival, the SBW schema continues to uphold tenets rooted in self-sacrifice and self-silencing. For centuries, Black women navigated labels and images, socially constructed to the detriment of their identity and overall psychosocial, socio-emotional, and interpersonal development (Davis & Tucker-Brown, 2013). The SBW schema is anchored in the goal of protecting self, partner, and family, yet silently disempowers emotional vulnerability and resilience (Abrams et al., 2019; Walker-Barnes, 2009). Since emancipation, most Black women have been expected to engage in workforce and family leadership as primary contributors (Dozier, 2010) to aid systemically oppressed household economic development (Collins, 2012; Staples, 1985). For example, a familiar narrative of Black women depicts a single-parent family structure, with the Black woman serving as the sole breadwinner for her household, working all day and coming home to prepare a meal for her family and either eating last or not eating at all. For many, this scenario can be observed as common sacrificial behavior of parents. However, scenarios such as this also present a pattern of sacrifice that can be observed in other areas of a Black woman's life. While honorable in her efforts to provide for her family, a common SBW narrative suggests, "I have to be strong for my family," which may be to the detriment of her physical and psychological well-being. The necessity of strength remains relevant to the current lived experiences of all Black women who endure daily systemic societal injustices (Davis, 2015).

The contemporary manifestation of the SBW schema remains consistent with the original definition. The current reported physical and psychological practices of strength expose the continued use of suppression, internalization, and desensitization to the inevitable vulnerabilities of feelings and emotions (Woods-Giscombé, 2010). Conclusively, using these stress responses in the context of a romantic relationship highlights the potential for difficulty in developing healthy intimate relationships. Further, while many Black women achieve highly in their academic and professional pursuits, they must also bear witness to the Black men in their lives succumbing to societal acts of violence and forceful oppression, which is incredibly painful (Davis & Maldonado, 2015; McDaniel et al., 2011; Smiley & Fakunle, 2016). Black women watch as their Black male partners suffer from high levels of incarceration and violence. Black women also experience violence at the hands of police and at times Black men. These traumatic experiences feed into the SBW schema. Black women in low-income communities, in particular, are often shown stoically discussing the losses of their Black sons, brothers, and husbands at press conferences, moving quickly into action and advocacy, seeming to have little space or time to truly mourn the loss of their loved ones. Further solidifying the need for the SBW schema, the pressure to protect self and the Black community prevails as a responsibility for Black women.

Exploring further the nuances of Black female identity, professional Black women often utilize the SBW schema to advance, as this schema continues to protect Black women in the face of demanding professional interpersonal environments. Research on the psychological effects of workplace discrimination and sexual harassment for Black women exposes the psychological harm caused by recurrent encounters with racism and sexism (Buchanan & Fitzgerald, 2008; Hirsh & Lyons, 2010). Black women experience emotional wounds resulting from workplace discrimination that can result in feelings of isolation and bruised self-esteem and self-worth (Buchanan & Fitzgerald, 2008). Characteristics of the SBW can suppress these emotions and ultimately have the potential of transitioning into interpersonal constraints. The SBW schema, protective in its creation, can also inhibit openness and vulnerability, which are required for romantic relationships. The message of independence is a principle of the SBW in conclusively every fundamental area of life; however, when situated in a romantic relationship, researchers uncover a conflict of interpersonal messages.

2.3 The Strong Black Woman Schema in Romantic Relationships

The systemic oppression, racial trauma, and discrimination Black people endure negatively affects their interpersonal relationships (Cutrona et al., 2011). As previously mentioned, the SBW schema is in part a product of the oppression Black women experience and influences Black women in romantic relationships (Abrams et al., 2014; Watson & Hunter, 2016). The characteristics and coping strategies aligned with the SBW schema appear to hinder Black women from cultivating healthy, intimate, and vulnerable relationships with romantic partners. However, despite the challenges faced, many Black women demonstrate a commitment to the idea of Black romantic relationships and family (Johnson & Loscocco, 2015).

There is a high level of support for pursuing and cultivating loving romantic relationships in the Black community (Stackman et al., 2016). The SBW schema typically involves Black women fiercely protecting their partners, children, and family members from outside intrusion. This support is particularly pronounced in the Black Christian and Muslim communities and among middle- and upper-class Black people. For religious communities, marriage is highlighted as the anchor of the family; however, divorce and raising children outside of marriage is still common in the Black community. In middle- and upper-class communities, support for marriage may be tied to respectability politics and an attempt to demonstrate to white society that Black people have strong morals and values (Hill, 2006). However, Hill highlights the ways that Black women have exercised their agency by not getting married throughout their history in the United States. It is important to recognize that while partnership may be valued among Black women, marriage may not always be an advantageous decision for individual Black women, and in the Black community, child rearing, family, and romantic relationships do not always center around marriage (Hill, 2006). Further, Black women who adopt the SBW schema may be less likely to prioritize marital commitment, which might involve letting go of their independence and self-sufficiency and some of their power and control.

2.3.1 *Romantic Partnership Development*

In modern contexts, Black women often adopt the role of preserving Black love, Black families, and the Black community; many Black women hope to start their own Black families and have Black babies. Yet, parallel to the oppressions faced by Black women are the constrained experiences of their Black male partners. Black men and women have both shared and divergent experiences related to race and gender and romantic relationships between them have been influenced by sociohistorical factors as well (Cutrona et al., 2011; Pinderhughes, 2002).

Black women who are interested in partnering with men express concerns about finding suitable partners due to the belief that there are not enough eligible Black men to date (Henry, 2008). Researchers have connected high death rates of Black men, mass incarceration, and high unemployment rates among Black men to lower numbers of men who would be considered "marriageable" by Black women (Harknett & McLanahan, 2004; King & Allen, 2009; Mechoulan, 2011). In a study of middle-class African American men and women, King and Allen found that both men and women prioritized marrying a partner who is "reliable, monogamous, affectionate, financially stable" (p. 583) and preferred a partner who made a significantly higher income than they did. The education gap between Black men and women may cause tension and challenges in romantic partnerships between them (Burton & Tucker, 2009; Furdyna et al., 2008) and may make marriage to Black men who are less financially successful feel risky for Black women. Although the perception of the shortage of eligible Black male partners is more negative than reality, this perception often leads to feelings of anxiety among Black women who want to partner with Black men and may lead them to settle for relationship arrangements that they would not prefer (Gooden, 2016).

Adding to concerns about eligible and available Black men to partner are the Black men who partner and marry white or non-Black women. While the rates of interracial marriage among Black men are still relatively low, Black men are more likely to marry a non-Black partner than Black women are. Black women are criticized for their anger about Black men partnering with white women but in her qualitative examination of this dynamic, Childs (2005) identified that Black women often see Black man–white woman partnerships as representing their struggle to find love relationships as well as the devaluing of Black women in mainstream American society. The combined pain of struggling to find Black male partners and witnessing Black men partner with non-Black women may increase Black women's uncertainty about the possibility of finding a loving partnership.

Black women's fears of being devalued as potential romantic partners by society are validated as Black women turn to dating apps and websites to meet potential partners and face additional barriers related to receiving fewer inquiries from people who are interested in dating them. Data from dating websites has demonstrated that Black women are the least desirable as compared to women of other races, which means that they receive the fewest matches and responses from potential dates. OKCupid (a popular online dating site) reported in a post that has since been deleted that Black women were rated lowest compared to women of other races and were rated only slightly positively by Black men (OkCupid, 2014). Further, heterosexual Black women are less likely to date people from other races both due to an allegiance to Black men and the Black community and because men of other races are less likely to express romantic interest in Black women on dating apps or in person. The process of engaging in online and in-person dating is often filled with stress, anxiety, and feelings of rejection for Black women. This stress during the dating process may cause Black women to utilize coping strategies found within the SBW schema and suppress their desire and openness to finding a loving partnership. Closing themselves off to potential partners and the possibility of relationships may help Black women to protect themselves emotionally but it will also communicate to potential partners that they are not interested or are emotionally unavailable for a relationship, making it more difficult for them to connect and find love.

As Black women try to date and find sustainable romantic partnership with Black men, they are often prejudged by a narrative that Black women are "too much" and that they do not need men. Indeed, SBWs do not fit into the patriarchal paradigm of wives and mothers and therefore may be overlooked as potential romantic partners. Although some of the strengths exhibited in the SBW schema may be harmful to Black women, there are aspects of their strength and independence that foster healthy, egalitarian relationships. Research has demonstrated that when they do marry, Black men and women are more likely to have egalitarian relationships than their white counterparts and egalitarian dynamics in marriages are linked to more contentment (Marks et al., 2008).

2.3.2   Romantic Partnerships with Black Men

Black women now earn college and graduate degrees at higher rates than Black men women and although this success supports Black families and Black communities (Collins, 2012; Staples, 1985), it can cause complicated dynamics in heterosexual relationships between Black women and men. The SBW schema has an outward display of unlimited capacity and unrelenting self-command; however, it internally reinforces a danger in vulnerability that represents the narrative "I can't let them see me sweat." Abrams and colleagues (2014) highlight that one implication of the SBW schema, which involves Black women feeling they can rely only on themselves, is that marriage and long-term partnership may feel impossible or unnecessary. In part because of different gender socialized messages, Black women who are in romantic relationships with Black men may minimize their success and hide their strengths to avoid emasculating their male partners (Gooden, 2016). Additionally, part of the SBW schema involves Black women putting themselves and their needs last and this dynamic may continue in the context of romantic relationships in which they overfunction for their partners (Gooden, 2016; Jones & Shorter-Gooden, 2003) while hiding their own needs in a way that is not healthy or sustainable. Further, although many people have relationship dynamics where one partner overfunctions and another partner underfunctions, this is often a reflection of codependency and does not serve as a healthy foundation for long-term partnership.

In her book *Communion: The Female Search for Love*, bell hooks (2002) challenges the idea that women are more equipped to be loving than men are. She argues that although women are socialized to express their longing for love, they may struggle to actually be loving. This seems to be true for women who adopt the SBW schema, which may leave them longing for love without understanding how to be loving once they are in a romantic relationship. Many Black women are taught how to give care, and this is often how women who fit with the SBW schema show love to partners and family. However, hooks (2002) distinguishes between loving and showing care. Notably, a mutual partnership involves both giving and receiving love and the SBW schema may prevent Black women from receiving and giving love outside of a caregiving framework. In romantic relationships, Black women are able to practice vulnerability and interdependence, to move away from complete self-sufficiency and giving without receiving, to a space of mutuality, shared responsibility, and love. Clinicians can support Black women in healing, releasing the SBW schema, and engaging in healthy, fulfilling relationships.

2.3.3 Romantic Partnership

When SBWs do find love in the context of romantic relationships, their socialization to be strong and independent may get in the way of cultivating intimate and interdependent relationships with their partners of any gender. It is important to note that not all Black women are interested in romantic partnership with Black men. Black women who identify as lesbian, bisexual, pansexual, and/or queer might not feel anxiety and stress related to finding a Black male partner. However, these women may be navigating concerns about how their family and community will respond to them partnering with a woman or someone who is transgender or gender nonconforming. The additional stress of coming out and finding partnership while potentially navigating rejection from family and community can negatively impact nonheterosexual women in their search for romantic love. In contrast to the findings about heterosexual Black women prioritizing the financial stability of potential partners, some research has shown that Black lesbian and bisexual women may be less concerned with the financial status of their partners than heterosexual women (Battle & Ashley, 2008). There is also evidence that throughout history Black women have expressed their independence in romantic and sexual relationships with women (Hill, 2006; hooks, 2002), which aligns with the SBW schema. It is conceivable that Black women who adopt the SBW schema and are interested in romantic relationships with other women and nonmale partners would encounter similar challenges to those of heterosexual women in navigating long-term intimate relationships.

2.4   Clinical Implications

2.4.1   Trust before Vulnerability

It is important for therapists to understand that Black women who adopt the SBW schema are likely to want to show their therapist that they are competent and have it all together (Shorter-Gooden, 2009). Therefore, therapists must be patient with these clients and give them time to get comfortable and develop enough trust to be vulnerable in sessions and share their true challenges (Gooden, 2016).

2.4.2   Unpack the Schema

Therapists working with Black women who present with the SBW schema should help their clients unpack this schema and how it manifests in their life and relationships. As part of this unpacking, it is essential for therapists to facilitate emotional healing for Black female clients. As mentioned previously, Black women may adopt the SBW schema in response to trauma and disappointment and as a way of protecting themselves against a world that can be harsh and unforgiving to Black women. The SBW schema may serve as a form of emotional armor that helps Black women to suppress their emotions, show their strengths to the world, and put aside their needs and desires as they work to support themselves and their loved ones (Abrams et al., 2014; Harrington et al., 2010). It is important for clinicians to begin by acknowledging the ways in which the SBW schema has been adaptive for their Black female clients in their personal, academic, and professional lives before guiding these women to examine the ways that this mode of being may influence seeking and engaging in the love and intimacy they may long for.

2.4.3   Assess and Process Trauma

Often, before clients are ready to be emotionally intimate with other people, they must practice emotional intimacy with themselves. One thing that may block Black women from being in touch with their own emotions is trauma. Some Black women have experienced trauma in relationships with Black men, which may complicate their engagement in intimate relationships with Black men. It is important for therapists to assess whether their Black female clients have experienced trauma and when the client is ready, to guide them to reprocess and heal from any trauma that they may have experienced, with a particular attention to relational trauma. When traumatic experiences have begun to be processed and healed, it will feel safer for Black women to allow themselves to feel and be present with their emotions.

2.4.4   *Teach Self-Compassion*

To further Black women's emotional healing and intimacy with themselves, clinicians are also encouraged to guide Black women through a process of listening to and making room for their emotions. Self-compassion and mindfulness practices can be very useful in helping Black women develop an intimacy with themselves and openness to feeling their own emotions without judgment. Women who adopt the SBW schema may be harsh and critical toward themselves and others, and it may be useful for clinicians to help Black female clients cultivate a kind and compassionate voice and way of responding to emotions, vulnerability, and mistakes. The theme of this aspect of the therapeutic work is helping Black women to develop a more loving and accepting relationship with themselves.

2.4.5   *Unconditional Self-Worth*

An important aspect of helping Black women establish a healthy relationship with themselves is supporting Black female clients in embracing their unconditional self-worth. This is particularly important for Black women who adopt the SBW schema and may believe that their worth is dependent on being self-sufficient and constantly meeting the needs of others. Unconditional self-worth will enable Black women to see themselves as worthy in the absence of overfunctioning for others and will help them to love themselves and be willing to be vulnerable with others. Supporting Black female clients in connecting to their unconditional self-worth will also help them to move into romantic relationships with confidence and will free them from the fear that they need to prove that they are worthy of love and respect. In order to support this process, clinicians can guide their Black female clients to examine and challenge the conditions they have placed on their self-worth, forgive themselves for things they feel make them unworthy, and practice self-acceptance and self-compassion. It can also be helpful for clinicians to encourage their Black female clients to find safe, supportive friendships or groups where they are accepted and supported in being their full selves.

2.4.6   Facilitate Self-Identity Construction

Once Black women are on the path to healing their relationships with themselves, they will be freer to unpack the SBW schema. Clinicians can guide Black female clients through a process that supports them in defining and valuing themselves beyond the scope of the SBW schema. In a seminal text on Black feminist thought, Patricia Hill Collins (1986) argues, "Regardless of the actual content of Black women's self-definitions, the act of insisting on Black female self-definition validates Black women's power as human subjects" (p. S17). Supporting Black women in defining themselves and how they would like to engage in the world and their relationships is empowering. Further, Collins (1986) asserts that it is important for Black women to identify the qualities and characteristics they value for themselves beyond what is expected of them in their families, communities, and mainstream society. Black women may want to continue embodying some of the characteristics of the SBW schema and clinicians can support Black female clients in examining the schema and identifying for themselves what serves them and what they wish to release.

2.5   Supporting Black Women in Loving and Dating

Although it is not necessary for Black women to experience complete healing to begin exploring the possibility of healthy romantic relationships, having a foundation of self-love and self-worth are important aspects of helping Black women to find and cultivate healthy, loving relationships (hooks, 2001). As clinicians support Black women in finding love, they should begin with helping Black women to acknowledge and release any feelings of pain, loss, and anger they continue to experience in response to past romantic relationships or relationships that never came to fruition. Additionally, given the challenge that many Black women experience in finding male partners, clinicians are encouraged to help their clients name and process feelings of pain, disappointment, frustration, and rejection related to difficulties they have had with dating in the past. These painful experiences may cause Black women to turn to the SBW schema to suppress their romantic and sexual desire and seek to embody an image of Black womanhood that is embraced in the Black community.

Many Black women experience hurt, rejection, and anxiety in their search for love and when these experiences linger, they can cause Black women to go into new relationships with negative narratives and the belief that they need to protect themselves from vulnerability with new partners. An important aspect of helping Black women move forward is guiding them to forgive themselves and past partners for negative experiences and potential attachment wounds they have had in past relationships. Clinicians are encouraged to guide Black women through a process of forgiveness that allows for their repair journey to recalibrate intimate relationship needs (Stanley et al., 2010). As part of this forgiveness process therapists should help clients to identify the wisdom they gained from past relationships and how they would like to use this wisdom to guide them in future relationships.

Once past relationships and dating experiences are forgiven, therapists can support Black women in preparing for healthy, loving romantic relationships by guiding them to create a vision for what they would like their romantic partnership to look like. Negative developmental experiences can cause Black women to view relationships with skepticism (Simons et al., 2012) and to make it more likely for Black women to find the relationships they most desire, it is important for them to craft a vision for what a healthy relationship would look and feel like for them. When Black women know what they do and do not want in a relationship they will be able to let go of relationships that are harmful or unsupportive and move past the belief that they should hold on to any relationship that is available to them for fear that they may not find another partner (Gooden, 2016; Jones & Shorter-Gooden, 2003). Creating a vision for the relationship they want will help Black women prepare for mutual, intimate, and supportive relationships. As part of this preparation, clinicians can also help Black women to reflect on the ways they may overfunction in relationships with family, friends, and partners and encourage them to interrupt this pattern. As part of interrupting this pattern, Black women may need to practice receiving help, love, and care from others; therapists can encourage them to practice this in the therapy session and through asking for the support that they want from friends and family.

Finally, as Black women prepare to engage in romantic relationships, the therapeutic relationship can be a powerful medium through which they can practice being vulnerable in an emotionally intimate relationship. Clinicians are encouraged to utilize the therapeutic relationship to help Black women feel safe in expressing their full selves and experiencing the positive benefits of unconditional acceptance. Therapists may find it useful to process and explore their Black female client's interpersonal experiences in therapy and connect those insights to how they might engage in romantic relationships to help foster insight and support them in engaging constructively in their relationships outside of therapy.

2.6 Conclusion

There is a long history of Black women adopting the SBW schema and it is important for clinicians working with Black women to understand this schema as it relates to Black women's mental health overall and to their experiences loving and dating. The SBW schema remains adaptive and necessary for many Black women as they seek to survive and succeed in the world. However, despite the ways that the SBW helps Black women cope with challenging life experiences, it can also make it more difficult for them to find and engage in healthy, loving partnerships.

Black women experience a number of challenges in their search for love, and this is particularly true for Black women who are interested in partnering with Black men. The pain of disappointment in dating and not finding the love that they are seeking, may cause Black women to turn to the coping strategies of emotional suppression and denying personal needs within the SBW schema. When they do find love, strong Black women may struggle to open up and be vulnerable with partners of any gender because they have become accustomed to suppressing their emotions and showing invulnerability and strength. Although these qualities may protect them in a world that often discriminates against Black women, they will hinder emotional intimacy with partners.

Despite the challenges present for women who adopt the SBW schema when they are dating and seeking a partner, there is great opportunity for these women to find deep love and connection. Black women can have healing experiences in their romantic relationships that allow them to let down their emotional walls and receive love and care from a partner. Clinicians have the opportunity to support Black women on this journey by guiding them to heal from past relational trauma, cultivate a healthy relationship with themselves, unpack the SBW identity, and create a vision for the loving relationships that they want.

Discussion Questions

1. What are some ways that society continues to reinforce the SBW schema for Black females?
2. How might you recognize if your client embodied the SBW schema?
3. How might traditional gendered ways of being create conflict in the context of a romantic relationship between a Black man and a Black woman if both partners adhere to their gendered socialization.
4. Given your understanding of SBW schema, would you recommend individual therapy for the Black woman or couples therapy for her and her partner to address relational conflicts? Why?

REFERENCES

Abrams, J. A., Hill, A., & Maxwell, M. (2019). Underneath the mask of the strong Black woman schema: Disentangling influences of strength and self-silencing on depressive symptoms among US Black women. *Sex Roles*, *80*(9–10), 517–526. https://doi.org/10.1007/s11199-018-0956-y

Abrams, J. A., Maxwell, M., Pope, M., & Belgrave, F. Z. (2014). Carrying the world with the grace of a lady and the grit of a warrior: Deepening our understanding of the "Strong Black Woman" schema. *Psychology of Women Quarterly*, *38*(4), 503–518. https://doi.org/10.1177/0361684314541418

Bailey-Fakhoury, C., & Frierson, M. (2014). Black women attending predominantly White institutions: Fostering their academic success using African American motherwork strategies. *Journal of Progressive Policy & Practice*, *2* (3), 213–228.

Barr, A. B., Culatta, E., & Simons, R. L. (2013). Romantic relationships and health among African American young adults: Linking patterns of relationship quality over time to changes in physical and mental health. *Journal of Health and Social Behavior*, *54*(3), 369–385. https://doi.org/10.1177/0022146513486652

Battle, J., & Ashley, C. (2008). Intersectionality, heteronormativity, and Black lesbian, gay, bisexual, and transgender (LGBT) families. *Black Women, Gender & Families*, *2*(1), 1–24.

Black, A. R., & Peacock, N. (2011). Pleasing the masses: Messages for daily life management in African American women's popular media sources. *American Journal of Public Health*, *101*(1), 144–150.

Brown, D. L., & Tylka, T. L. (2011). Racial discrimination and resilience in African American young adults: Examining racial socialization as a moderator. *Journal of Black Psychology*, *37*(3), 259–285. https://doi.org/10.1177/0095798410390689

Brown, T. L., Linver, M. R., Evans, M., & DeGennaro, D. (2009). African–American parents' racial and ethnic socialization and adolescent academic grades: Teasing out the role of gender. *Journal of Youth and Adolescence, 38* (2), 214–227. https://doi.org/10.1007/s10964-008-9362-z

Buchanan, N. T., & Fitzgerald, L. F. (2008). Effects of racial and sexual harassment on work and the psychological well-being of African American women. *Journal of Occupational Health Psychology, 13*(2), 137–151. https://doi.org/10.1037/1076-8998.13.2.137

Burton, L. M., & Tucker, M. B. (2009). Romantic unions in an era of uncertainty: A post-Moynihan perspective on African American women and marriage. *The Annals of the American Academy of Political and Social Science, 621*(1), 132–148. https://doi.org/10.1177/0002716208324852

Childs, E. C. (2005). Looking behind the stereotypes of the "angry black woman": An exploration of Black women's responses to interracial relationships. *Gender & Society, 19*(4), 544–561. https://doi.org/10.1177/0891243205276755

Collins, P. H. (1986). Learning from the outsider within: The sociological significance of Black feminist thought. *Social Problems, 33*(6), s14–s32. https://doi.org/10.2307/800672

(2012). Just another American story? The first Black first family. *Qualitative Sociology, 35*(2), 123–141. https://doi.org/10.1007/s11133-012-9225-5

Cutrona, C. E., Russell, D. W., Burzette, R. G., Wesner, K. A., & Bryant, C. M. (2011). Predicting relationship stability among midlife African American couples. *Journal of Consulting and Clinical Psychology, 79*(6), 814–825. https://doi.org/10.1037/a0025874

Davis, D. R., & Maldonado, C. (2015). Shattering the glass ceiling: The leadership development of African American women in higher education. *Advancing Women in Leadership, 35.* https://doi.org/10.21423/awlj-v35.a125

Davis, S. M. (2015). The "Strong Black Woman Collective": A Developing theoretical framework for understanding collective communication practices of black women. *Women's Studies in Communication, 38*(1), 20–35. https://doi.org/10.1080/07491409.2014.953714

Davis, S., & Tucker-Brown, A. (2013). Effects of black sexual stereotypes on sexual decision making among African American women. *Journal of Pan African Studies, 5*(9), 111–128.

Dozier, R. (2010). Accumulating disadvantage: The growth in the black–white wage gap among women. *Journal of African American Studies, 14*, 279–301. https://doi.org/10.1007/s12111-010-9122-5

Friend, C. A., Hunter, A. G., & Fletcher, A. C. (2011). Parental racial socialization and the academic achievement of African American children: A cultural-ecological approach. *Journal of African American Studies, 15*(1), 40–57. https://doi.org/10.1007/s12111-010-9124-3

Furdyna, H. E., Tucker, M. B., & James, A. D. (2008). Relative spousal earnings and marital happiness among African American and White women. *Journal of Marriage and Family, 70*(2), 332–344. https://doi.org/10.1111/j.1741-3737.2008.00485.x

Gooden, A. S. (2016). Black women in couples and families. In J. Lebow, A. Chamber, & D. C. Breunlin (Eds.), *Encyclopedia of couple & family therapy* (pp. 285–289). Springer International Publishing. https://doi.org/10.1007/978-3-319-49425-8_702

Harknett, K., & McLanahan, S. S. (2004). Racial and ethnic differences in marriage after the birth of a child. *American Sociological Review*, *69*(6), 790–811. https://doi.org/10.1177/000312240406900603

Harrington, E. F., Crowther, J. H., & Shipherd, J. C. (2010). Trauma, binge eating, and the "strong Black woman." *Journal of Consulting and Clinical Psychology*, *78*(4), 469–479. https://doi.org/10.1037/a0019174

Henry, W. J. (2008). Black female millennial college students: Dating dilemmas and identity development. *Multicultural Education*, *16*(2), 17–21.

Hill, S. A. (2006). Marriage among African American women: A gender perspective. *Journal of Comparative Family Studies*, *37*(3), 421–440. https://doi.org/10.3138/jcfs.37.3.421

Hirsh, E., & Lyons, C. J. (2010). Perceiving discrimination on the job: Legal consciousness, workplace context, and the construction of race discrimination. *Law & Society Review*, *44*(2), 269–298. https://doi.org/10.1111/j.1540-5893.2010.00403.x

hooks, b. (2001). *All about love: New visions*. Harper Perennial.

    (2002). *Communion: The female search for love*. Perennial.

Hurt, T. R., McElroy, S. E., Sheats, K. J., Landor, A. M., & Bryant, C. M. (2014). Married Black men's opinions as to why Black women are disproportionately single: A qualitative study. *Personal Relationships*, *21*(1), 88–109. https://doi.org/10.1111/pere.12019

Johnson, K. R., & Loscocco, K. (2015). Black marriage through the prism of gender, race, and class. *Journal of Black Studies*, *46*(2), 142–171. https://doi.org/10.1177/0021934714562644

Jones, C., & Shorter-Gooden, K. (2003). The Sisterella Complex: Black women and depression (pp. 120–146). In *Shifting: The double lives of black women in America*. HarperCollins.

Jones, M. K., Leath, S., Settles, I. H., Doty, D., & Conner, K. (2022). Gendered racism and depression among Black women: Examining the roles of social support and identity. *Cultural Diversity and Ethnic Minority Psychology*, *28*(1), 39–48.https://doi.org/10.1037/cdp0000486

King, A. E., & Allen, T. T. (2009). Personal characteristics of the ideal African American marriage partner: A survey of adult Black men and women. *Journal of Black Studies*, *39*(4), 570–588. https://doi.org/10.1177/0021934707299637

Kogan, S. M., Lei, M. K., Grange, C. R., Simons, R. L., Brody, G. H., Gibbons, F. X., & Chen, Y. F. (2013). The contribution of community and family contexts to African American young adults' romantic relationship health: A prospective analysis. *Journal of Youth and Adolescence*, *42*(6), 878–890. https://doi.org/10.1007/s10964-013-9935-3

Marks, L. D., Hopkins, K., Chaney, C., Monroe, P. A., Nesteruk, O., & Sasser, D. D. (2008). "Together, we are strong": A qualitative study of happy, enduring African American marriages. *Family Relations*, *57*(2), 172–185. https://doi.org/10.1111/j.1741-3729.2008.00492.x

McDaniel, A., DiPrete, T. A., Buchmann, C., & Shwed, U. (2011). The black gender gap in educational attainment: Historical trends and racial comparisons. *Demography*, *48*(3), 889–914. https://doi.org/10.1007/s13524-011-0037-0

Mechoulan, S. (2011). The external effects of black male incarceration on black females. *Journal of Labor Economics*, *29*(1), 1–35. https://doi.org/10.1086/656370

Nelson, T., Cardemil, E. V., & Adeoye, C. T. (2016). Rethinking strength: Black women's perceptions of the "Strong Black Woman" role. *Psychology of Women Quarterly*, *40*(4), 551–563. https://doi.org/10.1177/0361684316646716

OkCupid. (2014). *Race and attraction, 2009–2014*. Medium. https://theblog .okcupid.com/race-and-attraction-2009-2014-107dcbb4f060 [post no longer available]

Parks, S. (2010). *Fierce angels: The strong black woman in American life and culture*. Random House Publishing Group.

Pinderhughes, E. B. (2002). African American marriage in the 20th century. *Family Process*, *41*(2), 269–282. https://doi.org/10.1111/j.1545-5300.2002 .41206.x

Robinson, A. R. (2007). Why does the slave ever love? The subject of romance revisited in the neoslave narrative. *The Southern Literary Journal*, *40*(1), 39–57.

Shorter-Gooden, K. (2009). Therapy with African American men and women. In H. A. Neville, B. M. Tynes, & S. O. Utsey (Eds.), *Handbook of African American psychology* (pp. 445–458). Sage Publications.

Simons, R. L., Simons, L. G., Lei, M. K., & Landor, A. M. (2012). Relational schemas, hostile romantic relationships, and beliefs about marriage among young African American adults. *Journal of Social and Personal Relationships*, *29*(1), 77–101. https://doi.org/10.1177/0265407511406897

Smiley, C., & Fakunle, D. (2016). From "brute" to "thug:" The demonization and criminalization of unarmed Black male victims in America. *Journal of Human Behavior in the Social Environment*, *26*(3–4), 350–366. https://doi .org/10.1080/10911359.2015.1129256

Stackman, V. R., Reviere, R., & Medley, B. C. (2016). Attitudes toward marriage, partner availability, and interracial dating among Black college students from historically Black and predominantly White institutions. *Journal of Black Studies*, *47*(2), 169–192. https://doi.org/10.1177/0021934715623520

Stanley, S. M., Rhoades, G. K., & Whitton, S. W. (2010). Commitment: Functions, formation, and the securing of romantic attachment. *Journal of Family Theory & Review*, *2*(4), 243–257. https://doi.org/10.1111/j.1756-2589.2010.00060.x

Staples, R. (1985). Changes in black family structure: The conflict between family ideology and structural conditions. *Journal of Marriage and the Family*, 1005–1013. https://doi.org/10.2307/352344

Thomas, A. J., & King, C. T. (2007). Gendered racial socialization of African American mothers and daughters. *The Family Journal*, *15*(2), 137–142. https://doi.org/10.1177/1066480706297853

Walker-Barnes, C. (2009). The burden of the strong Black woman. *Journal of Pastoral Theology*, *19*(1), 1–21. https://doi.org/10.1179/jpt.2009.19.1.002

Wallace, D. M. (2007). It's a MAN thang": Black male gender role socialization and the performance of masculinity in love relationships. *The Journal of Pan African Studies*, *1*(7), 11–22.

Wang, M. T., & Huguley, J. P. (2012). Parental racial socialization as a moderator of the effects of racial discrimination on educational success among African American adolescents. *Child Development*, *83*(5), 1716–1731. https://doi.org/10.1111/j.1467-8624.2012.01808.x

Watson, N. N., & Hunter, C. D. (2016). "I had to be strong": Tensions in the strong black woman schema. *Journal of Black Psychology*, *42*(5), 424–452. https://doi.org/10.1177/0095798415597093

West, L. M., Donovan, R. A., & Daniel, A. R. (2016). The price of strength: Black college women's perspectives on the strong Black woman stereotype. *Women & Therapy*, *39*(3–4), 390–412. https://doi.org/10.1080/02703149.2016.1116871

Woods-Giscombé, C. L. (2010). Superwoman schema: African American women's views on stress, strength, and health. *Qualitative Health Research*, *20*(5), 668–683. https://doi.org/10.1177/1049732310361892

CHAPTER 3

Black Same-Gender-Loving Male Couples' Health within an Afrocentric Psychological Paradigm: The Influences of Spirituality and Religion

Jonathan Mathias Lassiter

The most intimate interpersonal relationships that many people experience are their romantic partnerships. Several psychological and public health studies have found that the quality of one's romantic relationships may have positive and negative influences on the individual holistic health of each partner and the couple as a unit (Braithwaite & Holt-Lunstad, 2017). However, general couples research has not included Black same-gender-loving male couples (BSGLMCs) in large enough numbers so that the studies' findings are relevant for them (Lebow & Diamond, 2019). Very little research has queried Black same-gender-loving (SGL) men's lives in the contexts of their relationships (Lassiter et al., 2021). Additionally, studies have seldom focused on culturally-relevant factors, such as spirituality and religion, in BSGLMCs' lives and how those factors influence their romantic relationships (Fincham & Beach, 2014). There is also a lack of cultural specificity in the examination of BSGLMCs (Lassiter et al., 2021). Often these relationships are assessed based on white Eurocentric (and often heterosexist) relationship norms. These oversights represent major gaps in our understanding of BSGLMCs.

I have attempted to fill these gaps by presenting an analysis of the intersections of BSGLMCs' romantic relationship health, spirituality, and religion within an Afrocentric (Black) psychological paradigm. This is accomplished with three distinct tasks. First, the scholarly literature related to the Afrocentric psychological paradigm (including the Ubuntu principle), spirituality, religion, and BSGLMCs' romantic relationships was reviewed. Second, based on the review, a conceptual framework describing the potential mechanisms through which both positive and negative experiences of spirituality and religion may influence BSGLMCs' relationship health was developed. Third, a discussion of how this conceptual framework might guide future research and clinical work with BSGLMCs was explicated.

3.1   Review of the Afrocentric Psychological Paradigm, Spirituality, Religion, and BSGLMCs

3.1.1   The Afrocentric Psychological Paradigm

Afrocentric psychologists have proposed that a holistic understanding of the health of African descended people (ADP; i.e., people who are recent descendants of people who originated on the African continent, are considered Black, and treated as Black in society) can be achieved only by acknowledging the culturally specific values of African life described in precolonial African philosophy and psychology (Azibo, 1996). Afrocentric psychology asserts that the nature of reality is spiritual and sacred (Akbar, 2003), meaning that reality is influenced by a pervasive extrasensory energetic force that has been called by many names including God, the Sacred, Infinite consciousness, etc. (Myers, 1993). Thus, this force is the environment in which life happens, an energy that one embodies, and a resource that one may utilize in all aspects of life. People are considered spirit-beings whose purpose is to unfold as a sacred entity by aligning with the spiritual world in one's before-life, present (earth) life, and eventually in one's after-life when they rejoin the non-physical spiritual world after one's physical death (Akbar, 2003).

Health for ADP is dependent on how well one aligns with the spiritual. Myers (1993) and other scholars (Montgomery et al., 1990) have proposed that one achieves optimal health when they embrace a consciousness or worldview in which the spiritual and material worlds are intertwined and seek to gain oneness with the Sacred. A person that has a strong sense of themselves as aligned with the Sacred and lives their life in such a manner has a healthy spiritual consciousness. Myers (1993) has described this healthy spiritual consciousness as an optimal worldview that helps one develop a sense of themselves as the physical manifestation of the Sacred, having intrinsic self-worth and infinite potential, making decisions in life from a both/and logical perspective, valuing equitable human relationships above all else, and maintaining a carefree, resilient orientation to life. If one does not have a well-developed spiritual consciousness, they are deemed to have a suboptimal worldview. A suboptimal worldview contributes to one being individualistic, competitive, and materialistic. In sum, ADP's health is determined by the strength of their spiritual consciousness. If ADP have weakened spiritual consciousness, then their health is compromised.

3.1.1.1   Ubuntu
The spiritual can be embodied and expressed through relationships. From an Afrocentric psychological perspective, positive interpersonal relationships are of the highest value and one of the primary methods of societal interdependence (Myers, 1993). Many southern African societies have posited that humanity and health develop through the embodiment of *Ubuntu*. The Ubuntu principle was first articulated by Bantu and southern African people in their language of Xhosa with the saying *umuntu ngumuntu ngabantu*, which translates to "a person is a person because of other people" (Mangena, n.d., para. 1). From this perspective, one comes to know themselves only through their relationships with others and there is a reciprocal nature to relationships. Thus, relationships are fundamental to identity development as well as personal and collective health.

Ubuntu recognizes that healthy human functioning is dependent on people developing and prioritizing consciousness, connection, and competency in their interpersonal relationships. Consciousness refers to one's level of spiritual consciousness (i.e., spiritual alignment). Connection refers to one's relationships with their spiritual nature, the spiritual nature of others, and the expression of the Sacred in their actions with others. Competency is one's ability to develop, choose, and effectively implement social, cognitive, behavioral, and affective skills to create and maintain equitable relationships and health. Taken together, these three Cs can help people achieve identity, connection to ancestral and cultural roots, and emotional stability of belonging through healthy interpersonal relationships (Wilson & Williams, 2013).

Consciousness. Consciousness is a state of awareness. Within the Afrocentric psychological paradigm, one's level of spiritual consciousness —or awareness and alignment with the spiritual—is most important and has implications for their holistic health. Holistic health is conceptualized to encompass both non-Western (e.g., interconnectedness, cultural knowledge) and Western (e.g., happiness, absence of disease) components of that combine in distinct ways to induce optimal functioning, quality of life, and well-being (Saylor, 2004). Spiritual consciousness may fluctuate along a continuum with optimal worldview (i.e., strong spiritual consciousness) at one end and suboptimal worldview (i.e., weak spiritual consciousness) at the other (Obasi et al., 2009), thus having differential influences on holistic health. An optimal worldview has been found to be associated with positive health outcomes. For example, the relationship between stress and depressive symptoms was weaker for Black Americans who endorsed higher levels of optimal worldview compared to those who endorsed having higher levels of a suboptimal worldview (Neblett et al., 2010). Additionally, optimal worldview was also found to be negatively associated with avoidant coping (e.g., denying one's stressors and their affective consequences) and depressive symptoms (Neblett et al., 2010). These findings indicate that having a well-developed spiritual consciousness may not only prevent poor health but also protect ADP from the negative effects of stress. Black SGL men's health is dependent on their ability to develop a spiritual consciousness and allow that consciousness to inform their actions, emotions, and thoughts. Given the fluid nature of spiritual consciousness, Black SGL men's health may change depending on their fluctuating levels of spiritual consciousness. Thus, maintaining health would depend on retaining an optimal worldview.

Connection. Healthy connection requires that one recognizes and honors the Sacred within themselves and others. It may be manifested in many ways. This chapter explores two Afrocentric articulations of healthy connection: interconnectivity/self-extension and the principle of *Ma'at*.

Interconnectivity/self-extension. From an Ubuntu perspective, people are direct extensions of the Sacred and are simultaneously connected to the living, the yet-to-be-born, ancestors, community of spirits, and the divine Sacred (Azibo, 1996). Given this paradigm, the self is an "unbroken circle ... encompassing an infinite past, an infinite future" (Azibo, 1996, p. 52) and all ADP. The self is a "collective phenomenon while respecting the uniqueness of the individual self as a component of the collectivity" (Akbar, 2003, p. 68). Thus, one's individual personality and goals are similarly as important as the characteristics of one's collective history and cultural roots. The health of the individual is tied to the health of one's community and the community's health relies on the individual being holistically healthy. This position within one's spiritual and cultural community provides a foundation for one to cultivate an identity as an integrated spiritual, cultural being with infinite potential for power and empowerment. Power and empowerment comes from being connected to the Sacred, embodying one's deep cultural roots of precolonial African values, and the ability to transcend the physical limitations of the present circumstances by projecting one's self forward into a psychological or spiritual moment of transcendence, which could then provide a vision for self/collective-enhancing action. Such a powerful and empowered, integrated identity can sustain the self and the collective (e.g., romantic relationship).

Principle of Ma'at. The principle of Ma'at is derived from the mythology related to the Kemetic goddess of the same name. Ma'at is the daughter of the sun god Ra and her name means "that which is straight" (Mark, 2016, para. 2). She is believed to be the personification of order, justice, and harmony. The principle of Ma'at is considered by many Afrocentric psychologists to be "a code of conduct and a standard of aspiration" that can be applied as a model of human transformation (Parham et al., 2016, p. 143). This model of human transformation, which is tied to the spiritual, requires that one live by seven virtues: truth, justice, harmony, righteousness/propriety, order, balance, and reciprocity (Mark, 2016; Parham et al., 2016). These virtues are thought to underlie the Sacred that interconnects all living things. Thus, as one lives according to the principle of Ma'at, one will live in a way consciously connected to the Sacred.

Several scholars have defined the virtues of Ma'at (Parham et al., 2016; Pinch, 2002). Truth is honesty in words, actions, and personality. Justice is interacting with others in a way that promotes fairness and equity. Harmony is alignment with the totality of the Sacred in one's self and in others so that interactions are authentic, mutually beneficial, and well functioning. Righteousness/propriety refers to living life in a way that is free from causing harm to self and others. Order requires that one arrange their life in a way that is free from emotional, physical, spiritual clutter that may impede one from fulfilling their divine purpose. Balance is a state of existence where one's internal and external processes are aligned with the Sacred and others so that new possibilities and ways of being can be generated (Lee, n.d.). Reciprocity entails giving as much as one receives in all ways. Black SGL men's ability to cultivate and express these virtues has health implications for themselves and their romantic relationships.

Competency. Competency may be interpreted as one's ability to develop, choose, and use social, cognitive, behavioral, and affective skills to effectively form and maintain healthy relationships and outcomes. Such skills can help Black SGL men make meaning of their lives, define reality, make decisions, and cope in ways that are spiritually aligned. When competency is high, one can develop and maintain a holistic identity (e.g., integrated spiritual, racial, sexual, gender identities) and Afrocentric cultural practices (e.g., prioritizing the Sacred in all of one's thoughts and actions; Wilson & Williams, 2013). Black SGL men have demonstrated competency in several ways in their lives and relationships.

Culturally-relevant social, cognitive, behavioral, and affective skills that help Black SGL men achieve competency via holistic identity development and Afrocentric cultural practices have been studied more in recent decades (Graham et al., 2009; Lassiter et al., 2020; Lassiter & Mims, 2022; Pitt, 2010a, 2010b; Walker et al., 2015). Scholars have found that Black SGL men demonstrate competency in their development of strong racial identities, which are associated with a range of positive health outcomes at the individual level such as higher levels of self-efficacy and emotional awareness (English et al., 2020). Furthermore, Black SGL men with higher levels of racial and sexual identity integration have reported lower levels of psychological distress compared to those with lower levels of integration (Crawford et al., 2002). Other scholars have found that cultivating integrated sexual and spiritual identities contributed to lower levels of identity fragmentation (e.g., tension between one's racial/cultural, religious/spiritual, and sexual identities) and cognitive dissonance (Lassiter, 2015; Pitt, 2010b). Recently, Lassiter and Mims (2022) examined psychological and behavioral mechanisms associated with Black SGL men's health within an Afrocentric framework. Black SGL men in their study reported that having higher levels of spiritual consciousness contributed to them being able to (a) cultivate more emotional awareness, (b) embrace their emotions without judgment, (c) regulate their emotions, (d) develop sacred motivations for health behavior, and (d) engage in health-promoting behaviors. This research suggests that several Afrocentric forms of consciousness, connection, and competency are evident in Black SGL men's lives.

3.1.2 *Spirituality in the Lives of Black SGL Men*

Given the spiritual nature of ADP's lives, it is not surprising that spirituality and religion are two significant cultural factors in Black SGL men's lives. References in this chapter to spirituality and religion are meant to describe one's experiences of the Sacred through a personal relationship (i.e., spirituality) and collective, institutional modalities (i.e., religion). These experiences have been found to contribute to both positive and negative outcomes for Black SGL men's individual and couple health (Lassiter, 2014).

Black SGL men have reported significantly higher levels of spiritual identification, beliefs, and practices compared to their sexual minority counterparts of other races and ethnicities (Lassiter, Saleh, Starks, et al., 2017). In addition, some Black SGL men have defined spirituality in both universal and culturally-specific ways that emphasize their African and Black American heritages. For example, Lassiter and his colleagues (2020) found that Black SGL men defined spirituality as "(a) relationship with something greater than themselves, (b) part of the themselves, (c) a guiding force in their lives, and (d) multidimensional in nature. The culturally-specific aspects of their spirituality were identified as being (a) an energetic union of masculine and feminine energy within their physical body, (b) a connection to their ancestors, (c) an integration of the divine and the sensual, and (d) the use of spirituality to combat intersectional oppression" (p. 27). This spirituality, grounded in Afrocentric values, has positive implications for Black SGL men's health.

Research studies have indicated that spirituality informs Black SGL men's lives by engendering positive health outcomes and by protecting them from the negative consequences of life stressors (Lassiter, Saleh, Grov, et al., 2019; Miller, 2005). In racially diverse samples of SGL men, spirituality has been found to be associated with higher levels of resilience and social support and negatively correlated with depressive symptoms and rejection sensitivity (Lassiter, Saleh, Grov, et al., 2019). Furthermore, spirituality buffered the negative effects of religion on mental health so that those with higher levels of spirituality and religion had better mental health outcomes than those with low levels of spirituality and high levels of religion. A few studies have found a negative association between spirituality and health among Black SGL men. For example, Carrico and colleagues (2017) found that higher levels of spiritual and religious activities were associated with greater odds of reporting stimulant use. Although the authors found a significant association, it should be interpreted with caution as the questions about spirituality activities were conflated with religious activities (i.e., how often did you consult a spiritual or religious leader). This conflation is common in psychological and public health research (Lassiter & Parsons, 2016). Thus, that study may not be purely measuring spirituality but some amalgamation of spirituality and religion. The overwhelming body of health research suggests that spirituality is a central component in Black SGL men's lives that helps them make meaning of their experiences and act in ways that bolster their health.

3.1.3   Religion in the Lives of Black SGL Men

Religion can be both a positive and negative influence in Black SGL men's lives. Scholars have highlighted the positive aspects of religion for Black SGL men (Foster et al., 2011; Quinn et al., 2016). These scholars have emphasized that religion and religious institutions can be a source of social support, financial assistance, and vocational training. Many religious organizations in Black communities provide examples of effective coping with anti-Black racism such as communal activism (Lassiter, 2014). However, for all their assets, religion and religious organizations can be detrimental to Black SGL men's health.

Religion may be used to hurt Black SGL men when it is interpreted in ways that promote homonegativity. Fifty-one percent of Black American people reported believing religious texts should be taken literally (Pew Research Center, 2014). This practice contributes to some Black people developing a negative view of same-sex attraction and sexual behaviors based on conservative interpretations of a few passages (Helminiak, 2000). Religious organizations that engage in literal (or fundamentalist) interpretations of religious texts often promote hostile environments for Black SGL men. Religious leaders and participants in these settings may condemn and berate Black SGL men via sermons, exclusion from religious events and rituals, direct and indirect homonegative comments (e.g., "God hates gays"), and pressure to suppress one's sexual attractions and behaviors (Lassiter, 2014). These religion-based homonegative experiences can have negative effects on Black SGL men's health directly by causing psychological distress and indirectly through diminishing the positive aspects of religion (Griffin, 2006; Poteat & Lassiter, 2019). Previous literature (Super & Jacobson, 2011; Ward, 2005) has identified two specific forms of religion-based minority stress (e.g., religious abuse, spiritual genocide) that can contribute to identity fragmentation and other negative health outcomes. Overall, religion can be a double-edged sword for Black SGL men.

3.1.3.1 *Religious Abuse*

Black SGL men are religiously abused when they are subjected to religious pressure to conform to heteronormative expressions of sexuality and gender (Super & Jacobson, 2011). Religious people and organizations may justify the use of force, threats, rejection, condemnation, and manipulation with homonegative interpretations of religious scripture that categorize same-sex attraction and behaviors as sin. Many Black SGL men have reported receiving messages that indicated that they could not be both a religious or spiritual person and a SGL person (Lassiter, 2015). Homonegative interpretations of religion have been found to contribute to loss of social and familial ties (Garrett-Walker & Torres, 2017; Quinn et al., 2016), rejection, social isolation, loneliness (Griffin, 2006), refusal of participation in sacred rituals, and denial of access to material resources provided by religious organizations such as food pantry services (Lassiter et al., 2019). Additionally, many Black SGL men have reported experiencing violence at the hands of relatives, peers, and community members who used homonegative interpretations of religious doctrine to justify their cruelty (Wilson et al., 2011). These religion-based homonegative acts are a form of religious abuse that can harm Black SGL men's understanding of themselves and their ability to trust and care for others.

Black SGL men's identities are often fragmented when they grow up in religiously abusive environments. They may develop beliefs that they are sinful, defective, and unlovable by others including the Sacred. This may contribute to internalization of a negative identity. Black SGL men may also come to think of themselves as not fitting in with the people around them who are rejecting them (e.g., Black, religious, communal) and they may reject those people and the characteristics they possess. This rejection of the ones who rejected them may serve to protect themselves from the emotional harms of being condemned and not accepted. Although being critical of people who cause harm upon one's self can be a healthy adaptive strategy, rejecting all characteristics associated with those people may result in Black SGL men rejecting the parts of themselves that they share with those persons. If Blackness, the Sacred, and communal bonds are devalued, then Afrocentric values (e.g., interconnectivity/self-extension) found in healthy forms of religion and spirituality may go undiscovered or perceived as suspect and averse. Religious abuse that promotes Black SGL men viewing themselves as sexually perverted religious outcasts and as adversarial to Blackness, the Sacred, and community ultimately leads to disconnection and an individualistic orientation.

3.1.3.2   Spiritual Genocide

Religious abuse may impede Black SGL men's ties to religious people and organizations as well as hinder their creation of holistic identities and genuine interdependent connections with romantic partners. Religious abuse can also lead to spiritual genocide. Ward (2005) described spiritual genocide as the ways in which homonegativity in religious institutions harm Black SGL men. I build on Ward's conceptualization and offer that spiritual genocide, fostered by religious abuse, is the psychospiritual disconnection from the Sacred that strips Black SGL men of their (conscious or unconscious) will to live through a process of subtle and overt attacks to their spirit-hood. Spiritual genocide leaves Black SGL men hollow and makes it difficult for them to cultivate or even acknowledge an understanding of themselves as part of the Sacred and inhibits development of loving relationships with themselves and others.

Spiritual genocide is more severe than religious abuse in its impact on Black SGL men. Whereas religious abuse contributes to Black SGL men perceiving themselves as sinful, defective, and unlovable, spiritual genocide leaves Black SGL men in an existential crisis where their value orientations and purposes are nebulous. Religious abuse could prompt Black SGL men to have a negative, anti-self identity. Spiritual genocide prompts a non-identity, one without roots in the Sacred. This could lead to a suboptimal worldview that is materialistic, individualistic, consumed with escaping or avoiding pain, and death focused (Myers, 1993). In sum, religion may be a positive force that helps Black SGL men develop more fully integrated identities and spiritual consciousness, or a negative force that fragments their identities and acts as a barrier to them developing a strong spiritual consciousness.

3.1.4   Romantic Relationships among BSGLMCs

Population-based statistics suggest that approximately 56,000 BSGLMCs reside in the United States (LGBT Demographic Data Interactive, 2019). This number is likely an underestimate given the complex nature of sexual orientation disclosure among Black Americans (Lassiter et al., 2019). Kastanis & Wilson (2014) found that Black SGL men tend to choose romantic relationships with other Black men slightly more than romantic relationships with white American or other racial and ethnic minority men (54 percent vs. 33 percent vs. 13 percent, respectively). Additionally, 41 percent of them (more than same-sex couples of other races and ethnicities) reported raising children with their partner. They also reported lower incomes and rates of obtaining a college degree or having health insurance compared to same-sex couples of other races and ethnicities (Kastanis & Wilson, 2014). These few statistics that we have about BSGLMCs paint a picture of couples who have limited socioeconomic resources and significant familial responsibilities. However, this socioeconomic picture does not mean that BSGLMCs' relationships cannot flourish despite hardships.

BSGLMCs often cultivate resilient romantic relationships that are characterized as loving, pleasurable, and affectionate. Calabrese and her colleagues (2015) found that 95.6 percent of the Black SGL men in their sample felt love for their main partner and 97 percent felt loved by their primary partner during their last sexual experience together. Most Black SGL men (88.9 percent) in the sample also openly verbalized their love for their partner during their last sexual experience together. It is important to note higher percentages of Black SGL men reported feeling and verbalizing love during their last sexual encounter compared to those who endorsed they had an orgasm (86.5 percent). These findings indicate that romantic relationships between BSGLMCs who are committed to each are more characterized by their shared love than sexual pleasure.

Love and affection are but a few of the benefits BSGLMCs experience in their relationships. Some studies have highlighted racially protective benefits of Black SGL men being in romantic relationships with other Black SGL men. For example, English and his colleagues (2020) found that Black SGL men who had romantic relationships exclusively with other Black SGL men reported fewer experiences of racial discrimination in sexual encounters, and in turn reported fewer depressive symptoms than men whose romantic partners were not exclusively Black. Romantic relationships may also be opportunities for Black SGL men to model sex-positive norms and provide examples of long-term romantic partnerships for other Black SGL men who may or may not be in their own relationships (Barry et al., 2018). BSGLMCs can have a wide range of benefits.

BSGLMCs have multiple strengths and challenges just like all other couples. Applewhite and Littlefield (2015) found that BSGLMCs used several strategies to preserve and improve their romantic relationships. They found that social support from family and friends, organizational networks (e.g., church), and salient Black institutions in their communities helped BSGLMCs thrive. Being intentional and thoughtful in decision making as well as utilizing direct communication were also strategies that facilitated feelings of love, stability, and support among BSGLMCs. Dishonesty, lack of support from partner and community, and substance abuse all were identified as barriers to BSGLMCs maintaining a healthy relationship. Poor communication also limited intimacy and longevity. In addition, due to anti-Black racism in non-Black sexual minority communities, Black love is sometimes stigmatized. This is partly because Black SGL men have been described by non-Black SGL people as vectors of disease (e.g., HIV) and oversexualized (Grov et al., 2015; Matthews et al., 2016). Taken together, these findings demonstrate that several factors can impact the success and failure of BSGLMCs.

3.2   Conceptual Framework of Afrocentric Articulations of the Sacred and BSGLMCs' Health

The influence of religion and spirituality on BSGLMCs' relationship health may be understood building upon the Ubuntu principle. Based upon this framework, religion and spirituality may positively or negatively impact Black SGL men's ability to prioritize connection, consciousness,

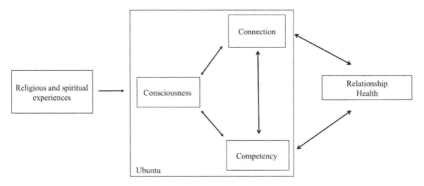

Figure 3.1   Conceptual framework of spirituality and religion's influence on Black
same-gender-loving couples' relationship health

and competency in their interpersonal relationships (Wilson, Olubadewo,
et al., 2016). Stated another way, religion and spirituality can promote or
hinder Black SGL men's ability to cultivate integrated holistic identities
that are spiritually conscious. This spiritual consciousness affects one's
ability to achieve substantive connection to self and romantic partner
and develop social, cognitive, behavioral, and affective skills that facilitate
personal and relational functioning with one's romantic partner. These
outcomes affect BSGLMCs' health.

Figure 3.1 depicts a conceptual framework to understand how spirituality and religion may influence BSGLMCs relationship health within an
Afrocentric psychological paradigm. This framework, supported by the
previously reviewed literature, proposes that many Black SGL men are
raised in environments where they have both positive and negative religious and spiritual experiences (Lassiter, 2014; Lassiter, Saleh, Starks,
et al., 2017). These experiences influence their level of spiritual
consciousness. Black SGL men who have positive religious and spiritual
experiences are likely to develop strong spiritual consciousness and an
understanding of themselves as integrated Black SGL men who can
unashamedly embrace their racial, sexual, spiritual, and gender identities
as they see fit (Lassiter, 2015). This translates to their romantic partners as
well. A strong spiritual consciousness facilitates Black SGL men in understanding their partners as being reflections of the Sacred and thus worthy
of compassion (Wilson & Williams, 2013). Spiritual consciousness under-
girds connection and competency in the romantic partnership.

Black SGL men who recognize themselves and their romantic partners
as part of the Sacred will seek deeper connection with their partners. In

fact, the Afrocentric psychological perspective would propose that Black SGL men with strong spiritual consciousnesses would perceive no separation between themselves and their partners. Thus, such spiritually conscious Black SGL men would live by a both/and logic that prioritizes both the health of his romantic partner and himself in a symbiotic manner. The romantic relationship between partners with strong spiritual consciousnesses is not only about having one's individual needs met but also focused on how each partner may serve as a model of human transformation for the other. The strengths and areas of improvement in one's partner are inspirations for growth for the other and vice versa. Such spiritual conscious orientations to the romantic relationship would result in Black SGL male partners connecting with each other in deeper, more substantive ways.

Strong spiritual consciousnesses may also translate to higher levels of competency within BSGLMCs. At the individual level, Black SGL men have utilized several skills including intellectual interrogation of nonaffirming religious messages, emotional awareness, emotional acceptance, emotional regulation, and health behaviors motivated by the Sacred to positively affect their health (English et al., 2020; Lassiter & Mims, 2022). At the couples-level, competency may look like BSGLMCs developing a relational spirituality in which the couples' relationship with the Sacred is a shared phenomenon that influences decisions related to the structure, maintenance, and evolution of their relationship (Mahoney, 2010). Competency may also look like joint decision making, direct communication that is open and honest, and joint problem-solving that leads to healthy relationship functioning (Applewhite & Littlefield, 2015; Tan et al., 2018). Other skills that may contribute to relationship health may include seeking and providing social support and words of affirmation to cope with the spiritual, racial, sexual, and gender discrimination that many Black SGL men experience simultaneously (English et al., 2020). A strong spiritual consciousness imbues Black SGL men with an understanding of themselves and their partners as reflections of the Sacred and worthy of compassion. Such a perspective provides the foundation for Black SGL men to develop competency in their romantic partnerships that contribute to BSGLMCs' relationship health.

Religious and spiritual experiences may also negatively impact BSGLMCs' relationship health. If Black SGL men experience religious abuse and spiritual genocide, they may develop anti-self and non-self identities, respectively, that either renders them averse to or disconnected from the Sacred. This contributes to one developing a suboptimal world-view or weak spiritual consciousness. With weak spiritual consciousnesses, Black SGL men are likely to approach romantic relationships as a process of getting their individual needs (e.g., material, sexual, emotional) met without a commitment to reciprocity. In this way, Black SGL men are thing oriented (e.g., receiving money, one-sided emotional support) and not person oriented (i.e., romantic partner). This approach to romantic partnerships will likely hinder connection. Competency will also be diminished as effective skills that contribute to healthy relationship functioning are likely to be un- or underdeveloped because the focus is on the self not the couple. Overall, BSGLMCs' relationship health will suffer.

This conceptual framework explicates a system of assumptions and beliefs that highlight the spiritual nature of life and its implications for BSGLMCs' relationship health. Positive and negative religious and spiritual experiences may foster or harm BSGLMCs' ability to actualize the Ubuntu principle through three central components (i.e., consciousness, connection, competency) and achieve relationship health. Given the high prevalence and importance of spirituality and religion in Black SGL men's lives, culturally-informed care requires that social scientists and psychotherapists develop a better understanding of the influence of these factors for BSGLMCs' relationship health. Furthermore, this framework is fundamentally rooted in an Afrocentric psychological paradigm that speaks specifically to the lived experiences and cosmological reality of ADP. It does not take an adaptive or accommodationist approach to BSGLMCs by attempting to use (white) Eurocentric norms and theories to describe and assess BSGLMCs. It centers African values, Black culture, and the spiritual in its explication of BSGLMCs' health.

3.3 Recommendations for Research and Clinical Work with BSGLMCs

The conceptual framework outlined in this chapter has implications for both social scientists and psychotherapists who work with BSGLMCs. The remainder of this chapter focuses on how this framework may guide empirical and clinical work with BSGLMCs who experience positive and negative spiritual and religious experiences. The recommendations are meant to inspire social scientists and psychotherapists to develop new research and clinical questions, theories, and approaches to working with BSGLMCs.

3.3.1   Research Recommendations

Previous scholars have called for more research that queries BSGLMCs (Mays et al., 2004; Wilson, Valera, et al., 2016). However, social scientists, as a whole, have yet to focus their attention on this population and its unique strengths and challenges (Jiwatram-Negrón & El-Bassel, 2014; Kousteni & Anagnostopoulos, 2020). Among studies that do center BSGLMCs, they often do so using either nonexplicit (or culturally neutral), (white) Eurocentric, or superficially culturally-adapted (e.g., inclusion of Black SGL male facilitators, inclusion of a discussion about race and racism) theories and approaches to guide their work (Applewhite & Littlefield, 2015; Tan et al., 2018). The conceptual framework described in this chapter provides myriad opportunities for empirical investigation within an Afrocentric psychological paradigm.

Although the framework presented in this chapter is bolstered by previous existing research studies that confirm individual components of it, it is still conceptual. Researchers may use the framework as a guidebook for testing and modifying the proposed associations between the constructs within it. The framework may also provide opportunities to develop culturally specific measures to operationalize the Ubuntu components (i.e., consciousness, connection, competency). With the exception of consciousness, these constructs have yet to be operationalized with an empirically-tested measure informed by the Afrocentric psychological paradigm. Although measures such as the African Self-Conscious Scale (Baldwin & Bell, 1985) and the Worldview Analysis Scale (Obasi et al., 2009) have been developed to assess consciousness, they have focused on racial and spiritual consciousness. Scales that operationalize holistic consciousnesses along the domains of spirituality, race, sexuality, and gender – as proposed by the framework – do not yet exist. Thus, there is plenty of space for researchers to engage in scale development and theory refinement related to BSGLMCs' relationship health within an Afrocentric paradigm.

There needs to be more diversity in research methods used with BSGLMCs. The conceptual framework provides possibilities for informing such use. The existing public health and psychological research has employed primarily individual-level qualitative and quantitative methods that explore BSGLMCs from the perspective of one partner (DuBois et al., 2018; Gonzales & Ortiz, 2015). There is little use of dyadic methods such as actor-partner interdependence model (Kenny & Ledermann, 2010) and dyadic qualitative analysis (Eisikovits & Koren, 2010; Morgan et al.,

2013). The use of image-based analyses is also rare. Methods such as cybercartography (i.e., the systematic observation, exploration, description, and categorization of Internet and social media websites and apps; Carballo-Diéguez et al., 2006) and photovoice (i.e., a methodology where participants are asked to photograph their daily experiences and environments as a tool for empowerment and policy change; Sitter, 2017) may also provide more expressive, non-text-based ways of understanding BSGLMCs. Mixed methods that integrate qualitative and quantitative data to provide a more comprehensive understanding of BSGLMCs are also lacking. Such diverse methods used with the conceptual framework outlined in this chapter will result in not only robust data but also a more culturally-relevant interpretation and application of that data.

Most research about Black SGL men and BSGLMCs has focused on HIV, sexual risk, and drug use (Wade & Harper, 2017). This focus on deficits continues to stigmatize these groups. The dearth of attention to cultural values, protective factors, resilience, and strengths-based approaches is conspicuous. The conceptual framework in this chapter can be used to direct future research that queries both risks and strengths among BSGLMCs. For example, this framework provides risk factors (i.e., religious abuse, spiritual genocide) and strengths (e.g., interconnectivity/self-extension, principle of Ma'at) that can be further explored for their contribution to BSGLMCs' relationship health. The explicated conceptual framework offers a bevy of possibilities for social scientists who want to move their work beyond deficit-based, (white) Eurocentric, individual-level understandings of health.

3.3.2   Clinical Recommendations

Na'im Akbar proclaimed that "renewal of the spiritual core of the Black man is the most effective therapy for his adjustment disorders" (Akbar, 2003, p. 25). Dr. Akbar's proclamation requires mental health providers who work with BSGLMCs to become well versed in culturally specific couples' treatment that is appropriately attuned to spiritual matters in BSGLMCs' lives. According to an Afrocentric psychological paradigm, BSGLMCs' relationship problems are due to one or more partners having a weak spiritual consciousness (i.e., holistic identity) that hinders the couple's ability to connect with each other and develop competency for maintaining relationship health. Negative spiritual and religious experiences are two such factors that may contribute to a weak spiritual consciousness. Some scholars have offered suggestions for assisting clients in healing from religious abuse and spiritual genocide so that they may build holistic identity that integrate their spiritual, racial, sexual, and gender identities (Bozard & Sanders, 2017; Lassiter, 2015). Additionally, other scholars have offered recommendations for how to utilize the Ubuntu principle in the psychotherapy room (Van Dyk & Nefale, 2005; Washington, 2010). These suggestions, while often conceptualized at the individual-level, may be modified to inform work at the couples-level.

3.3.2.1 Recommendations to Enhance Consciousness

Reconciliation of conflicting and fragmented identities must be primary in work with BSGLMCs where one or both partners have been the victims of religious abuse and spiritual genocide. Lassiter (2015) proposed several strategies that clinicians may teach and practice with their clients in the couple's session. These include helping BSGLMCs gain physical and emotional distance from homonegative religious and spiritual environments so that they may engage in critical interrogation of homonegative religious messages and experiences that communicate to them that they are antithetical to and disconnected from the Sacred. This critical interrogation may include questions about the veracity and theological basis for homonegative religious messages, queries about the motivation of the speaker of the nonaffirming messages, and seeking social support from other BSGLMCs who have strong spiritual consciousnesses (Lassiter, 2015; Pitt, 2010b). If one partner has a stronger spiritual consciousness than the other, the partner with the stronger spiritual consciousness may serve as a role model for the other partner and share strategies for reconciliation that they found effective in the past. These strategies move BSGLMCs toward stronger spiritual consciousnesses.

3.3.2.2 Recommendations for Enhancing Connection

Clinicians may help BSGLMCs connect with each other in healthier ways by engaging them in therapeutic exercises that assess for the current levels of interconnectivity and the principle of Ma'at in the relationship, and then help them improve these qualities. Empathy-building exercises that help couples engage in perspective-taking could assist in increasing interconnectivity by helping partners see themselves in each other and develop a deeper respect for the other's experiences. Clinicians may also find it beneficial to help BSGLMCs distinguish between the individual needs of each partner, the shared needs of the couple, and how conflicts in these may contribute to a lack of interconnectivity (Phillips, 1990; Wynn & West-Olatunji, 2008). This clarity may lend itself to helping

BSGLMCs make more informed decisions that will contribute to the growth of the couple and not only the individual. Therapeutic strategies that draw BSCLMCs attention to the values inherent in the principle of Ma'at can also increase connection within the romantic relationship. For example, couples could be encouraged to keep a journal to track how often they interact with each other in ways reflective of the principle of Ma'at (e.g., did you act with justice today and treat your partner fairly?). These types of exercises can facilitate deeper levels of connection in BSGLMCs.

3.3.2.3 *Recommendations for Enhancing Competency*

Clinicians working with BSGLMCs may find it useful to engage their clients in rituals (e.g., prayer, meditation, incantations, mind-body practices) that empower couples to advocate for themselves and develop health-inducing skills. Previous research has indicated that spiritual rituals done with or for a partner can have positive effects on relationship quality, satisfaction, and commitment (Fincham & Beach, 2014). Such rituals may help BSGLMCs to cultivate social, physiological, emotional, and cognitive spaces where they can develop and utilize other action-oriented strategies (e.g., emotional regulation, spiritually-informed health behaviors) that contribute to relationship health. These rituals may also be used to remind Black SGL men that they are spirit-beings inextricably tied to the Sacred and thus have infinite potential to influence themselves, their partner, and the world around them to the extent that they stay in contact with the Sacred even in a powerless situation (Washington, 2010). Clinicians may also assist BSGLMCs in developing new behavioral skills through the process of culturalization. Nobles and colleagues (2009) described culturalization as a behavioral change process that helps clients minimize negative social interactions and engage in healthy behaviors. This process consists of three techniques that clinicians may teach BSGLMCs: cultural realignment, cognitive restructuring, and character refinement. Cultural realignment would require that clinicians engage BSGLMCs in reeducating themselves about the positive and culturally aligned history and contemporary existence of healthy Black SGL men and BSGLMCs. This could be accomplished through bibliotherapy or other media consumption that centers the stories, histories, and cultures of BSGLMCs in a way that highlights their holistic identities. Cognitive restructuring with BSGLMCs may look like clinicians challenging couples to uncover and examine the functions of nonaffirming thoughts that create tension within the couple, and then change those thoughts. Character refinement would require the clinician to assist BSGLMCs in developing a consistent pattern of behavior that is congruent with the cultural realignment and cognitive restructuring that previously took place. These strategies are but a few examples of how competency may be enhanced within BSGLMCs.

3.4 Conclusions

BSGLMCs have seldom been the focus in public health and psychological research. When they have been included in such research, it has been overwhelmingly pathological, individual based, and informed by a (white) Eurocentric perspective. Such approaches have severely hindered our knowledge about BSGLMCs. This chapter offers an emergent conceptual framework through which to understand the influence of spiritual and religious experiences on BSGLMCs consciousness, connection, and competency that collectively influence their relationship health. This conceptual framework is rooted in an Afrocentric psychological paradigm that emphasizes the principle of Ubuntu in defining, studying, and treating BSGLMCs' relationship health. Several examples of how this conceptual framework may be leveraged in research and psychotherapeutic clinical work with BSGLMCs have been provided. This chapter represents a step toward heeding Piper-Mandy and Rowe's (2010, p. 14) directive to ADP and Afrocentric psychologists to "call ourselves into existence psychologically" through the explication of life within an Afrocentric paradigm that affirms our spiritual nature.

Discussion Questions

1. In what ways does Afrocentric psychology differ from Westernized European psychology? Why is Afrocentric psychology important?
2. How do the concepts of Ubuntu, consciousness, and connection impact BSGLMC's ability to cultivate healthy relationships?
3. Explain how spirituality and religion may influence BSGLMCs relationship health within an Afrocentric psychological paradigm.

REFERENCES

Akbar, N. (2003). *Akbar papers in African psychology*. Mind Productions.
Applewhite, S., & Littlefield, M. B. (2015). The role of resilience and anti-resilience behaviors in the romantic lives of Black same-gender-loving (SGL) men. *Journal of Black Sexuality and Relationships*, 2(2), 1–38. https://doi.org/10.1353/bsr.2016.0005

Azibo, D. (1996). *African psychology in historical perspective & related commentary.* Africa World Press.

Baldwin, J., & Bell, Y. (1985). The African self-consciousness scale: An Afrocentric personality questionnaire. *Western Journal of Black Studies, 9*(2), 61–68.

Barry, M., Threats, M., Blackburn, N., LeGrand, S., Dong, W., Pulley, D., Sallabank, G., Harpers, G., Hightow-Weidman, L., Bauermeister, J., & Muessig, K. (2018). "Stay strong! keep ya head up! move on! it gets better!!!!": Resilience processes in the healthMpowerment online intervention of young Black gay, bisexual and other men who have sex with men. *AIDS Care, 30*(S5), S27–S38. https://doi.org/10.1080/09540121.2018.1510106

Bozard, R., Jr., & Sanders, C. (2017). The GRACE model of counseling: Navigating intersections of affectional orientation and Christian spirituality. In M. M. Ginicola, C. Smith, & J. M. Filmore (Eds.), *Affirmative counseling with LGBTQI+ people* (pp. 313–327). American Counseling Association. https://doi.org/10.1002/9781119375517.ch23

Braithwaite, S., & Holt-Lunstad, J. (2017). Romantic relationships and mental health. *Current Opinion in Psychology, 13*, 120–125. https://doi.org/10.1016/j.copsyc.2016.04.001

Calabrese, S. K., Rosenberger, J. G., Schick, V. R., & Novak, D. S. (2015). Pleasure, affection, and love among Black men who have sex with men (MSM) versus MSM of other races: Countering dehumanizing stereotypes via cross-race comparisons of reported sexual experience at last sexual event. *Archives of Sexual Behavior, 44*, 2001–2014. https://doi.org/10.1007/s10508-014-0405-0

Carballo-Diéguez, A., Dowsett, G., Ventuneac, A., Remien, R., Balan, I., Dolezal, C., Luciano, O., & Lin, P. (2006). Cybercartography of popular Internet sites used by New York City men who have sex with men interested in bareback sex. *AIDS Education and Prevention, 18*(6), 475–489. https://doi.org/10.1521/aeap.2006.18.6.475

Carrico, A. W., Storholm, E. D., Flentje, A., Arnold, E. A., Pollack, L. M., Neilands, T. B., Rebchook, G. M., Peterson, J. L., Eke, A., Johnson, W., & Kegeles, S. (2017). Spirituality/religiosity, substance use, and HIV testing among young black men who have sex with men. *Drug and Alcohol Dependence, 174*, 106–112. https://doi.org/10.1016/j.drugalcdep.2017.01.024

Crawford, I., Allison, K. W., Zamboni, B. D., & Soto, T. (2002). The influence of dual-identity development on the psychosocial functioning of African-American gay and bisexual men. *Journal of Sex Research, 39*(3), 179–189. https://doi.org/10.1080/00224490209552140

DuBois, S., Guy, A., & Legate, N. (2018). Testing the partnership-health association among African American men who have sex with men. *Journal of Black Sexuality and Relationships, 4*(4), 33–51. https://doi.org/10.1353/bsr.2018.0010

Eisikovits, Z., & Koren, C. (2010). Approaches to and outcomes of dyadic interview analysis. *Qualitative Health Research*, *20*(12), 1642–1655. https://doi.org/10.1177/1049732310376520

English, D., Carter, J. A., Forbes, N., Bowleg, L., Malebranche, D. J., Talan, A. J., & Rendina, H. J. (2020). Intersectional discrimination, positive feelings, and health indicators among Black sexual minority men. *Health Psychology*, *39*(3), 220–229. https://doi.org/10.1037/hea0000837

Fincham, F. D., & Beach, S. R. (2014). I say a little prayer for you: Praying for partner increases commitment in romantic relationships. *Journal of Family Psychology*, *28*(5), 587–593. https://doi.org/10.1037/a0034999

Foster, M. L., Arnold, E., Rebchook, G., & Kegeles, S. M. (2011). "It's my inner strength": Spirituality, religion and HIV in the lives of young African American men who have sex with men. *Culture, Health, and Sexuality*, *13* (9), 1103–1117. https://doi.org/10.1080/13691058.2011.600460

Garrett-Walker, J. J., & Torres, V. M. (2017). Negative religious rhetoric in the lives of Black cisgender queer emerging adult men: A qualitative analysis. *Journal of Homosexuality*, *64*(13), 1816–1831. https://doi.org/10.1080/00918369.2016.1267465

Gonzales, G., & Ortiz, K. (2015). Health insurance disparities among racial/ethnic minorities in same-sex relationships: An intersectional approach. *American Journal of Public Health*, *105*, 1106–1113. https://doi.org/10.2105/AJPH.2014.302459

Graham, L. F., Braithwaite, K., Spikes, P., Stephens, C., & Edu, U. (2009). Exploring the mental health of Black men who have sex with men. *Community Mental Health Journal*, *45*, 272–284. https://doi.org/10.1007/s10597-009-9186-7

Griffin, H. (2006). *Their own receive them not: African American lesbians and gays in African American churches*. The Pilgrim Press.

Grov, C., Saleh, L. D., Lassiter, J. M., & Parsons, J. (2015). Challenging race-based stereotypes about gay and bisexual men's sexual behavior and perceived penis size and size satisfaction. *Sexuality Research and Social Policy*, *12*, 224–235. https://doi.org/10.1007/s13178-015-0190-0

Helminiak, D. (2000). *What the Bible really says about homosexuality*. Alamo Square Press.

Jiwatram-Negrón, T., & El-Bassel, N. (2014). Systematic review of couple-based HIV intervention and prevention studies: Advantages, gaps, and future directions. *AIDS and Behavior*, *18*(10), 1864–1887. https://doi.org/10.1007/s10461-014-0827-7

Kastanis, A., & Wilson, B. (2014). *Race/ethnicity, gender and socioeconomic well-being of individuals in same-sex couples*. The Williams Institute, UCLA School of Law. https://escholarship.org/uc/item/71j7n35t

Kenny, D., & Ledermann, T. (2010). Detecting, measuring, and testing dyadic patterns in the actor–partner interdependence model. *Journal of Family Psychology*, *24*(3), 359–366. https://doi.org/10.1037/a0019651

Kousteni, I., & Anagnostopoulos, F. (2020). Same-sex couples' psychological interventions: A systematic review. *Journal of Couple & Relationship Therapy, 2,* 136–174. https://doi.org/10.1080/15332691.2019.1667937

Lassiter, J. M. (2014). Extracting dirt from water: A strengths-based approach to religion for African American same-gender-loving men. *Journal of Religion and Health, 53*(1), 178–189. https://doi.org/10.1007/s10943-012-9668-8

(2015). Reconciling sexual orientation and Christianity: Black same-gender loving men's experiences. *Mental Health, Religion & Culture, 18,* 342–353. https://doi.org/10.1080/13674676.2015.1056121

Lassiter, J. M., Brewer, R., & Wilton, L. (2019). Black sexual minority men's disclosure of sexual orientation is associated with exposure to homonegative religious messages. *American Journal of Men's Health, 13*(1), 1557988318806432. https://doi.org/10.1177/1557988318806432

(2020). Toward a culturally-specific spirituality for Black sexual minority men. *Journal of Black Psychology, 46*(6–7), 482–513. https://doi.org/10.1177/0095798420948993

Lassiter, J. M., Dacus, J. D., & Johnson, M. O. (2021). A systematic review of Black American same-sex couples research: Laying the groundwork for culturally-specific research and interventions. *Journal of Sex Research, 59*(5), 555–567. https://doi.org/10.1080/00224499.2021.1964422

Lassiter, J. M., & Mims, I. (2022). "The awesomeness and the vastness of who you really are:" A culturally distinct framework for understanding the link between spirituality and health for Black sexual minority men. *Journal of Religion and Health, 61,* 3076–3097. https://doi.org/10.1007/s10943-021-01297-4

Lassiter, J. M., & Parsons, J. (2016). Religion and spirituality's influences on HIV syndemics among MSM: A systematic review and conceptual model. *AIDS and Behavior, 20*(2), 461–472. https://doi.org/10.1007/s10461-015-1173-0

Lassiter, J. M., Saleh, L., Grov, C., Starks, T., Ventuneac, A., & Parsons, J. T. (2019). Spirituality and multiple dimensions of religion are associated with mental health in gay and bisexual men: Results from the One Thousand Strong Cohort. *Psychology of Religion and Spirituality, 11*(4), 408–416. https://doi.org/10.1037/rel0000146

Lassiter, J. M., Saleh, L., Starks, T., Grov, C., Ventuneac, A., & Parson, J. (2017). Race, ethnicity, religious affiliation, and education are associated with gay and bisexual men's religious and spiritual participation and beliefs: Results from the One Thousand Strong cohort. *Cultural Diversity and Ethnic Minority Psychology, 23*(4), 468–476. https://doi.org/10.1037/cdp0000143

Lebow, J. L., & Diamond, R. M. (2019). Brief history of couple and family therapy. In B. H. Fiese, M. Celano, K. Deater-Deckard, E. N. Jouriles, & M. A. Whisman (Eds.), *APA handbook of contemporary family psychology: Family therapy and training* (pp. 3–18). American Psychological Association. https://doi.org/10.1037/0000101-001

Lee, L. (n.d.). *Kemetic teachings: Principles of Maat.* Retrieved October 13, 2022, from https://www.spiritquestwithlinda.com/blog/principles-of-maat

LGBT Demographic Data Interactive. (2019, January). *LGBT data & demographics.* Williams Institute, UCLA School of Law. https://williamsinstitute.law.ucla.edu/visualization/lgbt-stats/

Mahoney, A. (2010). Religion in families 1999 to 2009: A relational spirituality framework. *Journal of Marriage and Family, 72*(4), 805–827. https://doi.org/10.1111/j.1741-3737.2010.00732.x

Mangena, F. (n.d.). Hunhu/ubuntu in the traditional thought of southern Africa. *International encyclopedia of philosophy.* Retrieved October 13, 2022, from https://www.iep.utm.edu/hunhu/

Mark, J. J. (2016, September 15). Ma'at. *World history encyclopedia.* https://www.ancient.eu/Ma%27at/

Matthews, D., Smith, J., Brown, A., & Malebranche, D. (2016). Reconciling epidemiology and social justice in the public health discourse around the sexual networks of Black men who have sex with men. *American Journal of Public Health, 106*(5), 808–814. https://doi.org/10.2105/AJPH.2015.303031

Mays, A., Cochran, S., & Zamudio, A. (2004). HIV prevention research: Are we meeting the needs of African American men who have sex with men? *Journal of Black Psychology, 30*(1), 78–106. https://doi.org/10.1177/0095798403260265

Miller, R. (2005). An appointment with god: AIDS, place, and spirituality. *Journal of Sex Research, 42,* 35–45. https://doi.org/10.1080/00224490509552255

Montgomery, D., Fine, M., & James-Myers, L. (1990). The development and validation of an instrument to assess an optimal Afrocentric world view. *Journal of Black Psychology, 17,* 37–54. https://doi.org/10.1177/00957984900171004

Morgan, D. L., Ataie, J., Carder, P., & Hoffman, K. (2013). Introducing dyadic interviews as a method for collecting qualitative data. *Qualitative Health Research, 23*(9), 1276–1284. https://doi.org/10.1177/1049732313501889

Myers, L. J. (1993). *Understanding an Afrocentric world view: Introduction to an optimal psychology.* Kendall/Hunt Publishing Company.

Neblett, E. W., Seaton, E. K., Hammond, W. P., & Townsend, T. G. (2010). Underlying mechanisms in the relationship between Africentric worldview and depressive symptoms. *Journal of Counseling Psychology, 57*(1), 105–113. https://doi.org/10.1037/a0017710

Nobles, W., Goddard, L., & Gilbert, D. (2009). Culturecology, women, and African-centered HIV prevention. *Journal of Black Psychology, 35*(2), 228–246. https://doi.org/10.1177/0095798409333584

Obasi, E. M., Flores, L. Y., & James-Myers, L. (2009). Construction and initial validation of the Worldview Analysis Scale (WAS). *Journal of Black Studies, 39*(6), 937–961. https://doi.org/10.1177/0021934707305411

Parham, T., Ajamu, A., & White, J. (2016). *Psychology of Blacks: Centering our perspectives in the African consciousness* (4th ed.). Routledge.

Pew Research Center. (2014). *The religious landscape study.* https://www
.pewforum.org/about-the-religious-landscape-study/

Phillips, F. B. (1990). NTU psychotherapy: An Afrocentric approach. *The Journal of Black Psychology, 17,* 55–74.

Pinch, G. (2002). *Egyptian mythology: A guide to the gods, goddesses, and traditions of ancient Egypt.* Oxford University Press.

Piper-Mandy, E., & Rowe, T. (2010). Educating African-centered psychologists: Towards a comprehensive paradigm. *Journal of Pan African Studies, 3*(8), 5–23.

Pitt, R. (2010a). "Killing the messenger": Religious Black gay men's neutralization of anti-gay religious messages. *Journal for the Scientific Study of Religion, 49*(1), 56–72. https://doi.org/10.1111/j.1468-5906.2009.01492.x

(2010b). "Still looking for my Jonathan": Gay Black men's management of religious and sexual identity conflicts. *Journal of Homosexuality, 57*(1), 39–53. https://doi.org/10.1080/00918360903285566

Poteat, T., & Lassiter, J. M. (2019). Positive religious coping predicts self-reported HIV medication adherence at baseline and twelve-month follow-up among Black Americans living with HIV in the southeastern United States. *AIDS Care, 31*(8), 958–964. https://doi.org/10.1080/09540121.2019 .1587363

Quinn, K., Dickson-Gomez, J., & Kelly, J. (2016). The role of the Black church in the lives of young Black men who have sex with men. *Culture, Health & Sexuality, 18*(5), 524–537. https://doi.org/10.1080/13691058.2015.1091509

Saylor, C. (2004). The circle of health: A health definition model. *Journal of Holistic Nursing, 22*(2), 98–115. https://doi.org/10.1177/0898010104264775

Sitter, K. C. (2017). Taking a closer look at photovoice as a participatory action research method. *Journal of Progressive Human Services, 28*(1), 36–48.

Super, J. T., & Jacobson, L. (2011). Religious abuse: Implications for counseling lesbian, gay, bisexual, and transgender individuals. *Journal of LGBT Issues in Counseling, 5,* 180–196. https://doi.org/10.1080/15538605.2011.632739

Tan, J., Campbell, C., Conroy, A., Tabrisky, A., Kegeles, S., & Dworkin, S. (2018). Couple-level dynamics and multilevel challenges among Black men who have sex with men: A framework of dyadic HIV care. *AIDS Patient and STDs, 32*(11), 459–467. https://doi.org/10.1089/apc.2018.0131

Van Dyk, G. A. J., & Nefale, M. C. (2005). The split-ego experience of Africans: Ubuntu therapy as a healing alternative. *Journal of Psychotherapy Integration, 15*(1), 48–66. https://doi.org/10.1037/1053-0479.15.1.48

Wade, R., & Harper, G. (2017). Young black gay/bisexual and other men who have sex with men: A review and content analysis of health-focused research between 1988 and 2013. *American Journal of Men's Health, 11*(5), 1388–1405. https://doi.org/10.1177/1557988315606962

Walker, J. J., Longmire-Avital, B., & Golub, S. (2015). Racial and sexual identities as potential buffers to risky sexual behavior for Black gay and bisexual emerging adult men. *Health Psychology, 34*(8), 841–846. https://doi .org/10.1037/hea0000187

Ward, E. (2005). Homophobia, hypermasculinity and the US African American church. *Culture, Health & Sexual Orientation, 7*, 493–504. https://doi.org/10.1080/13691050500151248

Washington, K. (2010). Zulu traditional healing, Afrikan worldview and the practice of ubuntu: Deep thought for Afrikan/Black psychology. *Journal of Pan African Studies. 3*(8), 24–39.

Wilson, D., Olubadewo, S., & Williams, V. (2016). Ubuntu: A framework for African American male positive mental health. In W. Ross (Ed.), *African American male series. Counseling in African American males: Effective therapeutic interventions and approaches* (pp. 61–80). Information Age Publishing.

Wilson, D., & Williams, V. (2013). Ubuntu: Development and framework of a specific model of positive mental health. *Psychology Journal, 10*(2), 80–100.

Wilson, P., Valera, P., Martos, A., Wittlin, N., Munoz-Laboy, M., & Parker, R. (2016). Contributions of qualitative research in informing HIV/AIDS interventions targeting Black MSM in the United States. *Journal of Sex Research, 53*(6), 642–654. https://doi.org/10.1080/00224499.2015.1016139

Wilson, P., Wittlin, N., Muñoz-Laboy, M., & Parker, R. (2011). Ideologies of Black churches in New York City and the public health crisis of HIV among Black men who have sex with men. *Global Public Health, 6*(Suppl. 2) S227–S242. https://doi.org/10.1080/17441692.2011.605068

Wynn, R., & West-Olatunji, C. (2008). Culture-centered case conceptualization using NTU psychotherapy with an African American gay male client. *Journal of LGBT Issues in Counseling, 2*(4), 308–325. https://doi.org/10.1080/15538600802501995

PART II

Foundations for Healthy Coupling

CHAPTER 4

The Foundations for Strong and Healthy Relationships between Black Men and Women: Purposes, Practices, and Processes

Daryl M. Rowe & Sandra Lyons Rowe

4.1 Introduction and Overview

Over the past twenty-five years, we have been presenting, writing, and providing clinical services to address the unique characteristics, strengths, and challenges of creating and sustaining healthy marital relationships between men and women of African ancestry (Rowe & Rowe, 2009; Rowe & Rowe, 2013). Central to this work has been grounding our thinking within the emerging field of African-centered psychology (Grills et al., 2016; Piper-Mandy & Rowe, 2010; Rowe & Webb-Msemaji, 2004) that has been critical to our professional, clinical, and scholarly experiences with heterosexual couples of African ancestry. In addition to the increased clinical work with couples, another outgrowth of this work has been the development of Conversations in Marriage© (CIM), a community empowerment program that promotes marriage education through a series of semistructured conversations or seminars. CIM was developed in 2002 to address the disturbing decline of marriage within the African American community (Rowe & Rowe, 2002). CIM grew out of more than 30 years of combined experience providing counseling and psychotherapy with heterosexual couples, families, and individuals of African ancestry. From these experiences, several assumptions have facilitated the development of culturally specific foundations that we have operationalized through examining particular purposes, practices, and processes for strengthening healthy relationships between heterosexual Black women and men, as follows:

1. In working with heterosexual couples of African ancestry, we've found that it is essential to explicitly incorporate cultural issues, both broadly and specifically, into the sets of strengths and challenges our couples must contend with, in addition to each partner's unique personal history.

85

2. In addition to customary challenges of managing personal differences, family stressors, health changes, and economic fluctuations, couples of African ancestry operate within the confines of a stratified oppressive social system that exacerbates each of these customary challenges.

3. Providing an overview of the cycle of healthy relationships for couples of African ancestry can help normalize unique obstacles and instill a sense of hope that sustaining and satisfying relationships are within reach.

4. Highlighting the legacy of healthy families of African ancestry, within the context of community needs and community survival, can often be more effective than simply stressing one couple's specific marital health; that is, it is often beneficial to help Black couples place their relational outcomes within a broader sociocommunal context.

5. Participatory, familiar discussions that mirror the storytelling style more consistent with African American culture (Murrell, 2002) can often facilitate more disclosure and openness from clients versus more detached reflective observation and exercises. Examples of how the purposes, practices, and processes can be utilized by Black couples are addressed in each section of the chapter.

6. Lastly, introducing and incorporating African proverbs can stimulate more engagement, prompt more insights, provide guidance, convey wisdom, and foster a sense of shared purpose into practices and processes for sustaining healthy marriages among couples of African ancestry. Key proverbs are included within each section of the chapter to highlight significant learning intentions.

4.2 Defining Culture

A people with power looks for the source of problems within themselves.

(African Proverb)

Although culture is an elusive construct to define, and there have been countless definitions offered (Kroeber & Kluckhohn, 1952; Lonner & Malpass, 1994; Nobles, 1986), Kleinman's (1996) definition provides a powerful, elegant framing, as follows, "Culture is constituted by, and in turn constitutes, local worlds of experience" (p. 16). In other words, that which we know as culture emerges out of everyday experience – it is not something that is esoteric and mysterious – it literally reflects our personal and collective or communal everyday patterns of daily life experiences. Culture reflects our *common sense*(s), communication with others, *routines* – rhythms, rituals, roles – and *responsibilities* and rules of everyday community or communal life that we take for granted as commonplace, normal, and natural (although these aspects are natural only within specified bounds of place and time). These common senses – the shared *roles, rules, responsibilities, routines,* and *rituals* – can serve as a basis for unpacking key foundations for healthy marriages within the African American community. Thus, cultural influences lead persons to develop specific belief or value systems, common language, and norms (Belgrave & Allison, 2006). Furthermore, direct or vicarious experiences of oppression moderate how persons may or may not choose to honor cultural influences or seek to change influences judged not to be positive.

Briefly, from a contemporary perspective, psychoeducational approaches for marital enrichment assume that longer-term marital therapy may not be necessary, feasible, or consistent with the readiness of the couples; and the overall aims are the prevention of relational difficulties and the promotion of more enduring and fulfilling marital relationships (Ripley & Worthington, 2002).

However, as Parks (2003) argues, the need for cultural competency requires a reexamination of more indigenous traditions grounded in African/African American folk beliefs and healing practices. Thus, the general psychoeducational approach has been modified consistent with African-centered metatheory (Rowe & Rowe, 2009). The basis for the structure of CIM is rooted in the social theory of African centeredness. Briefly stated, African centeredness locates African values and ideals at the center of any discussion involving African people, culture, and behavior (Asante, 1987). It reflects a model for living that emphasizes both an individual and collective social consciousness. Traditional African psychology has been defined as "a place – a view, a perspective, a way of observing" (Akbar, 2003, p. ix) – seeing humans as spirit, resilient and capable of restoration; as a framework for understanding the nature of human being-ness grounded in collective African cultural principles (Nobles, 1986); and as a combination of dynamic knowledge and ancestral experience (Grills, 2004). It includes practices and processes, grounded in observation and practical experience, that are passed down from generation to generation, orally or through symbols. A proverb that captures the essence of these ideas is: "It is not the eye that understands but the mind."

Therefore, African psychology includes (a) a theory of human being-ness, (b) a set of practices and processes aimed at connections, and (c) a system for determining and facilitating human functioning. According to Nobles (1998),

> African centeredness represents a concept which categorizes a *"quality of thought and practice"* which is rooted in the cultural image and interest of people of African ancestry and which represents and reflects the life experiences, history and traditions of people of African ancestry as the center of analyses. (p. 190)

Nobles' definition is critical because it shifts the debate from merely conceptual issues to the meanings and methods of African-centered psychology, because it places emphasis on the *quality* of thought and practice (Rowe & Webb-Msemaji, 2004). As such, psychology centered in African thought and practice reflects African people's intimate knowledge of their subjective human experiences as they interact with the world – nature, the cosmos, geographical location, others, and oneself. Parks (2003) relates these notions to more postmodernist thought, suggesting that African centered ideas reflect a cultural narrative wherein reality is interdependent or co-constructed by the person, community, and world.

However, as Nobles (1986) argued, the efforts to articulate African psychology are still in flux, thus:

> the work we do is constantly changing and we continue to inform our efforts by the need to transform psychology ... [current efforts] ... should not be taken as an example of "the African (Black) psychology," at least not in the sense of the complete or developed African (Black) psychology. Most of the work of Black psychologists should be seen as "African (Black) psychology becoming." (original quotations, pp. 109–110)

Thus, Rowe and Webb-Msemaji (2004) suggest that the term *African centered* best reflects how to encapsulate the various efforts for discussing the psychology of persons of African ancestry at this point in history. By "centered," they suggest that the current level of understanding is not sufficiently refined to have formal distinct boundaries for what comprises African cultural thought and practices *and* that scholars examining these issues should intentionally *locate* their theories, methods, and practices within the ever-deepening investigation into and reclamation of African cultural ways. They suggest four criteria for assessing parameters of African-centered psychology, as follows: (a) utilizes African cultural patterns and styles for understanding human behavior; (b) reflects the various ways African peoples have sought to understand, articulate, and project themselves to themselves, others, and the world; (c) emphasizes values that are more collective and situational, assumptions that are more integrative, and methods that are more affective and metaphorical; and (d) relies on African sources, that is, oral literature (proverbs, songs, tales/stories), praise songs and moral teachings, spiritual system "scripts," prayers, and the dynamic interdependence of community, nature, and spirit.

Similarly, Nobles (2004) suggests that African-centered psychology must address the oral tradition – how beliefs and traditions are handed down from one generation to the next. As a result, we contend that an additional domain of African-centered psychology can be discerned through a descriptive analysis of moral language; the sanctions used to enforce morality; and a review of proverbs, tales, and myths, which refer to the moral beliefs of the peoples. As Chinua Achebe (1964) indicates, conversation, particularly as handled by elder members of traditional African society, is one of the greatest repositories of African wisdom that portrays authentic African life and experience.

Thus, the theoretical grounding of CIM extends out of the earliest methods of instruction among persons of African ancestry – the use of proverbs to situate persons in life dilemmas. West African proverbs serve to stimulate discussion about key marital struggles and strategies for ameliorating those challenges. African proverbs are collections of metaphorical statements, usually short and to the point, which convey general truths about life, people, and community (Ackah, 1988). Traditionally, they have been used to instruct members into the customs and traditions of particular communities. A Yoruba proverb states:

> A proverb is a horse which can carry one swiftly to the discovery of ideas.

According to Dzobo (1992), proverbs can be used for four primary purposes: (a) to *express truths* that are difficult to comprehend; (b) as *guides for conduct* – as bases for determining the unacceptability of certain forms of behavior; (c) as *commentary on human behavior* – proverbs help to delineate the styles humans reflect in negotiating life; and (d) to *express values* – to reflect the centered values characteristic of Africans, from the psychological, moral, spiritual, humanistic, economic, and intellectual to the material. African proverbs are shared that are congruent with the core of each conversation's focal point. Proverbs are brief, serving as simple ways to convey elegant truths; are flexible, such that they can be used across a variety of situations and points in time; are profound, by stimulating further reflection and calling for deeper thinking about commonplace occurrences; and are communicative, by promoting conversation (Monye, 1996). Proverbs in such settings are like the seasonings, used to strengthen points made by different participants in the conversation. An African proverb states: "Knowledge is like a garden: if it is not cultivated it cannot be harvested." CIM stresses that marriage is the garden and the challenge is to recreate cultivation skills that allow the gardens of African American marriages to harvest healthy families – "it is legend that the nations start in the family" (Madhubuti, 1998, p. 3) – and to reestablish the foundation of healthy communities.

Most of the following insights have been informed through conversations that we've had with couples either in therapeutic settings or through our CIM program. These discussions have reflected a participatory process wherein couples explored strategies to help them improve their relationship skills, institute different standards for determining the viability of their relationships and foster long-term commitment to sustaining healthy marriages for the betterment of African American communities.

4.3   Challenges Affecting Relationships between Black Men and Women

The fragility and vulnerability of African American marriage has been well documented during the past forty years (Belgrave & Allison, 2006; James, 1998; Lawson & Thompson, 1994; Patterson, 1998; Staples, 1981; Tucker & Mitchell-Kernan, 1995). Various positions have been put forth underscoring the salience of competing factors: (a) economic issues, related to both the declining employment status of African American men and the increasing economic independence of African American women (Cherlin, 1998; James, 1998); (b) unequal sex ratio, related to multiple factors – higher death rates from disease, poor health care, violent crime, high rates of drug and alcohol abuse, gang activity, incarceration, and sexual orientation – that further reduce the number of desirable males available for marriage (Darity & Myers, 1995; James, 1998; Pinderhughes, 2002); (c) sociocultural issues, related to both the retention of African cultural values and delicate adaptations to hostile societal oppression, restrictions, and shifts (Parham et al., 2000; Patterson, 1998); and (d) relational struggles, tied to gender role flexibility, and couple communication, fidelity, power, and intimacy (Boyd-Franklin & Franklin, 1999; Bryant & Wickrama, 2005; Patterson, 1998).

Tucker and James (2005) provide an overview of characteristics of African American domestic relationships that, although somewhat dated, suggests important trends that impact marriage between African American heterosexual men and women. First, they suggest that there is increasing variation in family forms, with under 40 percent of Black children living with both biological parents, suggesting increasing stressors on parents as they manage multiple roles alone. Second, they report that more African Americans are embracing singlehood and/or not marrying at increasing rates, due to later and less marriage, more divorce, and less remarriage. Indeed, some have estimated that upwards of 65 percent of first marriages of African American women end in divorce (Raley & Bumpass, 2003). Third, couples are more likely to cohabitate, although the proportion of cohabitating African American couples is still less than 25 percent. A critical challenge is that while children are still being born, cohabitation often occurs without clarity of specific commitments and responsibilities. These data reflect troubling trends that have been growing over the past forty + years. For example, in 1960, a married couple was found in approximately 78 percent of African American households, decreasing to 64 percent in 1970; and by the late 1980s, only 48 percent of African American households included both a husband and a wife (Pinderhughes, 2002).

In summary, there are several implications of Tucker and James' (2005) review of the literature, as follows: (a) African American women are carrying more of the economic burden of maintaining families; (b) African Americans are becoming more and more isolated at critical junctures of caregiving, especially raising children and caring for elders; (c) with the increasing emphasis on singlehood and higher costs of living, generally, people are working more, leaving less and less time for cohesive family activities; and (d) African American fathers are increasingly less likely to live with their biological children. Our position is that strengthening marriages can serve to help reverse some of these trends, especially if we focus on developing culturally adaptive characteristics of marriage that resonate with broader African American values.

4.4 Cycle of Healthy Relationships: Foundations and Purposes

There are a number of principles that serve as foundations upon which we can build healthy, sustainable, heterosexual marital relationships with persons of African ancestry, although we suspect that some of these characteristics may be useful for a range of relationships that seek long-term viability and sustainability.

We believe that the first key principle for building sustainable healthy marriage is *choice*. From our experiences, how one decides to connect and with whom are two of the most important decisions to make in forming a long-lasting, viable partnership. Implicit is the presumption that one would want to be more deliberate and intentional in choosing potential partners than is often seen today. An African proverb that reflects this deliberative process is, "You have to spend time in a meadow to know it." The idea is that it takes a period of time to explore the facets and features of another person to determine how the two of you fit together and whether you share sufficient common purposes. Determining *fit* is a reason that choice is the foundation of sustainable relationships and why long-term, sustainable relationships typically build slowly.

So contrary to the pressure to move quickly and superficially, by swiping left or right, we believe that moving more slowly, with intention and deliberation; developing common interests or seeking connections with potential partners with whom you share interests; and sharing major values, perspectives, and philosophies of life are more important to have with potential partners that you're trying to get to know and become known by.

Second, we believe that ongoing, fluid *communication* is a critical principle for sustaining long-term relationships. We argue that couples always communicate – with what they say, what they do, what they don't say, and what they don't do. All of our behaviors communicate to our significant others something about our interests, intentions, insights, intrigues, and intimacies. The challenge we have is how we invite our significant others into the intricacies of our communications. Ideally, our goal is to strive to become more transparent about our interests and intentions, as well as our intrigues and intimacies. Our overarching aim is to more openly share the details of how we make meaning of the world with the person with whom we seek long-term connection and companionship. Simply put, communication in marriage is like oil in a car: no matter how fancy the car, if you don't keep the oil fluid and renewed, the machinery of the car will break down. Similarly, if you don't keep communication flowing within a relationship, no matter how well the relationship starts, or how much you may have in common, the relationship will stop functioning well.

We've found that conversations are different ways of learning – allowing for multidirectionality, active involvement, and egalitarianism versus unidirectionality, passivity, or inequality. Good conversations invite our partners to join in, wind along, dip in and out – sometimes superficially, sometimes deeply – and then circle back and enter the discussion again (Rowe & Rowe, 2009). Each time, partners can uncover more about themselves, others, and processes of sustaining healthy marriages. They can be tightly structured or organized, or more flowing or spontaneous, moving quickly sometimes and more slowly at other times. Conversations allow partners to grasp meaning out of expression, providing a hint into their understanding of African American marriage. The goal of these conversations is to support and encourage each partner in her/his quest to be better men and women together, reflected by the proverb, "The one who begins a conversation does not foresee the end." Fluid communication is foundational to sustaining long-term marriage.

Next, we believe that *compassionate cooperation* is an essential principle for sustaining long-term relationships. Typically, in expressing one's commitment to the journey of marriage, each partner co-promises some form of ongoing love, honor, and fidelity to their shared union; said simply, we agree to *compromise* or cooperate with compassion with our partners about various issues, big and small. Implicit in this idea of compassionate cooperation is that sustainable marriages are grounded in friendship. We believe that marriage is more than two individuals coming or falling together because they are attracted to each other; sustainable marriage is a higher calling. It brings two persons together, with similar purposes that can combine to bring their shared gifts to benefit the broader community (Somé, 1999).

Emphasis is placed on community because community is the outgrowth of marriage, and marriage is the basis of family. Traditionally, marriage has been the marker of adulthood and the focus of existence; the point where all members of a given community meet – the departed, the living, and those yet to be born (Mbiti, 1970). Marriage establishes and maintains family, creates and sustains the ties of kinship, and is the basis of community. Hence, from a historical perspective, marriage was seen as a requirement for society, a duty; indispensable for community – the root of civilization (Gyekye, 1996). From such a perspective, marriage is and has to be bigger than mere personal happiness – marriage is about building community and preserving civilization.

An appropriate African proverb for reinforcing compassionate compromise is, A friend is like a source of water during a long voyage. The aim is to cultivate a relationship with a partner who has your back, is supportive and encouraging, with whom you share similar interests, gives you a reality check and with whom you develop a deeper intimacy; these are features of a solid friendship.

Lastly, we believe that *commitment* is a key principle upon which we build healthy, long-term, sustainable marriages between African American men and women. Commitment is the glue that binds us together for the long and winding journey of marriage. This glue is mostly a decision, a resolution, a choice to be together and stay together through better and worse. Thus, choice and commitment fit together like hand in glove. As we suggest, commitment means taking the longest view of marriage possible; we started with a forty-year contract. Commitment means not leaving the side or back door open; not allowing for an "out" or escape clause. An African proverb that speaks to the power of commitment is, "If you are building a house and a nail breaks, do you stop building, or do you change the nail?"

Commitment means that the "we" is more important than the "I," underscoring the importance of having a shared identity and purpose and taking time to ascertain such commonalities. Commitment, as we use it, requires a certain amount of satisfaction in sacrifice, where we do things largely and regularly for our partner's benefit. Commitment means that our marriage sits as our top priority – as we share with our clients regularly, "24/7, 365 (twenty-four hours per day, seven days per week, three hundred and sixty-five days per year), with no time off for good behavior." Commitment means that we will be there for each other in the future and that we can count on each other in the present. Additionally, commitment implies that we regularly engage in renewal rituals. As Somé (1999) suggests,

> Marriage is a renewal of vows for those who have already married. It's a way of family coming together, a way of . . . [communities] . . . coming together, and it's an opportunity to celebrate the hearing of a call that two souls or two spirits heard and answered. (p. 78)

The implication is that couples sustain their commitment through regular renewal of their vows, whether yearly, or when someone else is marrying. Thus, implied in the principle of commitment is the importance and necessity of celebrating and creating ceremonies to mark or note the progress of our continued marriage journey; such ceremonies can be healing and reinforce opportunities to express our ongoing commitment and connection.

"The pot will smell of what is put into it" is a centering African proverb to bolster the principle of commitment.

As we suggested earlier, marriages are not private – marriages belong to the community (Rowe & Rowe, 2009). We think this is a powerful idea for transforming marriage within the African American community; it reinforces our contention that public *commitment* is essential to the long-term sustainability of marriage. The idea of community places emphasis on the shared responsibility of community members to safeguard the voices of its members, such that the community hears each person – valued and affirmed – and cultivates each person's gifts that then are freely given to the world (Somé, 1999). Thus, community serves to anchor persons to something bigger than only their partners or spouses, providing a higher sense of purpose and belonging. It is this commitment to something bigger than mere happiness, a commitment to strengthening community through the cultivation of long-term marriage that becomes a foundational ground for restoring vitality within communities of persons of African ancestry.

4.5   Cycle of Healthy Relationships: Strategies and Practices

As previously mentioned, our understanding of culture gives us insights into developing viable, sustaining relationships reflected through the commitment to marriage. Sustainable marriage culture is grounded in shared *common sense*(s) or practices, which include ongoing communication with one's partner, shared *routines* – rhythms, rituals, roles – and shared *responsibilities* and *rules* of everyday marital life, situated in community, that we take for granted as commonplace, normal and natural. These common practices – the shared *roles, rules, responsibilities, routines*, and *rituals* – can serve as a basis for building sustainable, fulfilling healthy marriages.

The idea behind *roles* has less to do with what each partner does within the context of their marriage, because, if the commitment is long, as intended, roles can and will change as we age and mature as partners; the key is that both partners have clarity about their roles within their sustaining, evolving journey together. Effective roles for marriage require shared understandings about household obligations – how responsibilities for maintaining a household from the simple to the profound; job-related undertakings – how money is earned, saved, and distributed over time and across circumstances; parenting duties – whether children are planned for, how they are cared for across all of the various parenting responsibilities (health, education, recreation, socialization); caregiving tasks – how extended family members and friends are handled; and life management activities – how decisions are managed for short-term, intermediate, and long-term planning that impacts the growth and development of the marriage and family (Tucker & James, 2005).

Marital *rules* refer broadly to the shared expectations or actions that partners adopt and implement to create a sense of order within their marriage (Bryant & Wickrama, 2005). Sustainable marriages need clear rules that exert social control over how partners behave within and over the course of long-term marriage. Typically, marital rules relate to sexual fidelity – the expectation that sexual relationships are exclusive and that transgressions to that exclusivity requires some form of reparation for the ruptured trust; financial fidelity – the expectation that monies earned within the marriage are shared between the partners and that spending or borrowing above an agreed upon threshold is negotiated prior to spending or borrowing; communication fidelity – the expectation that a certain negotiated amount of conversation between partners stays private; and role fidelity – the expectation that the roles delineated between the partners at various stages of the marriage are adhered to and honored by each partner.

Marital *responsibilities* refer to the detailed tasks each partner adopts and fulfills consistent with the roles and rules (Tucker & James, 2005). Thus, responsibilities are variable versus fixed, fluid instead of unchanging over the course of marriage. Effective responsibilities vary based on the tenure of the marriage – early, transitional, intermediate, late; whether the marriage has added children – birth, adopted, foster; work-/school-related activities – full-time versus part-time work/school, in-home versus out-of-home duties, fixed versus flexible schedules; and living arrangements – renters, shared community environments, home ownership, each of which may require differing sets of regular tasks to divide among partners.

Marital *routines*, as we think about them, relate to two different divisions: daily/weekly routines and relationship routines (Bryant & Wickrama, 2005). Daily/weekly routines refer to how we structure our time day to day and/or week to week. Raising children typically is a transformation of routines that many marriages are unprepared for. When children join marriages, the daily routine becomes much more structured in that certain tasks must be accomplished regardless of whatever else is going on. Daily routines, with children, look more or less like waking, exercise, grooming, breakfast, snack, chores, lunch, snack, chores, dinner, story-time, baths, bedtime, and chores with work life and connections with others squeezed in between. Typically, this is a full plate for most marriages and brings with it considerable stressors. It is at this juncture in the journey of marriage where successful marriages recognize that, as the old Nigerian Igbo proverb states, "It takes a village to raise a child" and partners seek support to handle the ongoing tasks of raising children and sustaining marriage.

Lastly, marital *rituals* are critical practices for sustainable long-term African American marriages. Rituals create processes that *remind*, *reveal*, and *reinforce* each partner's connection and authenticity to each other and to their marriage. We've identified several strategies or repetitive processes for sustaining healthy marriages including connecting, conversational, continuity, commitment, forgiveness, and rejuvenation rituals. Briefly, examples of connecting rituals include checking in with each other during the day through emails, phone calls, and/or texts – connecting rituals tend to remind us that we are working to maintain a flexible link to our partners and helps us accommodate ongoing changes that may impact us day to day. Examples of conversational rituals include setting aside time, regularly and frequently, to discuss dreams, goals, challenges, and accomplishments, within marriage. Examples of continuity rituals include weekly and monthly shared activities, from mundane tasks like chores and errands (gardening and groceries) to support and respite (backrubs, listening to music, dancing, etc.). Commitment rituals include remembrances or celebrations of birthdays, anniversaries, and renewing vows, for example. Forgiveness rituals include sending letters, cards, flowers; engaging in shared prayer, meditation, quiet spaces, dinners/meals, and walks. Lastly, rejuvenation rituals might include weekend retreats, vacations, and/or shared exercise. To summarize, marriage rituals are regular, repetitive processes that serve to remind partners to practice behaviors that lead to long-term, sustainable healthy marriages. A key proverb that might capture the thrust of these rituals is, "The person who goes to draw water does not drink mud." Said simply, practicing good relational habits builds strong marriages.

4.6   Cycle of Healthy Relationships: Methods and Processes

Although, there have been numerous methods and processes identified for strengthening African American marriages (Belgrave & Allison, 2006; Bryant & Wickrama, 2005), our work suggests that there are four key processes that need to be flexibly implemented to feed the marital relationship: *alone* time, *couple* time, *family* time, and *communal* time. We believe that each partner needs her/his solitary time – time spent with personal grooming, exercise, meditation, reading, friendships, hobbies, and interests – through which s/he works to develop, strengthen and cultivate his/her gifts to share with the broader society. Couple time is the time that partners spend deepening their insights into and knowledge of each other. These are the spaces where couples work on keeping their communication open, fluid, and transparent; where couples identify, develop, and strengthen common interests and activities. Although couple time is often operationalized as *date nights*, we think dates nights are more lazy examples of couple time, because they overemphasize the shared activities instead of strengthening the shared interests and deepening insights. A simple analogy for thinking about the aim of couple time is the ongoing sharing of *instruction manuals* for how each of us best works, entrusted into the hands of our partners with whom we are on this journey of marriage.

Family time is a routine whereby we seek to have constructive time between parents and children. This is a critical routine because it serves to reinforce the decision to commit to the journey of marriage and family. It is through family time that primary values are passed on to children, future plans are discussed and operationalized, and shared expectations are transmitted and reinforced. There are numerous examples of constructive family time, ranging from mealtimes, family chore days, and commuting times to game/arts/crafts nights, to various sporting activities, to civic/community activities, to camping, hiking, bicycling activities, and to differing types of vacations. Each of these types of activities can serve to strengthen and reinforce family and marital bonds.

Lastly, *communal* times involve regular, periodic time with other families who are on the journey of long-term marriage. Through these shared spaces partners have an opportunity to gain perspective about the strengths and limits of their marriage journey by witnessing how their particular challenges stack up against the struggles others may have. Such perspective-taking can serve as a chance to examine shortcomings, bolster virtues, and recommit themselves to their long-term journey of marriage. Thus, these common routines – alone time, couple time, family time, and communal time – form the foundation for how African American couples, committed to sustainable, long-term marriage journeys, can keep their unions viable, healthy, and stable building blocks of workable communities of Black families.

4.7   Summary and Implications

We believe that marriage is one of the critical threads that bind or hold communities together – they help to establish a sense of family and belonging that are valuable to African Americans, as a system of support within a larger society that is still inhospitable. Thus, our aim has been to emphasize the community empowerment functions of marriage, versus mere personal happiness; we want you to be weavers of a stronger community for our children. Marriage is our obligation to our ancestors, community, families, and nation; the responsibility of serious adults concerned with their duties to our children. We believe that marriage is a process, not a commodity – not something we obtain, but someone we become. Marriage brings two people together and creates a unit: the individuals each have their own needs and often the marriage (unit) has its needs. Sometimes the needs of the unit are different from the needs of the individuals. For the long-term journey of sustainable marriage, at times, the needs of the marriage unit must take precedence over the whims and wishes of the individuals. Thus, we believe that marriage is hard work; it gets easier only when one practices it. Our overarching aim is to make marriage – once again – normal and commonplace; a joining together that we do unashamedly and unapologetically. In closing, we leave you with this African proverb, "If you want to go fast, go alone, if you want to go far, go together."

Discussion Questions

1. What must the therapist be mindful of as they attempt to explicitly incorporate cultural issues into their work with couples of African Ancestry?
2. How does a therapist working from an African centeredness methodology differ in their approach when working with couples of African Ancestry?
3. How might a therapist use African proverbs to help couples strengthen their relationship?
4. The authors assert, "our aim has been to emphasize the community empowerment functions of marriage, versus mere personal happiness." How does this statement compare to twenty-first century views of marriage and how does it impact your clinical work?

REFERENCES

Achebe, C. (1964). *Arrow of God.* Anchor Books.

Ackah, C. A. (1988). *Akan ethics: A study of the moral ideas and the moral behavior of the Akan tribes of Ghana.* Ghana Universities Press.

Akbar, N. (2003). *Akbar papers in African psychology.* Mind Productions & Associates, Inc.

Asante, M. K. (1987). *The Afrocentric idea.* Temple University Press.

Belgrave, F. Z., & Allison, K. W. (2006). *African American psychology: From Africa to America.* Sage Publications.

Boyd-Franklin, N., & Franklin, A. J. (1999). African American couples in therapy. In M. McGoldrick & K. V. Hardy (Eds.), *Re-visioning family therapy: Race, culture and gender in clinical practice* (pp. 268–281). Guilford Press.

Bryant, C. M., & Wickrama, K. A. S. (2005). Marital relationships of African Americans: A contextual approach. In V. C. McLoyd, N. E. Hill, & K. A.

Dodge (Eds.), *African American family life: Ecological and cultural diversity* (pp. 111–134). Guilford Press.

Cherlin, A. J. (1998). Marriage and marital dissolution among Black Americans. *Journal of Comparative Family Studies*, 29(1), 147–159.

Darity, W., & Myers, S. (1995). Family structure and the marginalization of black men: Policy implications. In M. Tucker & C. Mitchell-Kernan (Eds.), *The decline of marriage among African-Americans* (pp. 263–308). Russell Sage Foundation.

Dzobo, N. K. (1992). *African symbols and proverbs as source of knowledge and truth.* Council for Research in Values and Philosophy.

Grills, C. N. (2004). African psychology. In R. Jones (Ed.), *Black psychology* (4th ed., pp. 171–208). Cobbs & Henry Publishers.

Grills, C. N., Aird, E. G., & Rowe, D. M. (2016). Breathe, baby, breathe: Clearing the way for the emotional emancipation of Black people. *Cultural Studies ↔ Critical Methodologies*, 16(3), 268–274. https://doi.org/10.1177/1532708616634839

Gyekye, K. (1996). *African cultural values: An introduction.* Sankofa Publishing Company.

James, A. D. (1998). What's love got to do with it? Economic viability and the likelihood of marriage among African American men. *Journal of Comparative Family Studies*, 29(2), 373–386.

Kleinman, A. (1996). How is culture important for DSM-IV?. In J. E. Mezzich, A. Kleinman, H., Jr. Fabrega, & D. L. Parron (Eds.), *Culture & psychiatric diagnosis: A DSM-IV perspective* (pp. 15–25). American Psychiatric Press.

Kroeber, A. L., & Kluckhohn, C. K. M. (1952). Culture: A critical review of concepts and definitions. *Papers. Peabody Museum of Archaeology & Ethnology, Harvard University*, 47(1), viii, 223.

Lawson, E., & Thompson, A. (1994). Historical and social correlates of African-American divorce: Review of the literature and implications for research. *The Western Journal of Black Studies*, 18(2), 91–103.

Lonner, W. J., & Malpass, R. (1994). *Psychology and culture.* Allyn and Bacon.

Madhubuti, H. R. (1998). *Heartlove: Wedding and love poems.* Third World Press.

Mbiti, J. S. (1970). *African religions and philosophies.* Anchor Books, Doubleday.

Monye, A. A. (1996). *Proverbs in African orature: The Aniocha-Igbo experience.* University Press of America.

Murrell, P. C., Jr. (2002). *African-centered pedagogy: Developing schools of achievement for African American children.* State University of New York Press.

Nobles, W. W. (1986). *African psychology: Toward its reclamation, reascension & revitalization.* The Institute for the Advanced Study of Black Family Life and Culture, Inc.

(1998). To be African or not to be: The question of identity or authenticity – some preliminary thoughts. In R. L. Jones (Ed.), *African American identity development* (pp. 183–206). Cobb & Henry Publishers.

(2004). African philosophy: Foundation for Black psychology. In R. Jones (Ed.), *Black psychology* (4th ed., pp. 57–72). Cobbs & Henry Publishers.

Parham, T. A., White, J. L., & Ajamu, A. (2000). *The psychology of Blacks: An African-centered perspective* (3rd ed.). Prentice-Hall.

Parks, F. (2003). The role of African American folk beliefs in the modern therapeutic process. *Clinical Psychology: Science and Practice, 10*(4), 456–467.

Patterson, O. (1998). *Rituals of Blood: Consequences of Slavery in two American Centuries.* Basic Civitas Books.

Pinderhughes, E. B. (2002). African American marriage in the 20th century. *Family Process, 41*(2), 269–283.

Piper-Mandy, E., & Rowe, T. D. (2010). Educating African-centered psychologists: Towards a comprehensive paradigm. *Journal of Pan-African Studies, 3*(8), 5–23.

Raley, R. K., & Bumpass, I. (2003). The topography of the divorce plateau: Levels and trends in union stability in the United States after 1980. *Demographic Research, 8,* 245–260.

Ripley, J. S., & Worthington, E. L, Jr. (2002). Hope-focused and forgiveness-based group interventions to promote marital enrichment. *Journal of Counseling & Development, 80*(4), 452–463.

Rowe, D. M., & Rowe, S. L. (2002). *Defining marriage.* Presented at Conversations in Marriage, a community forum of The Nubian Psychological Group, Los Angeles, CA.

(2009). Conversations in Marriage©: An African-centered marital intervention. In M. E. Gallardo & B. McNeill (Eds.), *Intersections of multiple identities: A casebook of evidence-based practices with diverse populations* (pp. 59–84). Routledge.

Rowe, D. M., & Webb-Msemaji, F. (2004). African-centered psychology in the community. In R. Jones (Ed.), *Black psychology* (4th ed., pp. 701–721), Cobb & Henry Publishers.

Rowe, S. L., & Rowe, D. M. (2013). Expert Interview. In K. M. Helm & J. Carlson (Eds.) *Love, Intimacy, and the African American Couple* (pp. 193–198). Routledge.

Somé, S. E. (1999). *The spirit of intimacy: Ancient teachings in the ways of relationships.* Berkeley Hills Books.

Staples, R. (1981). Race and marital status: An overview. In H. P. McAdoo (Ed.), *Black families* (pp. 173–176). Sage Publications.

Tucker, M. B., & James, A. D. (2005). New families, new functions: Postmodern African American families in context. In V. C. McLoyd, N. E. Hill, & K. A. Dodge (Eds.), *African American family life: Ecological and cultural diversity* (pp. 86–108). Guilford Press.

Tucker, M. B., & Mitchell-Kernan, C. (1995). Trends in African American family formation: A theoretical overview. In M. Tucker & C. Mitchell-Kernan (Eds.), *The decline of marriage among African-Americans* (pp. 8–26). Russell Sage Foundation.

CHAPTER 5

Considerations for Premarital Counseling and Education for Dating and Engaged Heterosexual African American Couples

Erica Holmes, Ronecia Lark, & Jessica M. Smedley

5.1 Introduction

Research continually finds that those who marry live longer, on average, and tend to be physically healthier than those who never marry, divorce, or become widowed (Dupre et al., 2009; Lawrence et al., 2019). In addition to physical health benefits, marriage has been demonstrated to positively impact wealth attainment, mental health, and social status (Rayley & Sweeney, 2009; Umberson et al., 2013; Williams et al., 1992; Zollar & Williams, 1987). Although these benefits have been documented, the Centers for Disease Control and Prevention (CDC) reported that marriage rates have steadily decreased overall in the United States (Curtin & Sutton, 2020). While there has been a decline in marriage for the general U.S. population, the decline is significant for African Americans, who reportedly have the lowest marriage rates and the highest divorce rate than any other ethnic group. Today, less than half of African Americans are married. The significant disparity in marriage rates between Blacks and other ethnic groups has not always been as prevalent. Once marriage was legalized post enslavement, African American men and women were married at substantial rates. However, by the late 1980s, the marriage rate for African Americans dropped drastically. Despite the decrease in African American marriages, when surveyed, African Americans continue to place a high value on marriage as well as desire marriage (Amato, 2011; Phillips et al., 2012).

Herein lies a contradiction between the value of and desire for marriage and a low number of marriages in the African American community. A true contextual understanding of the decline in African American marriage rates requires an examination of unique contributing factors through a historical and sociocultural lens, shedding light on how the legacy of institutionalized racism, discrimination, and oppression has profoundly shaped the African American family structure. This understanding lays the foundation for the development of effective prevention and early intervention resources to address unhealthy adaptations to the aforementioned experiences and teach skills proven to increase relational satisfaction.

5.2   African American Marriage Trends

Marriage trends have changed in recent years for all racial groups. In 2017, the U.S. marriage rate lingered around 50 percent (Parker & Stepler, 2017). The CDC reported that marriage rates have continually decreased overall in the United States. Marriage rates declined from 8.2 per 1,000 in the year 2000 to 6.5 per 1,000 in 2018 (Curtin & Sutton, 2020). Researchers have also reported a steady decline in marriages across race and ethnic groups. According to a Pew Research Center analysis of marriages from 1960 to 2010, marriage rates dropped from 74 percent in 1960 to 51 percent in 2010 for whites (32 percent decline), from 72 percent to 48 percent for Hispanics (34 percent decline), and from 61 percent to 31 percent for Blacks (50 percent decline) (Cohn et al., 2011). In 2016, 29 percent of African Americans were reported as married compared to 48 percent of whites and 44 percent of Hispanics. Surprisingly in 2019, a slight increase in marriage rates were reported at 57 percent for whites, 63 percent for Asians, 48 percent for Hispanics and 33 percent for Blacks (Horowitz et al., 2019). While there has been a decline in marriage for the general U.S. population, research clearly shows that African Americans have undergone the greatest decline over the years and continue to experience the lowest marriage rates.

Historical and cultural experiences have created a shift in current marriage trends for African Americans including marriage and divorce rates, attitudes about marriage, when to get married, and even whether or not to get married. Additionally, in general, more adults choose cohabitation as a present-day precursor to marriage. According to the US Census Bureau (Gurrentz, 2019), over 17 million unmarried adults live together (7 percent of the total adult population). This is a 38 percent increase since 1990 and an increase of 13 percent from 2009. While many adults are choosing to delay marriage and cohabitate, more African Americans choose to live together outside of marriage without considering it as a step toward marriage (Chambers & Kravitz, 2011). Relatedly, Black women who choose to marry do so much later in life compared to White and Hispanic women (Barr et al., 2013). It has also been noted that African

Americans are more likely to divorce than any other ethnic group. Further research has shown that almost 55 percent of Blacks divorce within the first fifteen years of marriage (Chambers & Kravitz, 2011; Copen et al., 2012). Dixon (2017) highlights that in 2013, the divorce rate for African Americans was at an all-time high of 67 percent. Furthermore, African Americans are also less likely to remarry after divorce.

The significant gap in marriage rates between Blacks and other groups has not always been as prevalent as it is currently. It is imperative to acknowledge that marriage patterns among African Americans have changed over time. Strong marriages and commitment to family life have always been central features of African American families. The strength and resiliency of the African American family could not be destroyed even by the illegality of Black marriages during enslavement. When given the legal right to marry, African Americans took advantage of this "privilege," which resulted in a high percentage of Blacks choosing to marry post enslavement. Blacks revered marriage and desired to reconnect with their African values and went to great lengths to legalize the informal marriages established while enslaved (Billingsley, 1992; Haines, 1996; Ruggles, 1994; Tucker & Mitchell-Kerman, 1995). It is reported that in 1880, 80 percent of African American families included a husband and wife (Billingsley, 1992). Researchers also note that between 1940 and 1960, African American families included marriages that were stable and thriving (Bryant et al., 2010; McAdoo, 2007). However, the 1970s marked a turning point for marriages in the African American community.

In 1960, at least 78 percent of African Americans were married. The number decreased to 64 percent by 1970 and to 48 percent by the late 1980s (McAdoo & Younge, 2009; Pinderhughes, 2002). Still today, less than half of African Americans are married. The current statistics on African American marriages might cause some to erroneously conclude that African Americans are incapable of commitment and do not know how to engage in loving, healthy, monogamous marriages. Some might even conclude that African Americans do not desire marriage. However, these assumptions are both simplistic and flawed.

A true contextual understanding of the decline in African American marriages requires an examination of such factors through a historical and sociocultural lens. The overall experiences of racism, discrimination, and oppression have profoundly shaped and significantly impacted the African American couple and must be considered when evaluating the overall state of African American relationships and marriages. The purposeful economic marginalization of Black men in the labor market, incarceration, and lack of access to education has created enormous disadvantages for Black families. Experiences of institutionalized racism, race-based trauma, and oppression impacts a couple's ability to foster and maintain relational intimacy and decreases the probability for African Americans to establish and sustain healthy marriages (Allen & Helm, 2013; Bryant et al., 2010; Dixon, 2009, 2014; Pinderhughes, 2002). These experiences color the ways that African Americans interpret and manage occurrences of marital conflicts found to be common in relationships.

5.3   Marital Conflict

African American couples face commonly identified marital challenges discussed in the literature. However, the social and historical context in which they live impact the meaning, significance, and implications of these challenges. Over the years, researchers have identified central themes that are frequently at the center of most marital conflict. These central themes include conflict over finances, ineffective communication, differences in parenting styles, relatives, unmet expectations, sex, and/or infidelity (Amato & Rogers, 1997; Henry & Miller, 2004; Miller et al., 2003). Additional sources of marital conflict are substance use issues, value or religious differences, fertility difficulties, and leisure activities (Henry & Miller, 2004).

According to Gottman (1994) any and all types of conflict can weigh heavily on a relationship and cause significant emotional distress. The impact of marital conflicts can range in severity, consequence, and outcome for the couple. Some issues are deemed more annoying than harmful and others more detrimental, leading to divorce (Amato & Rogers, 1997). The weight of marital challenges at either end of the continuum should not be minimized as any of the aforementioned factors can amass and lead to unintentional, detrimental outcomes, causing worsening implications for couples (Boyd-Franklin, 2003; Bryant et al., 2010; Raley & Sweeney, 2009). Additionally, if the conflict is deemed a minor annoyance but is connected to a deeper inner need or longing the conflict is likely to escalate and have serious negative consequences for the couple ultimately impacting marital satisfaction (Gottman, 1994; Miller et al., 2003).

5.4   Strain on African American Couples

In her work, *Salvation: Black People and Love*, bell hooks (2001) stated that there has not been a time when African American men and women have not been in a state of siege or oppression. Hence historical and sociocultural factors must be identified and taken into consideration when discussing marriage in the African American community. Oppressive social structures are directly related to the spuriously high divorce rate. Relatedly, a major factor in the never-married rates among African Americans is the imbalances that have occurred in the sex ratios of Black men and women due to the deaths (being killed and early deaths) of Black men and the spuriously high number who are incarcerated. This specific targeting of Black men has significantly impacted the numbers of marriageable Black men in the United States. Other factors that impact and serve as a foundation for these trends include internalized racism, invisibility syndrome, gender role strain, and economic disenfranchisement.

5.4.1   Internalized Racism and Stereotypes

Internalized racism involves both "conscious and unconscious acceptance of a racial hierarchy in which whites are consistently ranked above people of color" (Perez-Huber et al., 2005, cited in Johnson, 2008, p. 18). The manifestation of this acceptance includes attempted adaptations to white cultural ideals; thinking that supports the oppression, for example denying that racism exists; and a belief in negative racial stereotypes about the racial group to which one belongs. Internalized racism, inclusive of beliefs of negative stereotypes about one's own group, often pervades marital conflict in Black couples and reduces marital satisfaction (Taylor, 1990). Long histories of experiencing collective violence, oppression, and racism impact the psyche and are carried through generations, observed in parenting styles, interpersonal styles, and daily functioning.

African American women are often disparaged by their partners for being too independent, not being domestic enough, "too strong," outspoken, or emasculating (Allen & Helm, 2013). African American men are often criticized by their female counterparts for not helping care for the home, not being able to maintain a job or attain higher education, or being intimidated by their success. Demonstratively reinforcing stereotypes like these and many others can lead to relational dissatisfaction and disappointment, ultimately resulting in irreparable consequences. Beliefs about oneself and partner as inherently bad, immoral, and deficient will impact both what we believe we deserve and what we believe our partner is able to give.

5.4.2 Invisibility Syndrome

History demonstrates that the impact of enslavement on the Black family system was deeply profound, having yet to fully recover. The enslaved were not allowed to legally marry, did not have agency in choosing their partners, and were reduced to being used for reproduction with the intent of increasing the number of enslaved Blacks (Bethea & Allen, 2013). In her work, *Post-traumatic Slave Syndrome: America's Legacy of Enduring Injury and Healing*, DeGruy (2005) argued that the trauma from slavery essentially redefined the roles and purpose of the Black family, which were to ultimately serve white enslavers. She further stated that father roles are often assigned to the dominant male presence in a family's life. White enslavers were deemed the dominant male in the lives of the enslaved, shifting the notion of the father role to them rather than the Black male in the actual enslaved family system. This and other implications from American enslavement contributed to the "invisibility syndrome" experienced by African American men and women, causing a profound impact on the couple relationship (Boyd-Franklin, 2003).

The "invisibility syndrome" manifests in varied ways that are slightly different between men and women (Boyd-Franklin, 2003). The trope of the African American man as distrustful, intimidating, violent, and lazy evokes fear and disdain in white society. The resulting beliefs inform reactions to their presence and thus arouse feelings of invisibility in African American men. Beliefs about who "they" are and reactions to their mere existence negate the ability to be fully seen for who one is. Common present-day occurrences such as being ignored when hailing a cab or white women clutching their purses as they walk by remind Black men that it is the color of their skin that precedes them, not the content of their character. This invisibility leads to an internal struggle to define themselves and they may expend copious amounts of energy in an attempt to be seen. A deep fear of being misunderstood, labeled, or judged coupled with an internalization of negative racial stereotypes, may impact the ability to be emotionally available, secure, and vulnerable with another in a way that is healthy for a relationship.

For African American women, invisibility is a result of the double impact of racism and sexism. Stereotypes that began during enslavement have caused African American women to be viewed as less feminine, overly strong or assertive, and sexually promiscuous or aggressive (Bethea & Allen, 2013; Boyd-Franklin, 2003). They were often sexually violated during enslavement and beyond, were powerless over their immediate family systems, and were never given the grace of being viewed as emotional beings after they were observed coping "well" following traumatic experiences such as rape (hooks, 2001). Hence the trope of the "Strong Black Woman": the perception of Black women as "superhuman" and able to handle trauma without being severely emotionally or physically impacted. Resultantly, Black women may feel that their cries for help, their pain and woundedness are minimized or ignored leaving them feeling unseen and alone to bear the weight of their experiences. Current instances such as being labeled the "angry Black woman" when responding passionately to a topic of discussion or being called weak when crying reinforce this belief and may impact her ability to experience the full range of emotion and vulnerability necessary for true connection with her partner.

Invisibility of Black men and women manifests in ways that can have a significant impact on intimacy within the couple relationship (Lavner et al., 2018). Given their socialization in the same system of white supremacy, African American men and women may have difficulty truly "seeing" their partner as they struggle with their own internalized racism. Socialized beliefs about the inferiority of African Americans may cause partners to have overly negative reactions to and lowered tolerance for their partners behaviors akin to confirmation bias. One or both partners might be "waiting for the shoe to drop," preventing them from truly developing a mutual dependence in the relationship. This may leave both feeling misunderstood, insecure, and invisible.

5.4.3   Gender Role Strain

Over the years in the U.S. gender role norms have shifted for both men and women. Gender roles, in heterosexual relationships, determine how individuals conceptualize themselves and their expectations in relationships. Gender role expectations must be taken into consideration when exploring African American intimate relationships because their expectations may deviate from Western-European ideals and values due to historical context. The continuous increase in the number of women entering the workforce has necessitated a change in traditional ideas about gendered tasks, behaviors, and abilities inside and outside of the home. This shift has not been as drastic for African Americans. Due to American enslavement, the historical context within which African American gender roles evolved is drastically different from the context of any other racial group in this country. During U.S. enslavement, women worked alongside men performing various tasks obscuring delineation between the two (Dixon, 2017). Consequently, women were considered laborers and men were often put in positions to care for the household and children in the slave quarters. The oppressive conditions of enslavement required gender role flexibility to ensure that the needs of the family were met.

Post enslavement, African American women continued to engage the workforce and African American men continued to be involved in more domestic activities than either of their Euro-American counterparts (Farley & Allen, 1987; Hossain & Roopnarine, 1993).

Although these adaptations were born out of necessity and served to meet the needs of the family, socialization within a current U.S. context has emphasized more traditional gender roles as ideal and caused discrepant expectations within the couple. Attempting to form their own gender roles "Afro-Americans drew upon two sets of cultural resources: those they had developed during the period of slavery, and those of the Euro-American majority" (Patterson, 1998, p. 44). However, the values of the Euro-Americans can be at odds with traditional cultural values, situational adaptations and societal realities of the African American. As Johnson and Loscocco (2015) assert, the white conservative argument that if Black women and men would adopt more white middle-class gender role norms there would be less conflict and more marital stability is flawed. This argument negates the inherent strengths of flexible and cooperative gender roles and minimizes the strain of structural inequities on African American marriages. Additionally, these structural inequities continue to impact the attainment of white middle-class norms even if desired. It is the inherent tension between the desired and attainable that might create increased conflict between African American men and women.

5.4.4 *Economic Disenfranchisement*

Other residual impacts of enslavement on Black couple relationships tend to be social or economic in nature. Data from the Survey of Income and Program Participation (DeNavas-Walt & Proctor, 2015) suggests that Black households hold seven cents on the dollar compared to white counterparts. Further, the impacts of enslavement and ongoing instances of discrimination and institutional racism have resulted in Black families having a negative net worth (Darity et al., 2018). This impacts the ability to have resources in order to build wealth, which starts with access to equitable and affordable education, lending services, home-buying, or high-yield investment options. There are several myths that require awareness and debunking to truly address the impact on the Black marital relationship and family system (Darity et al., 2018). It is imperative to challenge myths that the racial wealth gap can be addressed within the Black community solely. The impact of institutional racism is correlated with and causal to the limited wealth attainment for Black men and women uniquely.

African American men are explicitly affected, as they are overrepresented in unemployment rates and incarceration rates. They are also less likely to successfully have support and access to higher education. Black men make up well over 50 percent of the prison population in the United States according to the Bureau of Labor Statistics and they experience unemployment rates almost double that of white counterparts (Bronson & Carson, 2019; U.S. Bureau of Labor Statistics, 2021). African Americans were a source of capital for white enslavers and have yet to earn wages that are comparable to those of their white counterparts. African Americans are often the most impacted by being unemployed or underemployed, have higher rates of challenges maintaining consistent housing, and are more likely to be arbitrarily stopped by law enforcement (Bethea & Allen, 2013; Boyd-Franklin, 2003; Lavner et al., 2018). These trends are directly correlated to the potential of sustaining a household, including access to and means of supporting a marriage and family. This can cause conflict in the marriage as the couple grapples with traditional patriarchal values. When this is not an option, the man can develop feelings of emasculation and insecurity and the woman may feel overwhelmed by financial responsibilities while continuing to engage in traditional household duties. This trend can result in the woman feeling as if the weight of the world is on her shoulders.

Further, African American families are more likely to be intergenerational and interdependent (Bryant et al., 2010). Varying generations within a family system may live in one household or in close proximity, adding additional financial responsibility and potential emotional stressors on the household. It is also not uncommon for Black families who have reached middle class status, or better, to be depended on by extended family members for support (Bryant et al., 2010).

5.5 Protective Factors for the African American Couple

Although African American couples face numerous challenges impacting the quality of their relationship, this does not negate the resilience and strength that have continued to persist. Research reveals that there are several factors that provide a nurturing foundation for sustainable, resilient relationships for African American couples. There is a strong cultural heritage that values community and collectivism, not lost during enslavement, which continues to fortify the individual. This sense of togetherness fosters love, hope, resilience and belonging that reinforces the value of connectedness. This notion, along with socialization in the United States, is indicative of the long history of African American couples being egalitarian in nature (Allen & Helm, 2013; Boyd-Franklin, 2003; Bryant et al., 2010). Although this trend may be informed by necessity due to generational wealth disparities, it is an example of a collaborative approach to marriage that informs greater marital satisfaction for African American men and women (Bryant et al., 2010).

In thinking about cultural strengths within the African American context one must consider racial identity. Experiences of racism have numerous deleterious impacts on one's sense of self, yet a positive sense of racial identity serves as a buffer and sense of pride and resilience for African Americans. Racial identity is imperative to one's sense of self, confidence in their racial presence in the world, and how comfortable they feel navigating in their skin (Bryant et al., 2010). Possessing differing levels of racial identity impacts how an individual will present in the couple relationship and how they will relate to their partner. Positive racial identity, often experienced as the notions of confidence, ancestral pride, and ability to positively relate to others in society each serve as a buffer, increase resilience, and can alleviate some emotional and social stressors.

Intimacy is often a common topic that arises when discussing marital relationships. While there are differing types of intimacy, spiritual intimacy is uniquely important for many Black couples. Historically, African Americans have been very spiritually and religiously engaged (Boyd-Franklin, 2003; Bryant et al., 2010). The Black church has historically served as a place of support, resilience, and hope for the Black community. It has traditionally been a sanctuary of safety and peace from a hostile, racist society. Churches were some of the first institutions built by Black people once freed from enslavement (Lincoln & Mamaya, 1990). Research on the Black church and its direct impact on the institution of marriage is limited, but there have been findings to suggest that Black couples who attend church together tend to experience higher marital satisfaction (Bryant et al., 2010).

The high rates of divorce in African American families can be discouraging, but it is encouraging to continue to witness Black couples that desire marriage. Hence there is a need for supportive interventions that encourage sustainability, fostering positive resilience and intimacy for Black couples. Proactively engaging in discussions and processing of common marital challenges within a cultural historical context can serve as protective factors to sustaining quality and longevity in a marital relationship. A premarital curriculum specifically designed for the African American couple can serve as that intervention.

5.6   Premarital Counseling as an Intervention

Premarital education is defined in varying ways throughout the literature. However, Clyde et al. (2020) defined it as "an educational program with curriculum specifically designed for couples preparing for or seriously considering marriage" (p. 150). Additionally, although there can be differences between premarital counseling and premarital education, the terms are often used interchangeably and are used together for the purposes of this chapter. Premarital education and counseling have been used as a preventative measure by both professionals and laypersons to increase relational skills and knowledge in an effort to enhance marital satisfaction and decrease divorce rates. Two meta-analysis studies, measuring overall effectiveness, found that premarital prevention program participants have shown gains in interpersonal skills, overall relationship quality, and communication (Carroll & Doherty, 2003; Fawcett et al., 2010).

Considering the unique experiences of African Americans and the documented impacts of those experiences on marital and relational dynamics, the development of a premarital curriculum to foster healthy relational connections and improve later marital satisfaction must be rooted within the sociocultural ecological context in which they live. The proposed premarital curriculum uses this sociocultural contextual history as a foundation upon which to build a framework that thoroughly and systematically identifies essential focus areas. Historically, premarital education objectively examined the impact of values, beliefs, and family history on relational functioning. However, there is a dearth of literature that addresses how cultural histories, such as experiences of racism, oppression, and inequality, affect coupling and overall relational behaviors. As highlighted throughout previous sections in this chapter, the impact of these systematic and institutional abuses of power are inextricably linked to the evolution of the African in America. As such, it is imperative that premarital education and counseling designed for African American couples not only remediate potential deficits and challenges but also fortify inherent relational strengths and adaptations developed in response to these adverse social conditions. In essence the authors assert that premarital education should seek to reduce risk factors and increase protective factors found to be correlated with marital satisfaction, and divorce.

5.6.1 Outline of Proposed Curriculum Considering the African American Context

5.6.1.1 Finances

Finances continue to rank as one of the most conflictual issues between all married couples regardless of race (Miller et al., 2003). However systematic and institutional racism have created economic and educational disparities along gender lines among African Americans (Lavner et al., 2018). Currently, African American women are the most educated group in the United States (National Center for Education Statistics, 2019). This coupled with wage disparities increases the possibility that the female might out earn her male partner. A 2013 analysis of U.S. Census Bureau data reported that 40 percent of all households with children under the age of 18 include mothers who are either the sole or primary source of income for the family. This represents a sharp increase from 1960 when the share was just 11 percent (Pew Research Center, 2013). Further the analysis revealed married Black mothers are more likely to be the primary bread-winner than to be mothers whose husbands have a higher income. The share of Black mothers among those who outearn their husbands is 10 percent, compared with 6 percent among couples where the husband is the primary breadwinner (Pew Research Center, 2013).

In the twenty-first century, one might overestimate strides made during the women's liberation movement and the fight for women's equality. Men and women in the United States continue to be socialized within two historic traditionally Euro-American worldviews and political systems: patriarchy and capitalism (Bell et al., 1990). Simply stated these systems emphasize a connection between (a) money and power and (b) power and men. Although disenfranchised since the first ships carrying enslaved Africans landed on U.S. shores, African American men, like all men in the country, are socialized to be the financial head of the household. However, systematic oppression, as discussed previously in this chapter, creates significant barriers to attainment and these barriers can cause unnamed and unacknowledged conflict within the couple.

Hence premarital counseling and premarital education for African American couples must not only address general ideas about money management but also explore deep, potentially unacknowledged, feelings about disparities in educational attainment and financial earnings if they exist. Additionally, the curriculum must assess beliefs about egalitarianism within the relationship and the potential need for nontraditional gender roles.

5.6.1.2 Religion/Spirituality

Africans have always had a sense of the Divine and deeply held religious beliefs continue to be a mainstay in the majority of African American households. While the United States is generally considered a highly religious nation, African Americans stand out as the most religiously committed racial or ethnic group in the country, including level of affiliation with a religion, attendance at religious services, frequency of prayer and religion's importance in life. According to the U.S. Religious Landscape Study (Saghal & Smith, 2009), conducted by the Pew Research Center's Forum on Religion & Public Life, African Americans were the most likely to report a formal religious affiliation compared with other racial and ethnic groups, with fully 87 percent of African Americans describing themselves as belonging to one religious group or another and 88 percent indicating they were absolutely certain that God exists.

Additionally, a 2015 Pew Research Center study found that although the majority of African Americans made up the overwhelming majority of historically Black Protestant congregations (94 percent), Black representation was found across all major religions. Specifically, their survey found that Blacks represented 6 percent of Catholics, 3 percent of Buddhists, 6 percent of Evangelical Protestants, 2 percent of Hindus, 27 percent of Jehovah's Witnesses, 2 percent of Jews, 1 percent of Mormons, 28 percent of Muslims, and 8 percent of Orthodox Christians.

Religious/spiritual belief systems are indissolubly linked to and frame worldview and value systems, which have enormous implications for aspects of daily life, child rearing, rituals and traditions, celebrations, gender role expectations, dietary considerations, and numerous daily tasks and ways of being. Hence it is important for a premarital curriculum to assess religious beliefs, affiliation, practices, and involvement.

5.6.1.3 Blended Families

Over the past forty years there has been a continual shift from a traditional marriage and family system to a heterogeneous family system that consists of three major types of families: intact nuclear families, single-parent families, and stepfamilies (Boyd-Franklin, 2003; Cohn et al., 2011;

Parker, 2011). Today, nearly 40 percent of Americans are a part of a stepfamily (Parker, 2011). However, given the number of births outside of marriage, Black Americans have an increased probability of entering stepfamilies that far outnumbers the national average. According to the National Center for Health Statistics, in 2015, 77.3 percent of nonimmigrant Black babies were born to unwed mothers. While African Americans tend to have lower marriage rates and higher divorce rates than other racial groups, they also have a tendency to cohabitate at a greater rate than their counterparts (Chambers & Kravitz, 2011; Horowitz et al., 2019). This distinction is important because it recognizes that although many families do not meet the traditional definition of a "stepfamily" where the parties are joined legally, their daily existence mirrors that of a more formalized family system. This includes the likelihood of experiencing similar challenges and expectations that occur after marriage. Furthermore, the high rate of unwed births for African Americans creates an increased potential for a more "complex" stepfamily structure defined by both partners having children from previous relationships. This is compared to a "simple" stepfamily structure where only one partner has children from a previous relationship.

Given the aforementioned statistics regarding single-mother births, there is an increased likelihood that African American engaged couples will bring at least one child into the marriage. Therefore, it is imperative that these couples are provided pertinent information to increase their understanding and ability to navigate the nuances of blending family. Along with being given an opportunity to reflect on and express their own experiences with, beliefs about, desires for, and fantasies of stepfamilies.

5.6.1.4 Gender Roles and Expectations

Gender norms for men and women have slowly evolved over the decades, moving further away from a traditional gender role orientation. Yet, the United States continues to function based on overwhelmingly patriarchal values. African Americans have been socialized within this system, while simultaneously being barred from participation in its tenets, if so desired. Patriarchy dictates that the father is the supreme authority in the family (i.e., fathers are to financially support the household and are the final decision makers), and children (and the wife) belong to the father's family (i.e., the wife and children take on the father's last name). As previously discussed, during enslavement, the white enslaver took on the role of authority in the households of the enslaved, stripping enslaved men and women of their ability to fulfill their patriarchal roles within the family system. During enslavement, enslaved men and women were considered "genderless." Enslaved women were expected to carry out the same hard labor as the men (Dixon, 2017) and men were essentially powerless, considered childlike and effeminate.

Post enslavement, the inability of Black men to provide financially for their families due to institutionalized racism forced Black women to enter the workforce. Simultaneously, this necessitated for many men an increase in caretaking responsibilities of the home and children. The woman's role was masculinized, and the man's role was femininized (Bethea & Allen, 2013). Although African Americans are believed to have more flexible gender role orientations than other racial groups in the United States, this reversal of roles can cause internal dissonance. There can be internal struggles as each attempts to reconcile the socialized "ideal" with lived "reality." Institutionalized and systemic racism coupled with educational and economic disenfranchisement has impacted what is and continues to shape and influence future possibilities. Currently, there is an increased probability that women will be more "degreed," and outearn their male partners. Likewise, they may have very different gender role attitudes and expectations that they have never consciously explored but inherently ascribe regarding gender.

Premarital education and counseling for African Americans must assess gender role expectations, desires, and feasibility. Stereotypes of the Strong Black Woman and "weak, incompetent Black man" must be explored and their juxtaposition to socialization of the ideal traditional male–female gender roles.

5.6.1.5   Extended Families

Researchers and clinicians often overlook the purposeful and adaptive importance of the extended family composition and supportive kinship networks of African American households. African American families have often existed in and thrived because of significant reliance on extended family networks. Both traditional biological networks along with strong kinship bonds served to provide psychological, physical, financial, and spiritual support for families (Boyd-Franklin, 2003). This way of being is often at odds with more Westernized values which emphasizes individualism and focuses on self-sufficiency of the nuclear family.

Brown et al. (2008) posit that in general divorce is tolerated and accepted more within the Black community, than it is in the white community. A few researchers have asserted that this may be due in part to extended family ties and support within African American families, which makes marital disruption more manageable (LaTaillade, 2006; Orbuch et al., 2013). Alternatively, a 2006 qualitative study by Marks et al. suggests that embeddedness in extended networks is a source of stress for couples. Their study found that constant care taking for biological extended family, fictive kin and acquaintances serves as continuous stressors on marriages.

This highlights the need for premarital education and counseling for African Americans to discuss appropriate boundaries, assess connection to traditional values related to extended family/kinship involvement and develop a shared value system and plan/strategy for incorporating others into their new union.

5.6.1.6 Handling Conflict

Conflict in marriage is inevitable and several couples theorists assert that conflicts, if handled properly, provide opportunities for the couple to grow together and increase connection (Gottman & Silver, 1999; Ostenson & Zhang, 2014; Recker, 2010). Conflicts have also been identified as one of the most crucial factors impacting the quantity and quality of relationships among family members. Gottman (1994; Gottman & Silver, 1999) found that couples that are unhappily married, and more likely to divorce report that their interactions are more negative during conflict and their daily interaction with their spouse is more negative than happy compared to stable couples. The way in which one engages in and resolves conflict with their partner is extremely important and will have an enormous impact on relational satisfaction and survival.

Although every individual has unique life experiences, the historical impact of trauma on African Americans increases the likelihood of having been exposed to high conflict in their home, family, and community, as well as the larger society than other racial groups. Often these experiences were not coupled with healthy skills and tools for successful resolution. The traumatic responses to such exposure can be carried into future relationships causing repeated unhealthy ways of handling emotionally charged interactions.

In his book *Principia Amoris: The New Science of Love*, John Gottman (2014) draws upon the work of Harold Raush conjoined with his own research to identify five types of couples in conflict: Conflict-Avoiding, Validating, Volatile, Hostile, and Hostile-Detached. Although not specifically written about nor normed on African Americans, his typology allows for adaptation to understand them, and for them to understand themselves.

Premarital education and counseling for African Americans should include information about the impact of historical trauma, along with the role of conflict in marriage, that allows the couple to identify their conflict style and teach tools and skills to manage conflict in a healthy and productive manner.

5.6.1.7   *Intimacy*

Intimacy is an integral part of a relationship and has been intricately linked to relational and marital satisfaction. Intimacy usually encompasses shared vulnerability, communication, and openness. Five primary aspects of intimacy are discussed in the literature: experimental, sexual, mental, emotional, and spiritual (Kardan-Souraki et al., 2016). Although new relationships might have moments of intimacy, curating sustained intimacy is a gradual process that occurs over time and requires placidity and interaction. Within the African American community, differing cultural values about each of the five aspects of intimacy may affect the importance of each in the relationship and how they are conveyed. Factors such as attitudes and beliefs, cultural and religious messages, and socialized values, identity, and beliefs about masculinity and sexuality impact the ways in which Black individuals experience and expect any and all aspects of intimacy (Dogan et al., 2018).

Embedded within a larger social context, sociocultural norms may not support or may be in conflict with African American group norms about intimacy and connection. Consequently, researchers and clinicians have acknowledged several threats to intimacy for Black persons, such as racism and discrimination, negative stereotypes, gender ratio imbalance, poverty, and media and technology (Helm & Carlson, 2013).

African American experiences with these structural systems often impact beliefs about safety, vulnerability, and trust, which are foundational pillars for building intimacy. Furthermore, internalized oversexualized media messages about African American men and women can copiously emphasize sexual intimacy at the expense of emotional and spiritual intimacy, which many argue are more involvedly connected to long-term relational satisfaction. Premarital education and counseling for African Americans must provide information about the five aspects of intimacy and help the couple to develop skills in each.

5.7   Conclusion

This chapter detailed how the unique experiences of African Americans in the United States can influence their relational dynamics. Continued experiences of racism, discrimination, marginalization, economic disenfranchisement, etc. impact self-identity and other relatedness and color the lens through which life is filtered. Resultingly, an argument is made for the development of specific premarital interventions for dating and engaged African American heterosexual couples. Targeted interventions aimed at addressing the phenomenological lived experiences of the individuals to help them surmount potential relational challenges that might arise. Culturally specific premarital education and counseling can help couples develop insight and skills crucial to healthy and successfully marital relationships.

Discussion Questions

1. How might internalized racism impact marital satisfaction and marital success in African American couples?
2. Imagine that an engaged African American couple came to see you for premarital counseling. Write a paragraph explaining to them the importance of understanding sociohistorical context in their marriage.
3. Why do you think most couples, in general, do not seek premarital counseling/education? What unique factors contribute to low rates of premarital education for African American couples?
4. Reflect on how your own family history and socialization impact your thoughts about African American families and marriage. What biases do you need to be mindful of when working with these couples?

REFERENCES

Allen, T., & Helm, K. (2013). Threats to intimacy for African American couples. In K. Helm & J. Carlson (Eds.), *Love, intimacy, and the African American couple* (pp. 85–116). Routledge.

Amato, P. R. (2011). *Marital quality in African American marriages*. National Healthy Marriage Resource Center.

Amato, P. R., & Rogers, S. J. (1997). A longitudinal study of marital problems and subsequent divorce. *Journal of Marriage and Family, 59*(3), 612–624.

Barr, A. B., Culatta, E., & Simons, R. L. (2013). Romantic relationships and health among African American young adults: Linking patterns of relationship quality over time to changes in physical and mental health. *Journal of Health and Social Behavior, 54*(3), 369–385.

Bell, Y. R., Bouie, C. L., & Baldwin, J. A. (1990). Afrocentric cultural consciousness and African American male-female relationships. *Journal of Black Studies, 1*(2), 182–189.

Bethea, S., & Allen, T. (2013). Past and present societal influences on African American couples that impact love and intimacy. In K. Helm & J. Carlson (Eds.), *Love, intimacy, and the African American couple* (pp. 20–59). Routledge.

Billingsley, A. (1992). *Climbing Jacob's ladder: The enduring legacy of African American families*. Simon and Schuster.

Boyd-Franklin, N. (2003). *Black families in therapy: Understanding the African American experiences*. Guilford Press.

Bronson, J., & Carson, A. E. (2019). *Prisoners in 2017*. U.S. Department of Justice, Bureau of Justice Statistics. https://bjs.ojp.gov/library/publications/prisoners-2017

Brown, E., Orbuch, T. L., & Bauermeister, J. A. (2008). Religiosity and marital stability among Black American and White American couples. *Family Relations, 57*, 186–197.

Bryant, C., Wickrama, K. A., Bolland, J., Bryant, B., Cutrona, C., & Stank, C. (2010). Race matters, even in marriage: Identifying factors linked to marital outcomes for African Americans. *Journal of Family Theory & Review, 2*(3), 157–174.

Carroll, J. S., & Doherty, W. J. (2003). Evaluating the effectiveness of premarital prevention programs: A meta-analytic review of outcome research. *Family Relations, 52*, 105–118. https://doi.org/10.1111/j.1741-3729.2003.00105.x

Chambers, A., & Kravitz, A. (2011). Understanding the disproportionately low marriage rate among African Americans: An amalgam of sociological and psychological constraints. *Family Relations, 60*(5), 648–660.

Clyde, T. L., Hawkins, A. J., & Willoughby, B. J. (2020). Revising premarital relationship interventions for the next generation. *Journal of Marital and Family Therapy, 46*(1), 149–164. https://doi.org/10.1111/jmft.12378

Cohn, D., Passel, J., Wang, W., & Livingston, G. (2011, December 14). *Barely half of U.S. adults are married – a record low*. https://www.pewsocialtrends.org/2011/12/14/barely-half-of-u-s-adults-are-married-a-record-low/

Copen, C., Daniels, K., Vespa, J., & Mosher, W. (2012). *First marriages in the United States: Data from the 2006–2010 National Survey of Family Growth* (National Health Statistics Reports No. 49). National Center for Health Statistics. https://www.cdc.gov/nchs/data/nhsr/nhsr049.pdf

Curtin, S. C., & Sutton, P. D. (2020). *Marriage rates in the United States, 1900–2018*. Centers for Disease Control and Prevention. https://www.cdc.gov/nchs/data/hestat/marriage_rate_2018/marriage_rate_2018.htm#ref5

Darity, W., Hamilton, D., Paul, M., Aja, A., Price, A., Moore, A., & Chiopris, C. (2018). *What we get wrong about closing the racial wealth gap*. Samuel DuBois Cook Center for Social Equity; Insight Center for Community Economic Development. https://socialequity.duke.edu/wp-content/uploads/2020/01/what-we-get-wrong.pdf

DeGruy, J. (2005). *Post-traumatic slave syndrome: America's legacy of enduring injury and healing*. Uptone Press.

DeNavas-Walt, C., & Proctor, B. D. (2015). *Income and poverty in the United States: 2014*. Current Population Reports, P60-252. U.S. Census Bureau. https://www.census.gov/library/publications/2015/demo/p60-252.html

Dixon, P. (2009). Marriage among African Americans: What does the research reveal? *Journal of African American Studies, 13*(1), 29–46.

(2014). AARMS: The African American relationships and marriage strengthen in curriculum for African American relationships courses and programs. *Journal of African American Studies, 18*(3), 337–352.

(2017). *African American relationships, marriages, and families: An introduction.* Routledge.

Dogan, J., Hargons, C., Meiller, C., Oluokun, J., Montique, C., & Malone, N. (2018). Catchin' feelings: Experiences of intimacy during Black college students' sexual encounters. *Journal of Black Sexuality and Relationships, 5*(2), 81–107. https://doi.org/10.1353/bsr.2018.0021

Dupre, M. E., Beck, A. N., & Meadows, S. O. (2009). Marital trajectories and mortality among US adults. *American Journal of Epidemiology, 170*(5), 546–555.

Farley, R., & Allen, W. (1987). *The color line and the quality of life in America.* Russell Sage Foundation. https://www.russellsage.org/publications/color-line-and-quality-life-america

Fawcett, E., Hawkins, A., Blanchard, V., & Carroll, J. (2010). Do premarital education programs really work? A meta-analytic study. *Family Relations, 59*(3), 232–239. http://www.jstor.org/stable/40864536

Gottman, J. (1994). *Why marriages succeed or fail: What you can learn from the breakthrough research to make your marriage last.* Simon & Schuster.

Gottman, J. M. (2014). *Principia amoris: The new science of love.* Routledge/Taylor & Francis Group.

Gottman, J., & Silver, N. (1999). *The seven principles for making marriage work.* Three Rivers.

Gurrentz, B. (2019, September 23). *Unmarried partners more diverse than 20 years ago: cohabiting partners older, more racially diverse, more educated, higher earners.* U.S. Census Bureau. https://www.census.gov/library/stories/2019/09/unmarried-partners-more-diverse-than-20-years-ago.html

Haines, M. R. (1996). Long-term marriage patterns in the united states from colonial times to the present. *The History of the Family, 1*(1), 15–39.

Helm, K. M., & Carlson, J. (Eds.). (2013). *Love, intimacy, and the African American couple.* Routledge.

Henry, R. G., & Miller, R. B. (2004). Marital problems occurring in midlife: Implications for couples therapists. *The American Journal of Family Therapy, 32,* 405–417.

hooks, b. (2001). *Salvation: Black people and love.* Harper Perennial.

Horowitz, J., Graf, N., & Livingston, G. (2019, November 6). *Views on marriage and cohabitation in the U.S.* Pew Research Center. https://www.pewsocialtrends.org/2019/11/06/marriage-and-cohabitation-in-the-u-s/.

Hossain, Z., & Roopnarine, J. L. (1993). Division of household labor and childcare in dual-earner African-American families with infants. *Sex Roles. 29,* 571–583. https://doi.org/10.1007/BF00289205

Johnson, K. R., & Loscocco, K. (2015). Black marriage through the prism of gender, race, and class. *Journal of Black Studies, 46*(2), 142–171. https://doi.org/10.1177/0021934714562644

Johnson, R. N. (2008). *The psychology of racism: How internalized racism, academic self-concept, and campus racial climate impact the academic experiences and achievement of African American undergraduates.* [Unpublished doctoral dissertation]. Los Angeles.

Kardan-Souraki, M., Hamzehgardeshi, Z., Asadpour, I., Mohammadpour, R. A., & Khani, S. (2016). A review of marital intimacy-enhancing interventions among married individuals. *Global Journal of Health Science, 8*(8), 53109. https://doi.org/10.5539/gjhs.v8n8p74

LaTaillade, J. J. (2006). Considerations for treatment of African American couple relationships. *Journal of Cognitive Psychotherapy, 20,* 341–358. https://doi.org/10.1891/jcpiq-v20i4a002

Lavner, J. A., Barton, A. W., Bryant, C. M., & Beach, S. R. H. (2018). Racial discrimination and relationship functioning among African American couples. *Journal of Family Psychology, 32*(5), 686–691.

Lawrence, E., Rogers, R., Zajacova, A., & Wadsworth, T. (2019). Marital happiness, marital status, health, and longevity. *Journal of Happiness Studies, 20,* 1–23.

Lincoln, C. E., & Mamiya, L. H. (1990). *The Black church in the African American experience.* Duke University Press.

Marks, L. D., Swanson, M., Nesteruk, O., & Hopkins-Williams, K. (2006). Stressors in African American marriages and families: A qualitative study. *Stress, Trauma, and Crisis: An International Journal, 9,* 203–225.

McAdoo, H. P. (2007). *Black families* (4th ed.). Sage Publications.

McAdoo, H. P., & Younge, S. (2009). Black families. In H. Neville, B. Tynes, & S. Utsey (Eds.), *Handbook of American psychology* (pp. 103–115). Sage Publications.

Miller, R. B., Yorgason, J. B., Sandberg, J. G., & White, M. B. (2003). Problems that couples bring to therapy. A view across the family life cycle. *The American Journal of Family Therapy, 31,* 395–407.

National Center for Education Statistics. (2019). *Status and trends in the education of racial and ethnic groups 2018* (NCES 2019-038). U.S. Department of Education. https://nces.ed.gov/programs/raceindicators/indicator_ree.asp

Orbuch, T. L., Bauermeister, J. A., Brown, E., & McKinley, B. D. (2013). Early family ties and marital stability over 16 years: The context of race and gender. *Family Relations, 62*(2), 255–268. https://doi.org/10.1111/fare.12005

Ostenson, J. A., & Zhang, M. (2014). Reconceptualizing marital conflict: A relational perspective. *Journal of Theoretical and Philosophical Psychology, 34*(4), 229–242. https://doi.org/10.1037/a0034517

Parker, K. (2011, January 13). *A portrait of stepfamilies.* Pew Research Center. http://pewsocialtrends.org/2011/01/13/a-portrait-of-stepfamilies/

Parker, K., & Stepler, R. (2017, September 14). *As U.S. marriage rate hovers at 50%, education gap in marital status widens.* Pew Research Center. https://www.pewresearch.org/fact-tank/2017/09/14/as-u-s-marriage-rate-hovers-at-50-education-gap-in-marital-status-widens

Patterson, O. (1998). *Rituals of blood: Consequences of slavery in two American centuries.* Civitas/CounterPoint.

Pew Research Center. (2013, May 29). *Breadwinner moms: Mothers are the sole or primary provider in four-in-ten households with children; Public conflicted about the growing trend.* https://www.pewsocialtrends.org/2013/05/29/breadwinner-moms/

(2015). *Racial and ethnic composition. Religious Landscape Study.* https://www.pewforum.org/religious-landscape-study/racial-and-ethnic-composition/

Phillips, T., Wilmoth, J., & Marks. L. (2012). Challenges and conflicts. Strengths and supports: A study of enduring African American marriages. *Journal of Black Studies, 43*(8), 936–952.

Pinderhughes, E. (2002). African American marriage in the 20th century. *Family Process, 41*(2), 269–282.

Raley, R. K., & Sweeney, M. M. (2009). Explaining race and ethnic variation in marriage: Directions for future research. *Race and Social Problems, 7*(3), 132–142.

Recker, N. (2010). *Dealing with anger in a marriage.* Ohio State University Extension. http://ohioline.osu.edu/hyg-fact/5000/pdf/5191.pdf

Ruggles, S. (1994). The origins of African American family structure. *American Sociological Review, 59,* 136–151.

Saghal, N., & Smith, G. (2007). *A religious portrait of African-Americans.* Pew Research Center. https://www.pewforum.org/2009/01/30/a-religious-portrait-of-african-americans/

Taylor, J. (1990). Relationship between internalized racism and marital satisfaction. *Journal of Black Psychology, 16*(2), 45–53. https://doi.org/10.1177/00957984900162004

Tucker, M. B., & Mitchell-Kernan, C. (Eds.). (1995). *The decline in marriage among African Americans: Causes, consequences and policy implications.* Russell Sage Foundation.

Umberson, D., Thomeer, M. B., & Williams, K. (2013). Family status and mental health: Recent advances and future directions. In C. S. Aneshensel, J. C. Phelan, & A. Bierman (Eds.), *Handbook of the sociology of mental health* (pp. 405–431). Springer Dordrecht.

U.S. Bureau of Labor Statistics. (2021). *Labor force characteristics by race and ethnicity, 2020.* https://www.bls.gov/opub/reports/race-and-ethnicity/2020/home.htm

Williams, D. R., Takeuchi, D. T., & Adair, R. K. (1992). Marital status and psychiatric disorders among blacks and whites. *Journal of Health and Social Behavior, 33*(2), 140–157.

Zollar, A. C., & Williams, J. S. (1987). The contribution of marriage to the life satisfaction of Black adults. *Journal of Marriage and the Family, 49*(1), 87–92.

PART III

Adapting Major Therapeutic Approaches for Work with African American Couples

CHAPTER 6

Emotionally Focused Therapy with Black Couples

Yamonte Cooper

6.1 Overview of EFT

Johnson and Greenberg (1985) developed Emotionally Focused Therapy for couples (EFT) due to the lack of empirically validated couple interventions. EFT is an evidence-based couples therapy model grounded in attachment theory that has a demonstrated effectiveness rate of 70–73 percent in the reduction of relationship distress (Johnson et al., 1999). EFT is an experiential therapy with a foundation in humanistic and systemic processes that are instrumental in creating a secure attachment bond among couples.[1] The systemic component includes the conceptualization of negative, rigid interaction patterns and negative affect (i.e., negative interactional cycle) that are reinforcing (i.e., circular causality), which commonly cause distress in couple relationships and manifest as emotional disconnection and insecure attachment. The intrapsychic perspective and the interpersonal systemic perspective are both integrated within an experiential approach that utilizes interventions (e.g., both intrapsychic and interpersonal) that help distressed partners cultivate attachment security in their relationships through the creation of emotional accessibility, responsiveness, and engagement that are foundational to secure attachment. EFT focuses on the here and now as a present process-oriented therapy through the exploration of primary emotions (e.g., anger, shame, sadness, and fear) that are often obscured from awareness by reactive surface emotions and responses. Couples are encouraged to take a risk and share from a place of vulnerability their primary emotions with their partner during the session, which is considered a symbolic reach for connection. Their partner is encouraged to listen and respond in a

---

[1] This chapter is focused on heterosexual Black couples but has elements of application to other Black populations.

manner that creates emotional attunement. These new vulnerable responses elicit new experiences of self and other (e.g., working models of self and other) and gradually changes the rigid negative interactional cycle into a more flexible positive interactional cycle of secure attachment (Johnson, 2019, 2020; Wiebe & Johnson, 2016).

EFT includes nine steps within a three-stage progression that can be conceptualized as a developmental process. The first stage includes cycle *deescalation* where the negative interactional cycle that motivates the relational distress is made explicit. This includes the therapist tracking and reflecting the patterns of interaction and identification of negative cycles (e.g., demand/criticize/attack followed by defend/ distance/withdrawal) that constrain partner responses. Steps one through four are part of stage one (Johnson, 2004, 2019, 2020; Wiebe & Johnson, 2016).

Step one includes creating an alliance and conducting an assessment (e.g., nature of the problem, relationship/individual goals and agendas for therapy). Step two entails identifying the negative interactional cycle and attachment issues, and step three involves accessing the underlying emotions supporting the reactive moves in the cycle, which fosters mutual empathy that leads to deescalation. The problem is reframed in terms of the negative interactional cycle along with corresponding feelings and attachment needs in step four. Stage one concludes with couples having a meta-perspective on their interactions where the negative cycle is the problem in the maintenance of their relationship insecurity and emotional distress (Johnson, 2004, 2019, 2020; Wiebe & Johnson, 2016).

The second stage, *restructuring the bond*, includes the creation of new emotional experiences and interactions that produce a more secure connection. Steps five through seven take place during stage two. Step five includes promoting the identification with disowned needs, fears, aspects of self, and integrating these into interactions (i.e., deepening experience). Step six entails promoting the acceptance of the partner's experience and new interactional responses, and step seven involves facilitating the deeper expression of attachment emotions and needs as well as creating open emotional engagement (i.e., bonding events). Safety is created where attachment vulnerabilities (i.e., fears) and needs are shared with partners in session through structured enactments (also referred to as encounters). The responding partner is guided in responding in an emotionally attuned and supportive way that also includes the exploration of any blocks that may impede this process. Fears such as failure or rejection that undergird withdrawal or a lack of responsiveness are expressed and made explicit through newly formulated and expressed emotional responses that evoke new responses in the partner (e.g., compassion rather than anger and blaming) that represent an interactional shift in positions. An instrumental therapeutic change event within this process includes *withdrawer reengagement* where the previously withdrawing (i.e., conflict avoidant) partner expresses their attachment needs while becoming more open and responsive to their partner. A second instrumental therapeutic change event is *blamer softening* where the previously pursuing partner who would display blame and criticism begins to express their attachment needs and vulnerable primary emotions (e.g., hurt, sadness, fear, or shame) in a soft and clear manner that cultivates connection and their partner is encouraged to listen and respond in an emotionally attuned manner. A corrective emotional experience of secure connection is produced for both partners through the *blamer softening* change event. Both change events foster secure attachment through the creation of new constructive cycles of contact and caring where both partners can express their needs for comfort and care in a soft and emotionally congruent manner that elicits an empathetic response from their partner (Johnson, 2004, 2019, 2020; Wiebe & Johnson, 2016).

The third stage, *consolidation*, includes the application of the newly acquired secure attachment bond and improved relationship functioning in couple relationship problem-solving that translates into their everyday lives, which fosters a narrative of relationship resilience and mastery. Steps eight and nine occur during stage three. Step eight includes facilitating the emergence of new solutions to differences and problems and step nine entails consolidating new positions, cycles, and stories of secure attachment (Johnson, 2004, 2019, 2020; Wiebe & Johnson, 2016).

6.2   The EFT Tango

The EFT Tango is a core process within the EFT model and is referred to as a macro-intervention that encompasses a set of interventions that consists of five "moves." The EFT Tango occurs within a therapeutic alliance and is utilized throughout the three stages of *deescalation, restructuring the bond*, and *consolidation* in a dynamic fashion where pacing and intensity are adapted to the sensitivities and needs of the client. The Tango moves includes mirroring present process (move 1), affect assembly and deepening (move 2), choreographing engaged encounters (move 3), processing the encounter (move 4), and integrating and validating (move 5) (Johnson, 2019, 2020).

Mirroring the present process includes tracking and collaboratively identifying intrapsychic and interpersonal experiential processes (i.e., reinforcing cycles of affect regulation and interactions with partner). Affect assembly and deepening entail piecing together elements of emotion into a coherent whole that informs habitual engagement with self and others, which expands and deepens awareness and experiencing. The elements of emotion are the trigger or cue, initial perception, body response, primary emotion, meaning creation, and action tendency. Choreographing engaged encounters involves sharing the expanded or deepened inner experience with the partner in a structured manner that is guided by the therapist. This is indicative of a symbolic reach for their partner and prompts new experiences of self and other. Processing the encounter includes exploring and integrating with the client the new interactional responses including any stuck or negative responses from their partner. A meta-perspective is offered during move five (integrating and validating) where the whole process of the previous four moves is reflected and validated by the therapist with a focus on key significant moments and responses (i.e., new discoveries and positive interactional responses) that are indicative of the client's strength and courage. The client begins to develop a sense of confidence and competence that translates into intrapsychic and interpersonal (relational) experiences (Johnson, 2019, 2020).

6.3   The Role of the EFT Therapist

The role of the therapist is that of a process consultant where they are empathically attuned and validating of each partner. This creates safety for each partner to become more engaged with their experience as well as their partner's experience. Change does not occur due to insight, catharsis, or improved skills but due to the formulation and expression of new emotional experience that transforms the negative interactional cycle where attachment needs and emotions are foundational to the process. Insight or improved communication or problem-solving skills often occur as an after effect of EFT and the creation of a more secure bond and connection. The therapist remains near the *leading edge* of the client's experience and expands their experience with experiential interventions (micro-interventions) that include reflection, evocative questions, validation, heightening emotion, empathetic conjecture, and self-disclosure (Johnson, 2019, 2020; Wiebe & Johnson, 2016).

Systemic interventions include reframing (e.g., the problem is the negative interactional cycle and not a personality defect or partner difference as well as attachment needs and longings), tracking and reflecting interactional patterns that often exists within a self-perpetuating negative feedback loop, and restructuring and shaping new interactions. Moreover, therapists use scaffolding when attempting to engage clients with difficult emotions with deeper emotional engagement. The scaffolding creates safety and engagement, which form a working distance from powerful emotional experience that ultimately widens the emotional window of tolerance. This process focuses on nonverbal expression that indicates an emotional risk and is referred to with the acronym RISSSC (repeat, image, simple, slow, soft, and client's words) (Johnson, 2019, 2020; Wiebe & Johnson, 2016).

6.4   Transubstantive Error

EFT research has nearly exclusively focused on white, middle-class heterosexual couples. While EFT has demonstrated that it is an empirically supported couple therapy for white couples, there are no research studies utilizing EFT with Black couples. EFT asserts a universality in attachment needs and fears along with emotional expression, thus claiming application across cultures. This assertion is not only problematic but represents a Eurocentric perspective that can be harmful to Black couples. Matsumoto (1993) found significant ethnic differences in emotion judgments, display rules, and emotional expressions among a sample of Black, white, Asian, and Latino/a Americans. Attachment research has tended to focus on the Western middle-class as the norm and has lacked application with populations who have deviated (e.g., cultural values) from this constructed standard. Cross-cultural research on attachment is limited in scope as there is very little research on attachment distributions and ethnicity. According to Keller (2013), attachment theorists have not been responsive to developments in evolutionary sciences that require contextual variability to appropriately adapt attachment theory to populations outside of Western middle-class hegemony. Various cultural ecologies provide different views of the self that inform definitions of attachment relationships and include how relationships are defined and organized. According to van Ijzendoorn and Sagi-Schwartz (2008), attachment needs to be viewed from a network approach (e.g., multiple relationships) instead of a dyadic perspective with non-Western cultures.

Keller (2013) advocates for a new approach that departs from Bowlby's (1969) definition of attachment as an adaptive social construct that is necessary for survival and development and calls for an empirically supported interdisciplinary framework that incorporates differing cultures of attachment and integrates evolution, cultural conceptions of socialization, parenting, and child development (Cooper, 2023; Greenman & Johnson, 2013; Lopez et al., 2000; Magai et al., 2001; Nightingale et al., 2019; Tyrell & Masten, 2021; Wei et al., 2004; White, 1970; Wiebe & Johnson, 2016).

The research of Agishtein and Brumbaugh (2013) revealed that adult attachment patterns vary based on region of origin (i.e., country of origin), collectivism, acculturation, and ethnicity. Several research studies have indicated that Black Americans tend to demonstrate higher rates of avoidant attachment compared to white Americans. These interpretations are problematic as they use a Eurocentric theory (attachment theory) where the white middle-class is the norm and an ethnic group (Black Americans) with a vastly different culture is a deviation of the norm that displays nonnormative behaviors. These analyses are made without interrogating attachment theory, structural anti-Black racism, and cultural differences and without the incorporation of nonpathologizing contextual variables. According to Nobles (1976), the continued use of Western Eurocentric theories to explain Black life is part of systemic anti-Black racism that distorts Black reality and contributes to the degradation of Black people. The deficit orientations of Black families primarily consist of characterizations of poverty-acculturation, pathology, and victimization. Black families are thought to be a mimetic caricaturization of white families that represents a deviation from the normative culture. Nobles (1978) refers to this cultural hegemony as a transubstantive error where the behavior and or medium of one culture is defined and interpreted with meanings that are appropriate and consistent with another culture (Cooper, 2023; Greenman & Johnson, 2013; Lopez et al., 2000; Magai et al., 2001; Nightingale et al., 2019; Tyrell & Masten, 2021; Wei et al., 2004; White, 1970; Wiebe & Johnson, 2016).

The following sections include clinical considerations (e.g., racial realities of anti-Blackness) that must be integrated within the EFT therapy model to provide an appropriate adaptation that is a culturally responsive couple therapy. This includes institutional decimation and Black sex ratios, marriage, anti-Black racism, internalized stereotypes (anti-Blackness), Strong Black Woman (SBW), John Henryism, racial identity, and religion and spirituality.

6.5   Clinical Considerations

6.5.1   Institutional Decimation and Black Sex Ratios

This section focuses on heterosexual marriage markets. The figures of marriageability are likely to be impacted as approximately 4 percent of Black adults identify as LGBT. This section is a synthesis of the following sources: Alexis, 1998; Amato, 2005; Blumstein & Beck, 1999; Chetty et al., 2018; Cho et al., 2021; Cooper, 2023; Cox, 1940; Craigie et al., 2018; Curry, 2017, 2020; Darity, 1980; Darity et al., 2018; Darity & Myers, 1983, 1984a, 1984b, 1989, 1995; Fitzgerald & Ribar, 2004; Geronimus & Korenman, 1992; Hagan & Dinovitzer, 1999; Hamilton et al., 2009; Hampton, 1980; Hoffman et al., 1993; Holzer, 2007; Kaplan et al., 2008; Kearney & Levine, 2017; Koball, 1998; Landry, 1987; Lichter et al., 1991; McLanahan & Booth, 1989; McLanahan & Sandefur, 1994; Miller, 1991; Noël, 2014; Pettit, 2012; Pew Research Center, 2015; Rodgers & Thornton, 1985; Sampson, 1987; Schneider, 2011; Seltzer, 1994; South, 1996; Staples, 1985; Stewart & Scott, 1978; Strobino & Sirageldin, 1981; Watson & McLanahan, 2011; Willhelm, 1986; Wilson, 1987; Wolfers et al., 2015.

The reduction in the supply of economically able men to fill the roles of husband and father is the primary cause for the decline in two-parent families in Black communities. Black men are deemed to be of no use in the emerging economic order where they are socially unwanted, unneeded, and insignificant. Policies designed to contain or eradicate the unwanted and marginalized Black male population (institutional decimation) exacerbate the reductions in the supply of marriageable (unmarried males in the labor force or in school) mates. Black families headed by women saw an increase from 25 percent in the 1950s to nearly 50 percent in the 1990s. Poverty significantly impacts Black families headed by mothers. The fragile economic position of Black men and the inability of Black women to locate marriage partners in significant numbers has a compound effect on the high percentage of Black families headed by women. In addition, sex ratios (number of males and females in the general population) are a fundamental determinant of the increase in Black female-headed families. There are more Black women than men in every age group over fifteen, which creates a surplus of Black women particularly of childbearing ages fifteen to thirty. This sex gap is nonexistent in childhood as there are approximately as many Black boys as girls. But the gap begins to appear among teenagers and widens through the twenties and peaks in the thirties while continuing throughout adulthood.

According to the *New York Times*, there are 1.5 million Black men missing due to early death and hyperincarceration. This results in 83 Black men for every 100 Black women not incarcerated. Large sex gaps ratios were found in Ferguson, Missouri, and North Charleston, South Carolina. In addition, large numbers of Black men are missing from New York, Chicago, Philadelphia, Detroit, Memphis, Baltimore, Houston, Charlotte, North Carolina, Milwaukee, Dallas, and the states of Georgia, Alabama, and Mississippi. This sex gap is nearly nonexistent for whites (99 white men for every 100 white women not incarcerated) (Wolfers et al., 2015).

Premature deaths and hyperincarceration decimate Black communities and leave them without enough men to be fathers and husbands. Increasing incarceration levels over time were due to changes in policy and not changes in male behavior. Moreover, Black men (more than one out of six) who would have been between the prime-age years of twenty-five and fifty-four years old have disappeared from daily life. Approximately 900,000 are dead and approximately 600,000 Black men are incarcerated. According to Mason (2006), there are 71 Black males to 100 Black females compared to 119 white males to 100 white females among the civilian unmarried population. Adding full-time employment as a criterion for marriageable males decreases this figure to 46 Black males to 100 Black females compared to 90 white males to 100 white females. Marriage is an economic institution and not solely a romantic commitment. Therefore, the ability to be strong economic providers or breadwinners in the household is highly correlated with the attractiveness of males as marriage prospects. Further, unmarried Black males who are deemed marriageable are positioned with the ability to choose highly desired females due to the scarcity of marriageable Black males.

A large percentage of Black women have participated in the labor force out of necessity due to the scarcity of marriageable Black males. Charles and Luoh (2010) found that women increased both their schooling and labor supply in response to male incarceration. The comparative supply of marriageable males in 1980 was 40 percent for Black Americans and 60 percent for whites. By 2010, it had declined to 35 percent for Black Americans and 55 percent for whites. The ratio of marriageable males to unmarried females for Black Americans is 2:5 compared to 3:5 for whites. The sharp decline in the probability of marriage for Black women is exacerbated by the growing excess of women over men in every age group during the marriageable years. The cumulative probability of remaining unmarried increases as the sex ratio increases and surpasses the sex ratio increase.

Historically, over 90 percent of Black women were married by the age of forty-four. This figure decreased to 75 percent in the 1970s. By 1980, one third of Black women had never been married by the age of forty-four. Whites do not experience an excess of females over males until the age of forty-four, which is beyond major childbearing years. Therefore, the percentage of female-headed white families (never-married, single, teenaged mothers) is significantly lower than among Black Americans. The structures of Black families are influenced by the surplus of women. The sex ratio imbalances among Black Americans are affected by high infant and childhood mortality among males, high mortality rate among young Black males, and hyperincarceration. Black families are destroyed by hyperincarceration through the removal of fathers from homes, which leaves Black males disenfranchised (erosion of human capital, collateral consequences, etc.) and unemployed under America's racial caste system. Further, the family is left to deal with potential financial instability and emotional and psychological effects on the children and partner along with social stigma, which is an experience that is like the death of a parent or divorce. In addition, the marriageable pool of Black men is lowered due to the absence of jobs for Black men, which increases the prevalence of families headed by females in Black communities. The institutional decimation of Black men is established through the significant differential mortality rates between Black men and women, the increased institutionalization of Black men, and the withdrawal of Black men from the civilian labor force that includes their increased entry into the armed forces are all contributing factors that have severely impacted marriage and two-parent families.

Homicide is the greatest cause of death for Black men. The extreme rates of incarceration of Black men represent a human rights and public health issue. Black men have withdrawn from the civilian labor force, and some have entered the armed services at rates that doubled between 1970 and 1990; Black men are significantly more likely to reenlist compared to whites due to declining employment opportunities. Further, the least desirable jobs within the armed services are assigned to Black men who experience higher rates of unemployment upon reentry into civilian life. Thus, their entry into the ranks of the unemployed is temporarily postponed by military service. A surplus of unmarried women over marriageable men is created by these mechanisms of institutional decimation. The reverberating effects are long-term declines in fertility, increase in divorce, and increases in the percentage of women who have never been married by the age of twenty-four. Approximately 28 percent of Black

families were headed by females in 1970, increasing to 46 percent that
were female headed by 1990. In comparison, approximately 9 percent of
white families were headed by females in 1970, increasing to 13 percent by
1990. In 2011, 55 percent of all Black families were female headed
compared to 22 percent of all white families.

Testa and Krogh (1995) found that Black male employment is positively related to marriage rates. Black men in stable employment were
twice as likely to marry than unemployed men. The sharpest increase in
female-headed Black families occurred between 1970 and 1990. According
to Joe and Yu (1984), the number of female-headed Black families rose by
700,000 and the number of Black men out of the labor force or unemployed increased by the same number between the years of 1976 and 1983.
This trend was recognized in 1960 where approximately 75 percent of
Black men were working, and female-headed Black families accounted for
21 percent of all Black families during the same year. Only 54 percent of
all Black men were in the labor force and female-headed Black families
were at 42 percent by 1982. Moreover, the largest relative gains in the
decade following civil rights legislation were obtained by Black women.
They experienced economic and social gains in the late 1960s through the
1970s due to their occupational opportunities greatly expanding. Black
women comprise the majority of Black Americans who have moved into
the middle-class since the Civil Rights Movement. Black women were
brought closer to parity with white women due to the occupational,
economic, and social gains that also had the effect of health gains. This
translated into a larger increase in life expectancy (approximately three
years) more than any other race-sex group. Black men did not experience
uniformly positive occupational and socioeconomic gains following civil
rights legislation to the same degree as Black women. The inconsistent
pattern of gains and setbacks that Black men experienced was initiated in
the 1940s by an extensive move out of agricultural work into blue-collar
operative jobs, which was countered in the 1960s by rising unemployment
relative to white men. Therefore, the occupational changes in the 1960s
that translated into gains in the 1970s had different effects on racial
inequality for Black men and women. Black women experienced a decline
in income disparity because of their occupational distribution becoming
like their white counterparts, whereas income disparity increased among
Black men as the average occupational status of white men increased,
moving away from the average status of Black men including a sharp
decline in labor market participation among a rising segment of Black
men. Therefore, the impact of civil rights legislation on the occupational

and economic pathways for Black men was minimal including the residual improved health that would come about from these types of gains. According to Kaplan et al. (2008), employers' racial animus toward Black men (anti-Black misandry) and a preference for Black women instead is a potential explanation for these disparities. Frazier's (1939) research on Black families from 1860 to 1900 documented that most families he surveyed had a female head and Black women had higher employment rates compared to Black men, which predates civil rights legislation.

Because of their institutional decimation, marriage for many Black men becomes an economic burden. Many Black men are unable to meet the patriarchal expectations of being a financial provider and protector of their families simply due to not being able to financially afford marriage. According to Ogungbure (2019), the function of the American capitalist economy is to destroy Black families through the exclusion of Black males from the mechanism of wealth creation. The persistence of anti-Black misandry in America is reflected in the unemployment and underemployment of Black males where they are permanently removed from the labor market (institutional decimation). According to Willhelm (1986), enslaved Black Americans did not have a class position and Black Americans who are not in the labor market have no class standing as well. He articulates that they are not part of an underclass but a *declassed* people. He identifies this structural formation as conditional genocide since class position establishes life opportunities and it is questionable if a declassed Black person even has a chance for life. The rise of the female-headed family is a consequence of economic oppression that impacts Black family structure. The consequence is an apatriarchal Black male who is unable to head a household or participate in American capitalist society. The victimization of Black males within America's capitalist and patriarchal political economy through mechanisms of socioeconomic deprivation, institutionalization, and death has led to the destruction of the socioeconomic status of the Black family.

6.5.2 Marriage

The marital bond is represented by a complex set of relationships that encompass psychological, economic, and social components. Black Americans are the least likely to marry, marry later in life thus spending less time married than white Americans, and are the least likely to remain married. Black Americans view marriage positively and married Black men and women significantly value marriage as the optimal context for raising children, companionship, and financial security. Black marriages are distinct from white marriages based on high egalitarianism in the marital relationship, involvement from extended family, and mutual self-disclosure. Financial strain (economic oppression), adverse work conditions, family obligations (e.g., extended family, children), racial discrimination (i.e., anti-Black racism), and race-based stress create adverse life circumstances that can contribute to poor marital quality and higher rates of divorce among Black Americans. Cutrona et al. (2003) found that neighborhood-level economic disadvantage predicted lower warmth (e.g., support, endearment, physical affection, escalation of warmth, reciprocation of warmth, assertiveness, listener responsiveness, communication, and prosocialness) during marital interactions and financial strain predicted lower perceived marital quality among Black Americans. Diminished warmth has been attributed to several contexts that include stressful events that trigger negative emotions where individuals are more likely to express anger and dissatisfaction with one another. Stressed individuals may be preoccupied with their problems (i.e., taxing circumstances) and inattentive to the needs of their partner resulting in less warmth. Persistent long-term problems may cause an individual to become demoralized where there is a lack of energy to actively provide affection to their partner. Dixon (2009) attributes a shift in U.S. culture from child-centered families (familism) to adult-centered families (individualism) that prioritized self-actualization and leisure time for adults as a contributing factor to the marriage status of Black Americans. This cultural shift emerged during the 1980s ("Me-Generation") that emphasized single lifestyles and a focus on the self. In addition, capitalistic consumerism through a genre of hip-hop culture that promoted materialism (e.g., expensive automobiles, jewelry, and brand-named clothing) as the foundation of relationship formation is also cited as a contributing factor (Hampton, 1980).

Black Americans' expectations for marriage include commitment, love, friendship, partnership, trust, and covenant. Research from King et al. (2009) evaluated the personal characteristics of the ideal marriage partner among Black American adults and found that Black men and women desire well-educated, financially stable, monogamous, and affluent partners who are spiritual, religious, self-confident, and reliable. Respondents preferred ideal marriage partners who earned significantly more income than they did regardless of sex/gender. This preference appeared to be motivated by a desire for middle-class mobility and security. Honesty and sensitivity were the most important characteristics identified among respondents.

Female respondents placed a greater emphasis on their partner's financial and educational status than male respondents, which may reflect the economic position of Black women and a desire to avoid marrying someone who may threaten or impede their social and economic status. Both Black men and women in the study sought marriage partners whose incomes were substantially higher than their own income. Haynes (2000) found that Black men and women still expect the opposite sex to perform traditional sex/gender-specific roles even though they endorsed egalitarian marriages. Women desired provider husbands and fathers whereas men desired primary nurturers. Satisfaction and subsequent partner commitment are influenced by equity, power, whether a partner is in proximity to a romantic ideal, physical attraction, and sexual satisfaction. Marital dissatisfaction is associated with high expectations of spousal roles, particularly when spouses are expected to simultaneously inhabit the role of friend, confidant, satisfying sexual partner, parent, and counselor (Dixon, 2009; Holmes, 1997; Orbuch et al., 2002).

In addition, relationship dissatisfaction, sexual desire differences, less regard for one another, and sexual satisfaction are the primary predictors of infidelity among men and women. Vaterlaus et al. (2017) examined marital expectations in strong Black marriages and found that there was growth in marital expectations over time that began with unrealistic expectations that evolved into more realistic expectations as the marriages progressed. Foundational expectations in the marriages included open communication, congruent values, and positive treatment of spouse. Moreover, autonomy was identified as an important aspect of marital relationships. Autonomy is a sense of volition and choice that is independent of pressure or coercion. Autonomy is not detachment or independence. From an attachment perspective, autonomy is possible in a relationship context due to secure attachment and relationship intimacy (i.e., a secure base). An individual can be autonomous and adventurous knowing that their partner will be there upon their return. Lynch (2013) found that people who felt more autonomous and had partners who supported their autonomy were more willing to turn to their partners for emotional support and experienced more vitality within their relationships. Predictors of relationship stability among Black couples include partner supportiveness and warmth. Research from Cutrona et al. (2011) assessed predictors of relationship stability over a five-year period among heterosexual cohabiting and married Black couples raising an elementary-school-age child. They found that higher levels of education were associated with higher income, lower financial strain, and family structures that are more

stable (e.g., marriage instead of cohabitation and biological-family instead
of stepfamily status). The relationship quality and stability were influenced
by these variables. In addition, religiosity promoted relationship stability
through its affiliation with marriage, biological-family status, and relationship quality among women (Dixon, 2009; Holmes, 1997; Orbuch et al.,
2002; Vowels et al., 2022).

6.5.3   Anti-Black Racism

Anti-Black racism in the United States is a chronic, pervasive, cumulative,
and noxious pollutant that has structured Black life since slavery. Thus,
Black people who descend from U.S. enslavement are racially stratified as a
racial undercaste. External stressors such as anti-Black racism impact life
opportunities among Black Americans and create disparities between Black
and white Americans in economic and political power, civil rights, and
accessibility to resources. The establishment and sustainability of romantic
unions are negatively impacted by socially engineered (i.e., sociogenic)
conditions that include sociohistorical, sociocultural, and sociostructural
barriers that affect emotional processes (i.e., socioemotional processes)
among Black men and women within the coupling process and romantic
relationships. Awosan and Hardy (2017) found that daily experiences of
explicit and implicit anti-Black racism affected motivation, desire, commitment, and efforts to maintain secure long-term romantic relationships
among never married heterosexual Black men and women. Moreover,
Black men and women felt that their efforts to acquire a high-quality
long-term love relationship with one another were adversely impacted by
negative racial stereotypes and anti-Black racism. Research from Murry
et al. (2001) indicated that maternal psychological distress (e.g., depression
and anxiety) among Black mothers was directly and indirectly correlated
with parent–child relationship quality through an association with intimate partnership quality. Stronger connections developed between stressor
pileup and psychological distress, including between psychological distress
and the quality of intimate partnerships and parent–child relationships
when racial discrimination was greater. Research from Kogan et al. (2016)
revealed that a combination of harsh parenting (e.g., slapping, hitting,
shouting, low nurturance, and poor relationship quality) and racial
discrimination (i.e., anti-Black misandry) are significant factors in
commitment-related behavior among young Black men. It was hypothe-
sized that harsh parenting and anti-Black misandry inform working models
of relationships and negative emotions. This can also be conceptualized as

an avoidant attachment style within attachment theory (Awosan & Opara, 2016; Cooper, 2023; Fanon, 1952).

6.5.4   Internalized Stereotypes (Anti-Blackness)

Stereotypes of Black people routinely serve a dehumanizing function that justifies white dominance and violence. Stereotypes of Black Americans have an extensive history dating back to colonialism, enslavement, and Jim/Jane Crow. Black men are often described as hypermasculine, hypersexual (e.g., rapists), aggressive, immoral, and dangerous (e.g., criminals). These racist descriptions continue to proliferate theory and gender discourse and are even framed as progressive ideologies. Black women are often described as embodying either one or a combination of three primary caricatures (Mammy, Sapphire, and Jezebel) that are typically conceptualized as controlling images. Black women are portrayed as either highly maternal/nurturing, self-sacrificing (Mammy); angry, hostile, aggressive, domineering, threatening, loud, sassy, argumentative, masculine/emasculating (Sapphire); or seductive, sexually unrestrained, promiscuous (Jezebel). These caricatures of Black men and women act as pathological stigmatizing agents that elicit an endorsement continuum ranging from oppression to death. Acceptance of negative stereotypes about Black males and females can potentiate relationship problems. Acceptance of such stereotypes assigns a low value to potential relationship partners and serves as a basis of distrust and suspicion that influence bias evaluations of all future actions of partners in a relationship. An extensive body of literature exists that documents both popular and social science stereotypes about Black men and Black women. Internalized stereotypes of Black men and Black women is a significant issue in understanding Black male–female relationships. These stereotypes may represent a pattern that results in intolerable Black male–female relationships. Efforts to increase trust, vulnerability, and intimacy through the expression of feelings and affection can be thwarted through the internalization of negative stereotypes. Therefore, the existence of negative internalized stereotypes can cause numerous relationship problems (Bogle, 2001; Cazenave & Smith, 1990; Cooper, 2023; Curry, 2017, 2018; Jewell, 1983; Kelly & Floyd, 2001; Walum, 1977; West, 1995).

Cazenave and Smith (1990) examined sex/gender differences in the perception of Black male–female relationships and stereotypes with Black males and Black females of various socioeconomic status (SES) levels and backgrounds and found that a substantial minority view their male–female relationships as being essentially negative in nature. Respondents who described their intimate relationships in a negative manner tended to never have been married or were currently divorced and accepted negative stereotypes about Black men. Further, there was a greater acceptance of negative stereotypes about Black men than Black women. A clearly identifiable pattern emerged of negative views about Black men for both the male and female respondents. In addition, there was a tendency for both male and female respondents who held negative stereotypes about Black men or Black women to be more traditional in their views of appropriate sex/gender roles and to accept the belief that Black Americans have not prepared themselves to take advantage of available opportunities (i.e., internalized beliefs that are a part of symbolic racism).

Chestnut (2009) identified negative Black male stereotypes as follows: Black men are hypersexual, dominating toward women, disrespectful, and unfaithful. Negative Black female stereotypes were identified as follows: Black women are ashamed of themselves, lazy, lying and trifling, give up easily, are weak, selfish, and neglect their families. Chestnut's (2009) research on internalized stereotypes among Black couples found that Black women endorsed more negative stereotypes of Black men and Black women than males; older age was correlated with negative stereotypes of Black males and negative stereotypes of Black females; women who obtained a higher education (completed college) endorsed more negative stereotypes of Black females than those who did not complete high school; and being in a committed relationship and holding positive stereotypes were highly correlated to overall adjustment of Black couples. Taylor (1990) found that among Black couples, husbands and wives who reported more internalized racism tended to report less marital satisfaction. Research from Taylor and Zhang (1990) revealed that Black distressed couples were more likely than nondistressed couples to internalize negative stereotypes about Black people. Moreover, Kelly and Floyd (2001) discovered that the partners of Black women who endorsed strong beliefs in negative racial stereotypes reported limited trust and found their female partners to be undependable.

6.5.5   Strong Black Woman [Superwoman] Schema

The Strong Black Woman/Superwoman Schema (SBW/SWS) refers to the sociopolitical context of Black women that includes the climate of anti-Black racism, sexism, disenfranchisement, and limited resources during and after slavery in the United States (sociohistorical) that forced Black women to assume the roles of mother, nurturer, and breadwinner out of economic and social necessity. Embodying a Superwoman has been necessary for survival. The Superwoman emerged due to the compromised and disenfranchised position (anti-Black misandry) of Black men that severely restricted their ability to provide financial and emotional support to their partners and families. The Superwoman role can be an asset to and a vulnerability of Black women's health. Black women have been praised for their strength (i.e., resilience, fortitude, and perseverance) despite societal and personal challenges. The Superwoman has contributed to the survival of the Black population and is viewed as a positive character trait or asset. Woods-Giscombé (2010) found that the Superwoman role is multidimensional and includes characteristics, contributing contextual factors, perceived benefits, and perceived liabilities. The characteristics were an obligation to manifest strength, an obligation to suppress emotions, resistance to being vulnerable or dependent, determination to succeed despite limited resources, and an obligation to help others. The contributing contextual factors include a historical legacy of racial or sex/gender stereotyping or oppression, lessons from foremothers, history of disappointment, mistreatment or abuse, and spiritual values. The perceived benefits were the preservation of self/survival, preservation of the Black community, and preservation of the Black family. The perceived liabilities include strain in interpersonal (e.g., romantic) relationships, stress-related health behaviors (e.g., postponement of self-care, emotional eating, poor sleep), and embodiment of stress (e.g., anxiety, depressive symptoms, adverse maternal health).

Black women who embody the SWS tend to suppress negative emotion and have difficulty accepting emotional support. It is not uncommon for Black women to be socialized with the belief that if they need help, no one will be there to help them and that they must become self-reliant. This can manifest as a resistance to being vulnerable or dependent. The stereotype of Black men being unreliable reinforces this belief. The SWS can also be demonstrated through the obligation to help others and difficulty declining (i.e., saying "no") multiple roles and responsibilities including the postponement of self-care. According to Abdullah (1998), this represents *mammy-ism* (e.g., negative self-image and low self-esteem) when the self-sacrificing component of the SWS is combined with internalized anti-Blackness (e.g., self-devaluation and denigration of Black culture) and accommodation to whites (e.g., in the workplace). The SWS can be found in recent proclamations of Black Girl Magic (#BlackGirlMagic), which is intended to affirm the ingenuity of Black women but ultimately sanctions the SBW and conceals the vulnerability of Black women. The research of Allen et al. (2019) examined stress-coping among Black women using the SWS Scale. Their research revealed that feeling obligated to present an image of strength and suppressing emotions were protective while feeling an intense motivation to succeed and feeling obligated to helping others exacerbated health risks associated with anti-Black racism. They posit that suppressing anger may be health protective within the context of frequent or chronic experiences of anti-Black racism. Emotion suppression may prevent emotional engagement with contextual anti-Black racism, which serves as a buffer against its harmful effects (Woods-Giscombé, 2010).

6.5.6 John Henryism

John Henry is part of the Black American folktale and refers to the railroad worker/steel-driver in the nineteenth century and known among railroad and tunnel workers for his remarkable physical strength and endurance. The folktale narrative indicates that he used powerful blows to beat a mechanical steam drill with a nine-pound hammer in a steel-driving contest of man against machine and won the contest but died moments later from complete physical and mental exhaustion. The John Henryism framework was developed by James et al. (1983) and refers to prolonged high-effort active coping with chronic psychosocial stressors that are associated with an increased risk for adverse health outcomes (e.g., elevated blood pressure) (Bennett et al., 2004; Cooper, 2023; James, 1994; Link & Phelan, 2001).

John Henryism can be manifested by Black men who work extremely hard under pressure to disprove stereotypes of laziness and inability. It encompasses an individual's perception that he can meet the demands of his environment through hard work and determination and emphasizes environmental mastery (i.e., attempting to control environmental stressors with personal efficacy and locus of control). Said differently, John Henryism includes the belief that psychosocial environmental stressors (i.e., social and economic oppression, e.g., chronic financial strain, job insecurity, anti-Black racial micro/aggressions) can be managed through hard work and determination. The John Henryism framework includes the three main components of efficacious mental and physical vigor, a strong commitment to hard work, and a steadfast determination to succeed. Higher scores on John Henryism (using the John Henryism Scale for Active Coping/JHAC12) tend to indicate hypertension (high blood pressure) among Black men. Black male employees attempt to counteract anti-Black misandric micro/aggressions through hard work and the belief that they will be able to transcend their experiences and achieve security and upward mobility in their occupations (Bennett et al., 2004; Cooper, 2023; James, 1994; Link & Phelan, 2001).

Research from James et al. (1984) revealed that men with high John Henryism felt that being Black had hindered their chances for job success, were more psychologically involved with their jobs (e.g., job success), and experienced low job security and lack of support from supervisors. The toxic environments in which Black Americans live and work expose them to incessant psychosocial stress that make them vulnerable to John Henryism. The psychological stress generated from these conditions requires an inordinate amount of daily energy to manage. Anti-Black racism erodes their economic security and psychological well-being and functions as a pernicious psychosocial stressor. John Henryism has been negatively associated with happiness and is associated with an increase in depression (i.e., subjective well-being) primarily among Black men (Angner et al., 2011; Bennett et al., 2004; Cooper, 2023; Hudson et al., 2016; James, 1994; James et al., 1983; Link & Phelan, 2001).

6.5.7   Racial Identity

Racial identity encompasses the significance and meaning that Black Americans place on race in their self-definition. The capacity to identify racism is contingent upon a person's racial identity statuses (i.e., stages). Racial identity can function as a protective factor (e.g., lower psychological distress in response to perceived racial discrimination) against racial discrimination. Racial identity development is a process that is characterized by the rejection of white culture in one's self-definition and includes the internal development of a positive racial identity. Racial identity ego statuses are dynamic and conform to a developmental or progressive stage process that ranges from an external (i.e., dominant racial group identification; conformity) to an internal (i.e., own-racial-group identification; internalization) status. An externally focused racial identity status includes color-blind ideology, conformity, or beliefs that race is not a significant factor in an individual's everyday life or the life of others. Therefore, the capacity to recognize race-based encounters (i.e., racism; race-based trauma) is dependent upon an individual's internally defined racial identity status (Cooper, 2023; Sellers et al., 1998; Thompson & Carter, 1997).

The most widely used model of Black American racial identity is the Cross (1971, 1991) model of Nigrescence (to become Black). The

Nigrescence model contains five stages (also referred to as attitudes or statuses; preencounter, encounter, immersion/emersion, internalization, internalization-commitment) of racial identity development among Black Americans that is instrumental in developing a psychologically healthy Black identity.

The first stage of *preencounter* includes the belief that race is not a significant component of identity. This may include the idealization of whiteness (white hegemony) or emphasizing another aspect of identity such as sex/gender, class, or religion. The second stage of *encounter* includes a significant racialized experience or multiple racialized experiences, which prompts individuals to reexamine their identity or develop a Black identity. The third stage of *immersion/emersion* includes a rejection of white culture and the idealization of Black culture. There is a preoccupation with identifying with Black culture but an internal lack of commitment to endorse all Black cultural values and traditions. The fourth stage of *internalization* includes an internal state of security and satisfaction with being Black. A less idealized perspective of the meaning of race is adopted along with the integration of a less dichotomous view of being Black and white. The fifth stage of *internalization/commitment* includes translating internalized identities into action. These stages represent a dynamic process that is situational/contextual as well as stable that may involve the gradual emergence of stage characteristics and the ability to return to a previous stage while experiencing that stage in a distinctly different manner. Often a person is primarily operating in one stage while simultaneously engaged with characteristics from other stages (Cooper, 2023; Cross, 1971, 1991; Helms, 1990, 1995; Parham, 1989; Thompson & Carter, 1997).

The integration of group identity theory and the cultural experiences of Black Americans inform the Multidimensional Model of Racial Identity (MMRI). Phenomenology that includes an individual's self-perceptions of what it means to be Black is instrumental in studying racial identity. Black racial identity is defined by the MMRI as the significance and qualitative meaning that individuals attribute to their membership within the Black racial group in their self-concepts (Cooper, 2023; Sellers et al., 1998).

The following two questions are foundational to this definition: *How important is race in the individual's perception of self? What does it mean to be a member of this racial group?* The theoretical assumptions of the MMRI are that identities are situationally and contextually influenced as well as being stable properties of the person, individuals have a number of different hierarchically ordered identities (e.g., race in the context of other identities is able to be investigated), individual perception of racial identity is the most significant indicator of identity, and the status of a person's racial identity instead of its development is a primary focus of the MMRI. The MMRI includes four dimensions (*salience, centrality, regard,* and *ideology*) of racial identity and underscores the significance and the qualitative meaning of race in the self-concepts of Black Americans. Racial *salience* denotes the extent to which an individual's race is a relevant aspect of one's self-concept situationally and contextually. Racial *centrality* denotes the significance individuals assign to race. Racial *regard* denotes an individual's judgments about their race and includes *private regard* (perceptions of being Black American and views of other Black Americans) and *public regard* (an individual's assessment of how Black Americans are viewed by society). *Ideology* contains an individual's beliefs, opinions, and attitudes regarding how Black Americans should act and includes *assimilationist, humanist, oppressed minority,* and *nationalist perspectives. Assimilationist* ideology includes a focus on the similarities between Black Americans and American society. *Humanist* ideology describes an emphasis on the similarities among all humans. *Oppressed minority* ideology emphasizes the similarities between Black Americans and other oppressed populations. *Nationalist* ideology describes the uniqueness of the being Black experience (i.e., the Black American experience). Sellers et al. (2006) discovered that substantial racial centrality and private regard were related to greater psychological well-being. The Nigrescence model of racial identity development and the MMRI are important racial identity development models for understanding Black racial identity (Cooper, 2023; Sellers et al., 1998).

6.5.8   Religion and Spirituality

Religion refers to a formalized set of ideological commitments among a group (faith community) that includes an organized system of beliefs, rituals, and cumulative traditions whereas spirituality refers to the personal and subjective aspect of religious experience. Religious institutions and spirituality are instrumental aspects of cultural practices among Black Americans that serve as significant sources of strength and coping. Black Americans are significantly more religious on various measures (e.g., belief in God, frequency of prayer, and attendance at religious services) than the general population (e.g., 87 percent of Black Americans report a religious affiliation; 78 percent are Protestant, 59 percent report belonging to historically Black Protestant churches). Religion has a direct and indirect association with marital quality. Direct associations include an increase in the social support of norms and values of marriage and relationship-enhancing behaviors (e.g., partner forgiveness) whereas indirect outcomes include the cultivation of increased psychological well-being, temperance, and sexual fidelity (Jagers & Smith, 1996; LaTaillade, 2006; Pew Charitable Trust Forum, 2009a, 2009b).

Spirituality for Black Americans includes a sense of connection with one's ancestors, which contains beliefs in the unobservable and nonmaterial that governs life. Spirituality can serve as a protective factor against life stressors among Black couples exposed to economic deprivation, structural anti-Black racism, and oppression. Spirituality has long served as a form of affirmation and resistance to white hegemony among Black people in the United States. The corporate manifestation of spirituality through religion has provided Black couples with a few institutions (i.e., the Black church) that they can access and trust and receive instrumental and emotional support (Jagers & Smith, 1996; LaTaillade, 2006).

Black churches have historically been sources of support for Black communities by offering programs developed to enhance emotional, educational, and economic welfare; providing leadership opportunities (i.e., conferring status positions, e.g., deacons) that would not be available to Black people in U.S. society; and mobilizing political organization, activism, and resistance in response to anti-Black racism and oppression. Research from Fincham et al. (2011) examined spirituality and marital satisfaction among Black couples and found that husband religiosity was related to his own and partner satisfaction. In addition, they found that spirituality and religiosity operated independently despite conceptual overlap. Religiosity seemed to function as a couple variable with similar levels of religiosity among partners whereas spirituality functioned as an individual variable that was not shared among spouses. Higher levels of spirituality were associated with experiences of relationship quality. The level of spirituality and its association with negative marital quality were significantly higher among Black men (Jagers & Smith, 1996; LaTaillade, 2006).

The following section includes clinical implications that will assist therapists practicing EFT with integrating the clinical considerations into their therapeutic practice. This will afford therapists the ability to make appropriate modifications and adaptations of the EFT model and provide culturally responsive couple therapy.

6.6   Clinical Implications

There is a lack of definitive information on evidence-based practice with Black couples. The existing literature on therapy with Black couples is clinical, anecdotal, and theoretical and lacks empiricism. EFT is a Eurocentric theoretical model. The proposition of EFT as a universal therapy and attachment theory as universal is problematic and reveals the limitations of EFT and attachment theory. Universalism is a Eurocentric myth that is designed to legitimize Western civilization. The rejection of universalism requires that Black lived experience be recognized as a source of knowledge production. EFT and attachment theory will need to be significantly modified to be a culturally responsive therapy to the needs of Black couples. Adult attachment needs to be conceptualized from a network approach (e.g., multiple relationships/collectivism) instead of only a dyadic perspective. In addition, acculturation (i.e., racial identity), and race/ethnicity, institutional decimation and Black sex ratios, anti-Black racism, internalized stereotypes (anti-Blackness), SBW, John Henryism, and religion and spirituality are all important factors to consider in providing culturally responsive care and clinical interventions that inform treatment approaches with Black couples. The denial of structural racism has been associated with anti-Black racism. White and other non-Black therapists tend to frame acts of anti-Black racism as discrete interpersonal events that are unusual rather than a broad spectrum of routine acts that structure racial hierarchy and Black existence in the United States. Attempts to address systemic and structural anti-Black racism with EFT are outside the scope of EFT and include disavowing the true nature of anti-Black racism with an overreliance on attachment and supposed relationships that historically have been entanglements of dominance. The motivation for this position is to create an optimistic version of Blackness that humanizes whiteness, which is comforting for white therapists but is ultimately narrative fiction and has very little to do with the lived experiences of Black people. Anti-Black racism can be addressed by EFT only within the coupling (relationship) dynamics as anti-Black racism can exacerbate other forms of contextual stress within the relationship (Awosan & Hardy, 2017; Cooper, 2023; Shorter-Gooden, 2008; Utley, 2016; Yi et al., 2022).

Black Americans tend to be high on both individualism and collectivism in comparison to other Americans. The high individualism is likely due to self-reliance and beliefs that interdependence indicates weakness, which were influenced by U.S. society and survival needs. This may be demonstrated through a desire for personal uniqueness in a society that blocks achievement among Black Americans. Further, Black culture has managed to retain aspects of its collectivist African heritage that aid in survival such as turning toward Black communities for support. Therapists will need to validate individualistic and collectivistic coping responses within the relationship (Kelly & Hudson, 2017; Komarraju & Cokley, 2008).

Ross et al. (2019) found that socioeconomic risk moderates the demand/withdraw pattern (common negative interactional cycle in EFT) and wives' relationship satisfaction where high levels of withdrawal were beneficial to the relationship when socioeconomic risks were high. Demands can provide partners with opportunities to voice concerns while withdrawal can deescalate conflict and stabilize satisfaction. Behavioral withdrawal by men appeared to be maladaptive when couples had access to social and economic resources (i.e., relatively affluent) to enact desired changes; however, withdrawal proved to be adaptive when they lacked such resources (i.e., relatively disadvantaged thus unable to control and resolve their problems). Ross et al. (2019) contend that efforts to change couple communication without integrating the larger social and economic contexts of those behaviors may be counterproductive. Therefore, it is important to consider SES and the negative interactional cycle where EFT may need to be modified with Black couples who are experiencing socioeconomic risks.

Moreover, it is important to integrate a strengths-based perspective with a focus on relationship-enhancing characteristics such as demonstrating appreciation and affection, commitment, positive communication, enjoyable times together, spiritual/religious well-being and practices, the ability to effectively manage stress and crisis, egalitarianism, role flexibility, familial kin, community support, and a positive racial identity. These strengths can serve as resources for Black couples that reduce conflict, avert relationship distress and instability, and support positive treatment outcomes. Black families and couples perform important social and psychological functions and serve as a protective sanctuary from the impacts of anti-Black racism (e.g., daily micro/aggressions) where support is provided that is unavailable in the general society. Individual experiences with anti-Black racism are transformed into a family issue that elicits familial support and is recognized as a historical structural problem. But this can also cause vicarious trauma among family members and couples that can eventually damage the relational bond among romantic partners. These experiences can elicit feelings of sadness and a sense of inadequacy with the inability (powerlessness) of self-protection and protecting one's partner from the daily assaults of anti-Black racism that ultimately undermine romantic relationships among Black people. Consequently, therapists may consider recruiting respected extended family members, elders, community leaders, and clergy to collaborate in the treatment and serve as a support system for the couple. Couples therapy is limited in scope where the stability of Black couples' relationships will need to be enhanced through required changes in societal conditions (e.g., restorative justice through reparations) that limit or block economic opportunities and weaken relationship bonds (Awosan & Hardy, 2017; Cutrona et al., 2011; DeFrain & Asay, 2007; Jean & Feagin, 1998; Kelly & Boyd-Franklin, 2009; LaTaillade, 2006; Murry et al., 2001; Nobles, 1978).

Anti-Black stereotypes are a form of dehumanization that sanctions the domination of Black men and women. These stereotypes endorse the exploitation of Black women and the disposability of Black men. Stereotypes of Black men and women may be problematic and associated with low self-esteem and related anti-Black misandry, sexism, misogyny (i.e., hostile sexism), other anti-Black biases, and relationship mistrust and distress. Relationships have the potential to be improved by understanding precisely what these stereotypes are, who holds them, and their social origins. Therapists must be aware of the sexual myths and stereotypes they hold about Black men and women including perceptions that they might potentially project onto their clients regarding Black sexuality. The institutional decimation of Black males and its impact on Black sex ratios create a shortage of marriageable Black men, which positions highly sought-after Black men with the opportunity to attain a high-status spouse. Colorism through skin shade may be a marker of a high- or low-status spouse. Colorism is another form of anti-Blackness that is routinely demonstrated with greater social status being ascribed to Black women with lighter skin shade. This may manifest in some Black men preferring Black women with lighter skin, white women, or interracial relationships as well as some Black women preferring interracial relationships. In these instances, Black women with dark skin are devalued as well as Black men in general. Colorism also creates a standard of beauty that is primarily Eurocentric. Lighter skin, longer and straighter hair, a thin body, and European facial features are considered the standard of beauty where white femaleness is equated with femininity and attractiveness. This ideology can be reinforced daily through various forms of media and experienced as an assault on the personhood of Black women. Therefore, many Black women may struggle with self-image and feeling good about their physical appearance with attempts to meet a Eurocentric ideal. Feelings of shame and low self-worth can be elicited from these experiences (Cazenave & Smith, 1990; Cooper, 2023; Hamilton et al., 2009; Kelly & Boyd-Franklin, 2009; Shorter-Gooden, 2008; West, 1995).

It is not uncommon for discourse regarding Black men and women to covertly shape conversations and the therapy. This includes the assumption that Black men do not have the capacity to express feelings of love and commitment nor act on them and the assumption that Black women do not respect the efforts of Black men to demonstrate care for them or their children. Therapists tend to be heavily invested in the aspect of this discourse that relates to the emotional engagement of Black men and may perpetuate these ideas about Black men by endorsing the belief that Black men display stoicism and conceal emotions to not be perceived as weak or vulnerable and in control (i.e., Cool Pose). The Cool Pose thesis has a foundation in culture of poverty and criminology theories of Black male deviance. The research of Unnever and Chouhy (2021) revealed that Black males including poor Black males in urban areas were equally as likely as white males to feel pressure to conceal their feelings when they felt sad or anxious. Therefore, endorsing beliefs that Black men display some sort of unique emotional disposition (e.g., Cool Pose) or nonnormative emotional expression not only represents anti-Black misandry but is a form of dehumanization (i.e., speciation). Research indicates that Black men are more sex/gender progressive than white men and women and have exceeded the sex/gender consciousness of Black women in various measures, are more involved with their children than white or Latino fathers, and hold the most liberal sexual attitudes of all sex-race groups in the United States. But these data are obscured through myths and caricatures of Black men that are presented as factual truths. On a systemic level the ultimate solution to these problems requires fundamental changes in American social structure. But psychoeducational interventions and therapy have the potential to provide appropriate targeted interventions to individuals to reduce negative internalized stereotypes that can ultimately impact coupling dynamics. This includes challenging negative views of their in-group and their partners as well as normalizing their problems and providing education regarding the systemic and structural issues that contextually impact their relationship (Akinyela, 2008; Blee & Tickamyer, 1995; Cazenave, 1983; Cooper, 2023; Gooley, 1989; Harnois, 2010, 2014; Hunter & Sellers, 1998; Jackson, 2018; Jones & Mosher, 2013; Majors & Billson, 1993; Simien, 2007; Staples, 1978).

The SBW can be protective against anti-Black racism but can be problematic in an intimate relationship when Black women who embody the SBW are unable to acknowledge pain or vulnerable feelings, unable to request help, present an image of perfection (e.g., having it all together), or feel undeserving of support. Attachment and interdependency can be frightening and experienced as dangerous and weak, which can produce a sense of chronic loneliness and emotional isolation. The lack of attachment and interdependence can affect male partners and elicit a sense of inadequacy especially among men who desire an emotionally available partner who depends on them to provide comfort and support. The expression of depression becomes more acceptable through expressions of anger or somatic symptoms. In addition, the suppression of vulnerable emotions (e.g., sadness, fear, or shame) might manifest as anxiety or binge eating. The need to project an image of perfection can make it difficult and even intolerable to hear their male partners express dissatisfaction with any aspect of the relationship and can result in the silencing of the male partner (Shorter-Gooden, 2008).

It is important for the therapist to help Black women who embody the SBW to be able to integrate a sense of strength and capability along with being securely attached and interdependent (e.g., emotional support) with their partners. This involves them acknowledging their needs and taking a risk by allowing themselves to be vulnerable with their partners (Shorter-Gooden, 2008).

The embodiment of John Henryism (e.g., overworking or high-effort coping to control/manage their environment) among some Black men can impact intimate relationships and leave their female partners feeling neglected and even abandoned when there is a preoccupation with one's occupation. Further, the female partners can be left feeling deprioritized in the relationship and unimportant. It is essential that therapists working with Black men who embody John Henryism aid them in feeling empowered in their lives with active engagement in healthier coping mechanisms while exploring other rewarding aspects of their lives that is independent of their employment (Cooper, 2023).

Therapists can misinterpret and pathologize Black women who embody the SBW and Black men who embody John Henryism as attachment avoidant or any semblance of restrictive emotionality as some sort of personality defect or maladaptive adjustment instead of a socioemotional response to socially engineered conditions (i.e., anti-Black racism) that serves a protective and adaptive function.

Black men and women who hold positive racial identities commonly seek each other out as potential relationship partners due to a shared history and culture as well as overlapping experiences of anti-Blackness. Black couples typically feel safe with Black partners who understand what it is like to be Black in the United States (e.g., struggles with daily assaults on Black life) based on lived experience. Racial identity can potentially moderate the association between stressors and marital quality among Black Americans particularly in relationships where couples have a more internally defined racial identity status and greater racial centrality and private regard. Moreover, an externally defined racial identity status and low racial centrality and private regard as well as a racial identity mismatch between the husband and wife may potentially amplify social stressors that impact the marriage (Bryant et al., 2010).

The Multidimensional Inventory of Black Identity can be valuable in assessing a client's racial identity status. In addition, it is important that white therapists know their racial identity status. If the therapist is invested in this process, it can help them to move beyond a passive stance that is complicit and even endorses white supremacy (e.g., internalized whiteness) to an active stance that is commonly referred to as *antiracist* (e.g., relinquishing white privilege). An active stance will afford the white therapist with the ability to develop attunement and a working alliance with Black couples. This also applies to people of color knowing their racial identity status through the people of color racial identity development model (Helms, 1995, 2017; Hubbard et al., 2022; Sellers et al., 1998).

Spirituality is often important in the lives of Black people and may be important within a relationship. The therapist can create space and invite the couple to share their individual and collective beliefs and assist them in using their religious/spiritual resources in the therapeutic process. Couples may participate in prayer, which may indicate the importance of spirituality in their relationship and thus the therapist can incorporate it into their treatment. Spiritual behaviors such as prayer can utilized within the negative interactional cycle (i.e., conflict) of EFT, which emphasizes cooperative goals that can contribute to deescalation. Spirituality may be associated with the perception of fewer disagreements and the tendency to forgive, which benefits the relationship (Fincham et al., 2011; Shorter-Gooden, 2008).

Although Black women and men have overlapping experiences of anti-Black racism, they also have distinctly different experiences with anti-Black racism in a white patriarchal society where Black women are exploited, and

Black men are targeted with lethal violence and downward social mobility. Historically Black men have been antipatriarchal (i.e., apatriarchal) while not identifying with feminist ideology and the analytic impositions imposed by feminist articulations and interpretations of sex/gender (e.g., worldwide hierarchy of male dominance of women within and throughout every society). Therefore, it is important that therapists do not impose feminist or intersectional (intersectionality) ideology that includes notions of privilege, hypermasculinity, hypersexuality, criminality, or any other constructed caricature of Black male deviance upon Black couples and specifically Black men (Anderson, 2021; Boyd-Franklin & Franklin, 1998; Cooper, 2023; Curry, 2021; Oluwayomi, 2020; Sidanius et al., 2018; Sidanius & Pratto, 1999; Sidanius & Veniegas, 2000).

Other topics that were not covered in this chapter but might need to be addressed by the therapist when working with Black couples include bidirectional intimate partner violence and the sexual victimization of Black women and men (Cooper, 2023).

EFT will have to undergo a modification to ensure that it is a culturally viable and responsive couple therapy model when working with Black couples. It is important to remember that EFT is a Western Eurocentric couple therapy model and attachment theory is a Western Eurocentric theory. Therefore, the therapist will need to consistently interrogate these Western Eurocentric assumptions of universalism to prevent cultural hegemony, and this will always need to be a part of case conceptualization and treatment planning in the maintenance of responsive care. This includes the reconceptualization of adult attachment from a network approach (e.g., multiple relationships/collectivism) instead of just a dyadic perspective. Clinical considerations include race/ethnicity, institutional decimation and Black sex ratios, anti-Black racism, internalized stereotypes (anti-Blackness), SBW/SWS, John Henryism, racial identity, and religion and spirituality, which are all important factors in providing culturally responsive care and clinical interventions that strengthen treatment approaches with Black couples.

Discussion Questions

1. How would you ensure that attachment is conceptualized from a network approach instead of only a dyadic perspective when applying EFT to Black couples?
2. What factors are important to consider when articulating the expression of emotions among Black couples that avoids Eurocentrism?

3. How are Black marriages distinctly different than white marriages?
4. How can the Strong Black Woman/Superwoman Schema and John Henryism affect intimate relationships?
5. How can racial identity affect Black couples?

REFERENCES

Abdullah, A. S. (1998). Mammy-ism: A diagnosis of psychological misorientation for women of African descent. *Journal of Black Psychology*, 24(2), 196–210.

Agishtein, P., & Brumbaugh, C. (2013). Cultural variation in adult attachment: The impact of ethnicity, collectivism, and country of origin. *Journal of Social, Evolutionary, and Cultural Psychology*, 7(4), 384–405.

Akinyela, M. (2008). Once they come: Testimony therapy and healing questions for African American couples. In M. McGoldrick & K. V. Hardy (Eds.), *Re-visioning family therapy: Race, class, culture and gender in clinical practice* (pp. 356–366). Guilford Press.

Alexis, M. (1998). The economics of racism. *The Review of Black Political Economy*, 26(3), 51–75.

Allen, A. M., Wang, Y., Chae, D. H., Price, M. M., Powell, W., Steed, T. C., Rose Black, A., Dhabhar, F. S., Marquez-Magaña, L., & Woods-Giscombé, C. L. (2019). Racial discrimination, the superwoman schema, and allostatic load: exploring an integrative stress-coping model among African American women. *Annals of the New York Academy of Sciences*, 1457(1), 104–127.

Amato, P. R. (2005). The impact of family formation change on the cognitive, social, and emotional well-being of the next generation. *The future of children*, 15(2), 75–96.

Anderson, P. D. (2021, September 8). *The theory of intersectionality emerges out of racist, colonialist ideology, not radical politics – Rethinking the CRT debate part 3.* Black Agenda Report. http://www.blackagendareport.com/theory-intersectionality-emerges-out-racist-colonialist-ideology-not-radical-politics-rethinking

Angner, E., Hullett, S., & Allison, J. J. (2011). "I'll die with the hammer in my hand": John Henryism as a predictor of happiness. *Journal of Economic Psychology*, 32(3), 357–366.

Awosan, C. I., & Hardy, K. V. (2017). Coupling processes and experiences of never married heterosexual Black men and women: A phenomenological study. *Journal of Marital and Family Therapy*, 43(3), 463–481.

Awosan, C. I., & Opara, I. (2016). Socioemotional factor: A missing gap in theorizing and studying Black heterosexual coupling processes and relationships. *Journal of Black Sexuality and Relationships*, 3(2), 25–51.

Bennett, G. G., Merritt, M. M., Sollers, J. J., III, Edwards, C. L., Whitfield, K. E., Brandon, D. T., & Tucker, R. D. (2004). Stress, coping, and health outcomes among African-Americans: A review of the John Henryism hypothesis. *Psychology & Health*, 19(3), 369–383.

Blee, K. M., & Tickamyer, A. R. (1995). Racial differences in men's attitudes about women's gender roles. *Journal of Marriage and the Family, 57*(1), 21–30.

Blumstein, A., & Beck, A. J. (1999). Population growth in US prisons, 1980–1996. *Crime and Justice, 26*, 17–61.

Bogle, D. (2001). *Toms, coons, mulattoes, mammies, and bucks: An interpretive history of Blacks in American films*. Bloomsbury Publishing.

Bowlby, J. (1969). *Attachment and loss: Vol. I. Attachment*. Hogarth Press and the Institute of Psycho-Analysis.

Boyd-Franklin, N., & Franklin, A. J. (1998). African American couples in therapy. In M. McGoldrick (Ed.), *Re-visioning family therapy: Race, culture, and gender in clinical practice* (pp. 268–281). Guilford Press.

Bryant, C. M., Wickrama, K. A. S., Bolland, J., Bryant, B. M., Cutrona, C. E., & Stanik, C. E. (2010). Race matters, even in marriage: Identifying factors linked to marital outcomes for African Americans. *Journal of Family Theory & Review, 2*(3), 157–174.

Cazenave, N. A. (1983). Black male–Black female relationships: The perceptions of 155 middle-class Black men. *Family Relations, 32*(3), 341–350.

Cazenave, N. A., & Smith, R. (1990). Gender differences in the perception of Black male female relationships and stereotypes. In H. E. Cheatham & J. B. Stewart (Eds.), *Black families: Interdisciplinary perspectives* (pp. 149–170). Transactions Publishers.

Charles, K. K., & Luoh, M. C. (2010). Male incarceration, the marriage market, and female outcomes. *The Review of Economics and Statistics, 92*(3), 614–627.

Chestnut, C. (2009). *The study of internalized stereotypes among African American couples*. Drexel University.

Chetty, R., Hendren, N., Jones, M. R., & Porter, S. R. (2018). *Race and economic opportunity in the United States* (NBER Working Paper 24441). National Bureau for Economic Research.

Cho, S. K., Wilson, B. D. M., & Mallory, C. (2021, January). *Black LGBT adults in the US*. Williams Institute, UCLA School of Law. https://williamsinstitute.law.ucla.edu/publications/black-lgbt-adults-in-the-us

Cooper, Y. (2023). Racial trauma and Black men [Manuscript in preparation].

Cox, O. C. (1940). Sex ratio and marital status among Negroes. *American Sociological Review, 5*(6), 937–947.

Craigie, T. A., Myers, S. L., & Darity, W. A. (2018). Racial differences in the effect of marriageable males on female family headship. *Journal of Demographic Economics, 84*(3), 231–256.

Cross, W. E., Jr. (1971). The negro-to-black conversion experience. *Black World, 20*(9), 13–27.

  (1991). *Shades of black: Diversity in African-American identity*. Temple University Press.

Curry, T. J. (2017). *The man-not: Race, class, genre, and the dilemmas of Black manhood*. Temple University Press.

(2018). Killing boogeymen: Phallicism and the misandric mischaracterizations of black males in theory. *Res Philosophica, 95*(2), 235–272.

(2020). Conditioned for death: Analysing black mortalities from COVID-19 and police killings in the United States as a syndemic interaction. *Comparative American Studies an International Journal, 17*(3–4), 257–270.

(2021). Decolonizing the intersection: Black Male Studies as a critique of intersectionality's indebtedness to Subculture of Violence Theory. In R. Beshara (Ed.), *Critical psychology praxis* (pp. 132–154). Routledge.

Cutrona, C. E., Russell, D. W., Abraham, W. T., Gardner, K. A., Melby, J. N., Bryant, C., & Conger, R. D. (2003). Neighborhood context and financial strain as predictors of marital interaction and marital quality in African American couples. *Personal Relationships, 10*(3), 389–409.

Cutrona, C. E., Russell, D. W., Burzette, R. G., Wesner, K. A., & Bryant, C. M. (2011). Predicting relationship stability among midlife African American couples. *Journal of Consulting and Clinical Psychology, 79*(6), 814–825.

Darity, W. A., Jr. (1980). Illusions of black economic progress. *The Review of Black Political Economy, 10*(2), 153–168.

Darity, W. A., Jr., Hamilton, D., Paul, M., Aja, A., Price, A., Moore, A., & Chiopris, C. (2018). *What we get wrong about closing the racial wealth gap.* Samuel DuBois Cook Center on Social Equity and Insight Center for Community Economic Development.

Darity, W. A., & Myers, S. L. (1983). Changes in black family structure: Implications for welfare dependency. *The American Economic Review, 73*(2), 59–64.

Darity, W. A., Jr., & Myers, S. L., Jr. (1984a). Does welfare dependency cause female headship? The case of the black family. *Journal of Marriage and the Family, 46*(4), 765–779.

(1984b). Public policy and the condition of Black family life. *The Review of Black Political Economy, 13*(1–2), 165–187.

Darity, W. A., Jr., & Myers, S. L., Jr. (1989). Where have all the black men gone? *Black Excellence, 1*(2), 29–31.

(1995). Family structure and the marginalization of Black men: policy implications. In M. B. Tucker & C. Mitchell-Kernan (Eds.), *The decline in marriage among African Americans: Causes, consequences, and policy implications* (pp. 263–293). Russell Sage Foundation.

DeFrain, J., & Asay, S. M. (2007). Strong families around the world: An introduction to the family strengths perspective. *Marriage & Family Review, 41*(1–2), 1–10.

Dixon, P. (2009). Marriage among African Americans: What does the research reveal? *Journal of African American Studies, 13*(1), 29–46.

Fanon, F. (1952). *Black skin/White masks.* Grove Press.

Fincham, F. D., Ajayi, C., & Beach, S. R. (2011). Spirituality and marital satisfaction in African American couples. *Psychology of Religion and Spirituality, 3*(4), 259–268.

Fitzgerald, J. M., & Ribar, D. C. (2004). Welfare reform and female headship. *Demography*, *41*(2), 189–212.

Frazier, E. F. (1939). *The Negro family in the United States*. University of Chicago Press.

Geronimus, A. T., & Korenman, S. (1992). The socioeconomic consequences of teen childbearing reconsidered. *The Quarterly Journal of Economics*, *107*(4), 1187–1214.

Gooley, R. L. (1989). The role of Black women in social change. *The Western Journal of Black Studies*, *13*(4), 165–172.

Greenman, P. S., & Johnson, S. M. (2013). Process research on emotionally focused therapy (EFT) for couples: Linking theory to practice. *Family Process*, *52*(1), 46–61.

Hagan, J., & Dinovitzer, R. (1999). Collateral consequences of imprisonment for children, communities, and prisoners. *Crime and Justice*, *26*, 121–162.

Hamilton, D., Goldsmith, A. H., & Darity, W., Jr. (2009). Shedding "light" on marriage: The influence of skin shade on marriage for black females. *Journal of Economic Behavior & Organization*, *72*(1), 30–50.

Hampton, R. L. (1980). Institutional decimation, marital exchange, and disruption in Black families. *The Western Journal of Black Studies*, *4*(2), 132–139.

Harnois, C. E. (2010, March). Race, gender, and the Black women's standpoint. *Sociological Forum*, *25*(1), 68–85.

Harnois, C. E. (2014). Complexity within and similarity across: Interpreting Black men's support of gender justice amidst cultural representations that suggest otherwise. In B. C. Slatton & K. Spates (Eds.), *Hyper sexual, hyper masculine? Gender, race and sexuality in the identities of contemporary Black men* (pp. 85–102). Routledge.

Haynes, F. E. (2000). Gender and family ideals: An exploratory study of Black middle-class Americans. *Journal of Family Issues*, *21*(7), 811–837.

Helms, J. E. (1990). *Black and White racial identity: Theory, research, and practice*. Greenwood Press.

(1995). An update of Helm's White and people of color racial identity models. In J. G. Ponterotto, J. M. Casas, L. A. Suzuki, & C. M. Alexander (Eds.), *Handbook of multicultural counseling* (pp. 181–198). Sage Publications.

(2017). The challenge of making Whiteness visible: Reactions to four Whiteness articles. *The Counseling Psychologist*, *45*(5), 717–726.

Hoffman, S. D., Foster, E. M., & Furstenberg, F. F., Jr. (1993). Reevaluating the costs of teenage childbearing. *Demography*, *30*(1), 1–13.

Holmes, J. (1997). Attachment, autonomy, intimacy: Some clinical implications of attachment theory. *British Journal of Medical Psychology*, *70*(3), 231–248.

Holzer, H. J. (2007). *Reconnecting young black men: What policies would help?* National Urban League.

Hubbard, S. A., Lakey, B., Jones, S. C., & Cage, J. L. (2022). Black racial identity, perceived support, and mental health within dyadic relationships.

Journal of Black Psychology. Advance online publication. https://doi.org/10
.1177/00957984221079209

Hudson, D. L., Neighbors, H. W., Geronimus, A. T., & Jackson, J. S. (2016).
Racial discrimination, John Henryism, and depression among African
Americans. *Journal of Black Psychology, 42*(3), 221–243.

Hunter, A. G., & Sellers, S. L. (1998). Feminist attitudes among African
American women and men. *Gender & Society, 12*(1), 81–99.

Jackson, B. A. (2018). Beyond the cool pose: Black men and emotion management strategies. *Sociology Compass, 12*(4), e12569.

Jagers, R. J., & Smith, P. (1996). Further examination of the Spirituality Scale.
Journal of Black Psychology, 22(4), 429–442.

James, S. A. (1994). John Henryism and the health of African-Americans.
Culture, Medicine and Psychiatry, 18(2), 163–182.

James, S. A., Hartnett, S. A., & Kalsbeek, W. D. (1983). John Henryism and
blood pressure differences among black men. *Journal of Behavioral Medicine,
6*(3), 259–278.

James, S. A., LaCroix, A. Z., Kleinbaum, D. G., & Strogatz, D. S. (1984). John
Henryism and blood pressure differences among black men. II. The role of
occupational stressors. *Journal of Behavioral Medicine, 7*(3), 259–275.

Jean, Y. S., & Feagin, J. R. (1998). The family costs of white racism: The case of
African American families. *Journal of Comparative Family Studies, 29*(2),
297–312.

Jewell, K. S. (1983). Black male/female conflict: Internalization of negative
definitions transmitted through imagery. *Western Journal of Black Studies, 7*
(l), 43–48.

Joe, T., & Yu, P. (1984). *The "flip-side" of Black families headed by women: The
economic status of Black men.* Center for the Study of Social Policy.

Johnson, S. M. (2004). *The practice of emotionally focused couple therapy: Creating
connection* (2nd ed.). Routledge.

  (2019). *Attachment theory in practice: Emotionally focused therapy (EFT) with
individuals, couples, and families.* Guilford Press.

  (2020). *The practice of emotionally focused couple therapy: Creating connection*
(3rd ed.). Routledge.

Johnson, S. M., & Greenberg, L. S. (1985). Differential effects of experiential and
problem-solving interventions in resolving marital conflict. *Journal of
Consulting and Clinical Psychology, 53*(2), 175–184.

Johnson, S. M., Hunsley, J., Greenberg, L., & Schindler, D. (1999). Emotionally
focused couples therapy: Status and challenges. *Clinical Psychology: Science
and Practice, 6*(1), 67–79.

Jones, J., & Mosher, W. D. (2013). *Fathers' involvement with their children:
United States, 2006–2010* (National Health Statistics Report No. 70).
National Center for Health Statistics.

Kaplan, G., Ranjit, N., & Burgard, S. (2008). Lifting gates – lengthening lives:
Did civil rights policies improve the health of African-American women in
the 1960s and 1970s? In R F. Schoeni, J. S. House, G. A. Kaplan, & H.

Pollack (Eds.), *Making Americans healthier: Social and economic policy as health policy* (pp. 145–169). Russell Sage Foundation.

Kearney, M. S., & Levine, P. (2017, March 13). The *"marriage premium for children" depends on family resources*. Brookings Institution. https://www.brookings.edu/blog/social-mobility-memos/2017/03/13/the-marriage-premium-for-children-depends-on-family-resources

Keller, H. (2013). Attachment and culture. *Journal of Cross-Cultural Psychology, 44* (2), 175–194.

Kelly, S., & Boyd-Franklin, N. (2009). Joining, understanding, and supporting Black couples in treatment. In M. Rastogi & V. Thomas (Eds.), *Multicultural couple therapy* (pp. 235–254). Sage Publications.

Kelly, S., & Floyd, F. J. (2001). The effects of negative racial stereotypes and Afrocentricity on couple relationships. *Journal of Family Psychology, 156,* 110–123.

Kelly, S., & Hudson, B. N. (2017). African American couples and families and the context of structural oppression. In S. Kelly (Ed.), *Diversity in couple and family therapy: Ethnicities, sexualities, and socioeconomics* (pp. 3–32). Praeger/ABC-CLIO.

King, A. E., & Allen, T. T. (2009). Personal characteristics of the ideal African American marriage partner: A survey of adult Black men and women. *Journal of Black Studies, 39*(4), 570–588.

Koball, H. (1998). Have African American men become less committed to marriage? Explaining the twentieth century racial cross-over in men's marriage timing. *Demography, 35*(2), 251–258.

Kogan, S. M., Yu, T., & Brown, G. L. (2016). Romantic relationship commitment behavior among emerging adult African American men. *Journal of Marriage and Family, 78*(4), 996–1012.

Komarraju, M., & Cokley, K. O. (2008). Horizontal and vertical dimensions of individualism-collectivism: A comparison of African Americans and European Americans. *Cultural Diversity and Ethnic Minority Psychology, 14*(4), 336–343.

Landry, B. (1987). *The new black middle class*. University of California Press.

LaTaillade, J. J. (2006). Considerations for treatment of African American couple relationships. *Journal of Cognitive Psychotherapy, 20*(4), 341–358.

Lichter, D. T., LeClere, F. B., & McLaughlin, D. K. (1991). Local marriage markets and the marital behavior of black and white women. *American journal of Sociology, 96*(4), 843–867.

Link, B. G., & Phelan, J. C. (2001). Conceptualizing stigma. *Annual review of Sociology, 27*(1), 363–385.

Lopez, F. G., Melendez, M. C., & Rice, K. G. (2000). Parental divorce, parent-child bonds, and adult attachment orientations among college students: A comparison of three racial/ethnic groups. *Journal of Counseling Psychology, 47,* 177–186.

Lynch, M. F. (2013). Attachment, autonomy, and emotional reliance: A multilevel model. *Journal of Counseling & Development, 91*(3), 301–312.

Magai, C., Cohen, C., Milburn, N., Thorpe, B. McPherson, R., & Peralta, D. (2001). Attachment styles in older European American and African American adults. *The Journals of Gerontology: Series B: Psychological Sciences and Social Sciences, 56B*(1), S28–S35.

Majors, R., & Billson, J. M. (1993). *Cool pose: The dilemma of Black manhood in America*. Simon and Schuster.

Mason, P. (2006). *Reproducing racism: Reconstructing the political economy of race and persistent stratification economics*. Working paper, Florida State University.

Matsumoto, D. (1993). Ethnic differences in affect intensity, emotion judgments, display rule attitudes, and self-reported emotional expression in an American sample. *Motivation and Emotion, 17*(2), 107–123.

McLanahan, S., & Booth, K. (1989). Mother-only families: Problems, prospects, and politics. *Journal of Marriage and the Family, 51*(3), 557–580.

McLanahan, S., & Sandefur, G. D. (1994). *Growing up with a single parent: What hurts, what helps*. Harvard University Press.

Miller, E. (1991). *Men at risk*. Jamaica Publishing House.

Murry, V. M., Brown, P. A., Brody, G. H., Cutrona, C. E., & Simons, R. L. (2001). Racial discrimination as a moderator of the links among stress, maternal psychological functioning, and family relationships. *Journal of Marriage and Family, 63*(4), 915–926.

Nightingale, M., Awosan, C. I., & Stavrianopoulos, K. (2019). Emotionally focused therapy: A culturally sensitive approach for African American heterosexual couples. *Journal of Family Psychotherapy, 30*(3), 221–244.

Nobles, W. W. (1976). African science: The consciousness of self. In L. M. King, V. J. Dixon, & W. W. Nobles (Eds.), *African philosophy: Assumptions and paradigms for research on Black persons* (pp. 163–174). Fanon Research and Development Center.

Nobles, W. W. (1978). Toward an empirical and theoretical framework for defining black families. *Journal of Marriage and Family, 40*(4), 679–688.

Noël, R. A. (2014, November). *Income and spending patterns among black households: Beyond the numbers*. U.S. Bureau of Labor Statistics. https://www.bls.gov/opub/btn/volume-3/income-and-spending-patterns-among-black-households.htm

Ogungbure, A. (2019). The political economy of niggerdom: WEB Du Bois and Martin Luther King Jr. on the racial and economic discrimination of black males in America. *Journal of Black Studies, 50*(3), 273–297.

Oluwayomi, A. (2020). The man-not and the inapplicability of intersectionality to the dilemmas of black manhood. *The Journal of Men's Studies, 28*(2), 183–205.

Orbuch, T. L., Veroff, J., Hassan, H., & Horrocks, J. (2002). Who will divorce: A 14-year longitudinal study of black couples and white couples. *Journal of Social and Personal Relationships, 19*(2), 179–202.

Parham, T. A. (1989). Cycles of psychological nigrescence. *The Counseling Psychologist, 17*(2), 187–226.

Pettit, B. (2012). *Invisible men: Mass incarceration and the myth of black progress.* Russell Sage Foundation.

Pew Charitable Trust Forum. (2009a). *African-Americans and religion.* http:// www.pewforum.org/2009/01/30/african-americans-and-religion

(2009b). *A religious portrait of African Americans.* http://www.pewforum.org/ 2009/01/30/a-religious-portrait-of-african-americans

Pew Research Center. (2015, December 17). *Parenting in America: Outlook, worries, aspirations are strongly linked to financial situation.* https://www .pewresearch.org/social-trends/2015/12/17/parenting-in-america/

Rodgers, W. L., & Thornton, A. (1985). Changing patterns of first marriage in the United States. *Demography, 22,* 265–279.

Ross, J. M., Karney, B. R., Nguyen, T. P., & Bradbury, T. N. (2019). Communication that is maladaptive for middle-class couples is adaptive for socioeconomically disadvantaged couples. *Journal of Personality and Social Psychology, 116*(4), 582–597.

Sampson, R. J. (1987). Urban black violence: The effect of male joblessness and family disruption. *American Journal of Sociology, 93*(2), 348–382.

Schneider, D. (2011). Wealth and the marital divide. *American Journal of Sociology, 117*(2), 627–667.

Sellers, R. M., Copeland-Linder, N., Martin, P. P., & Lewis, R. L. H. (2006). Racial identity matters: The relationship between racial discrimination and psychological functioning in African American adolescents. *Journal of Research on Adolescence, 16*(2), 187–216.

Sellers, R. M., Smith, M. A., Shelton, J. N., Rowley, S. A., & Chavous, T. M. (1998). Multidimensional model of racial identity: A reconceptualization of African American racial identity. *Personality and Social Psychology Review, 2* (1), 18–39.

Seltzer, J. A. (1994). Consequences of marital dissolution for children. *Annual Review of Sociology, 20*(1), 235–266.

Shorter-Gooden, K. (2008). Therapy with African American men and women. In H. A. Neville, B. M. Tynes, & S. O. Utsey (Eds.), *Handbook of African American psychology* (pp. 445–458). Sage Publications.

Sidanius, J., Hudson, S. K. T., Davis, G., & Bergh, R. (2018). The theory of gendered prejudice: A social dominance and intersectionalist perspective. In A. Mintz & L. G. Terris (Eds.), *The Oxford handbook of behavioral political science* (pp. 1–35). Oxford University Press.

Sidanius, J., & Pratto, F. (1999). *Social dominance: An intergroup theory of social hierarchy and oppression.* Cambridge University Press.

Sidanius, J., & Veniegas, R. C. (2000). Gender and race discrimination: The interactive nature of disadvantage. In S. Oskamp (Ed.), *Reducing prejudice and discrimination* (pp. 47–69). Lawrence Erlbaum Associates Publishers.

Simien, E. (2007). A Black gender gap? Continuity and change in attitudes toward Black feminism. In W. Rich (Ed.), *African American perspectives on political science* (pp. 130–150). Temple University Press.

South, S. J. (1996). Mate availability and the transition to unwed motherhood: A paradox of population structure. *Journal of Marriage and the Family, 58*(2), 265–279.

Staples, R. (1978). Masculinity and race: The dual dilemma of Black men. *Journal of Social Issues, 34*(1), 169–183.

(1985). Changes in black family structure: The conflict between family ideology and structural conditions. *Journal of Marriage and the Family, 47*(4), 1005–1013.

Stewart, J. B., & Scott, J. W. (1978). The institutional decimation of Black American males. *The Western Journal of Black Studies, 2*(2), 82–92.

Strobino, D. M., & Sirageldin, I. (1981). Racial differences in early marriages in the United States. *Social Science Quarterly, 62*(4), 758–766.

Taylor, J. (1990). Relationship between internalized racism and marital satisfaction. *Journal of Black Psychology, 16*(2), 45–53.

Taylor, J., & Zhang, X. (1990). Cultural identity in maritally distressed and non-distressed Black couples. *The Western Journal of Black Studies, 14*(4), 205–213.

Testa, M., & Krogh, M. (1995). The effect of employment on marriage among black males in inner-city Chicago. In M. B. Tucker & C. Mitchell-Kernan (Eds.), *The decline in marriage among African Americans* (pp. 59–95). Russell Sage Foundation.

Thompson, C. E., & Carter, R. T. (1997). An overview and elaboration of Helms' racial identity development theory. In C. E. Thompson & R. T. Carter (Eds.), *Racial identity theory: Applications to individual, group, and organizational interventions* (pp. 15–32). Routledge.

Tyrell, F. A., & Masten, A. S. (2021). Father–child attachment in Black families: Risk and protective processes. *Attachment & Human Development, 24*(3), 1–13.

Unnever, J. D., & Chouhy, C. (2021). Race, racism, and the Cool Pose: Exploring Black and White male masculinity. *Social Problems, 68*(2), 490–512.

Utley, E. A. (2016). Humanizing blackness: An interview with Tommy J. Curry. *Southern Communication Journal, 81*(4), 263–266.

van Ijzendoorn, M. H., & Sagi-Schwartz, A. (2008). Cross-cultural patterns of attachment: Universal and contextual dimensions. In J. Cassidy & P. R. Shaver (Eds.), *Handbook of attachment: Theory, research and clinical applications* (pp. 713–734). Guilford Press.

Vaterlaus, J. M., Skogrand, L., Chaney, C., & Gahagan, K. (2017). Marital expectations in strong African American marriages. *Family Process, 56*(4), 883–899.

Vowels, L. M., Vowels, M. J., & Mark, K. P. (2022). Is infidelity predictable? Using explainable machine learning to identify the most important predictors of infidelity. *The Journal of Sex Research, 59*(2), 224–237.

Walum, L. R. (1977). *The dynamics of sex and gender: A sociological perspective.* Rand McNally.

Watson, T., & McLanahan, S. (2011). Marriage meets the joneses relative income, identity, and marital status. *Journal of Human Resources*, *46*(3), 482–517.

Wei, M., Russell, D. W., Mallinckrodt, B., & Zakalik, R. A. (2004). Cultural equivalence of adult attachment across four ethnic groups: Factor structure, structured means, and associations with negative mood. *Journal of Counseling Psychology*, *51*, 408–417.

West, C. M. (1995). Mammy, Sapphire, and Jezebel: Historical images of Black women and their implications for psychotherapy. *Psychotherapy: Theory, Research, Practice, Training*, *32*(3), 458–466.

White, J. L. (1970, September). Toward a Black psychology. *Ebony*, 43–50.

Wiebe, S. A., & Johnson, S. M. (2016). A review of the research in emotionally focused therapy for couples. *Family Process*, *55*(3), 390–407.

Willhelm, S. M. (1986). The economic demise of blacks in America: a prelude to genocide? *Journal of Black Studies*, *17*(2), 201–254.

Wilson, W. J. (1987). *The truly disadvantaged: The inner city, the underclass, and public policy*. University of Chicago Press.

Wolfers, J., Leonhardt, D., & Qualy, K. (2015, April 20). 1. 5 million missing black men. *The New York Times*. https://www.nytimes.com/interactive/2015/04/20/upshot/missing-black-men.html

Woods-Giscombé, C. L. (2010). Superwoman schema: African American women's views on stress, strength, and health. *Qualitative Health Research*, *20*(5), 668–683.

Yi, J., Neville, H. A., Todd, N. R., & Mekawi, Y. (2022). Ignoring race and denying racism: A meta-analysis of the associations between colorblind racial ideology, anti-Blackness, and other variables antithetical to racial justice. *Journal of Counseling Psychology*. Advance online publication. https://doi.org/10.1037/cou0000618

Use of the Gottman Method with African American Couples Impacted by Post-Traumatic Slave Syndrome

Satira Streeter Corbitt

From the time the first Africans were stolen from their homes and sold into slavery, there have been concerted efforts to destroy their sense of self and connection to each other. The system of slavery sought to destroy existing relationships and slavery undermined the ability to make new ones. More than 400 years later these efforts continue to persist and so do the resulting challenges faced by descendants of American enslavement who strive to create healthy relationships. Slavery, "breeding," Jim Crow, the prison industrial complex, and police brutality have all operated to weaken the Black family, create divisions between African American men and women, and destroy the African American community. This is exhibited by the fact that African Americans have higher rates of divorce and single parent–headed households, and lower rates of marriage and marital stability than other racial groups in the United States (National Healthy Marriage Resource Center, n.d.).

This chapter explores the trauma and challenges African American couples face along with the relevance of Dr. Joy DeGruy's theory of Post-Traumatic Slave Syndrome (PTSS) in the conceptualization of clinical assessment. In direct response to the horrific trauma of legalized slavery and segregation and the continued impact of systemic racism and oppression from which African Americans suffer, no evidence-based couples therapy method has been created, funded, or researched. However, among the most utilized couples therapies in the United States, the Gottman Method has the most trauma-aligning theories and exercises (Gottman & Gottman, 2017) and those tools are explored along with how they can be aligned with culturally responsive care. A case conceptualization of an African American couple that has been impacted by Post-Traumatic Slave Syndrome and treated using Gottman Method interventions are also presented.

Despite these challenges, Black love endures, and many couples are able to cultivate a true sense of happiness, solidarity, and support for their families and their greater communities. Strong villages, supportive religious institutions, and self-determination have all been attributed to this success (DeGruy, 2017). Relatedly, research has shown that these relationships can be enhanced by the incorporation of therapy and culturally relevant psychoeducational programs that help couples establish healthier unions and satisfaction through improved relationship skills and communication (Mikle & Gilbert, 2019). Unfortunately, there are many barriers to African American couples seeking therapeutic help including cost, location outside of African American communities, time, child care, stigma, and limited office hours (Davis et al., 2008). The biggest barrier to therapy, however, is the therapists themselves. There has been a long-standing healthy cultural suspicion of seeking therapy within the African American community because of the racist roots of psychology and the helping professions overall (Guthrie, 2004). Psychiatrists Grier and Cobbs (1968) coined the term, "Healthy Cultural Paranoia" in their classic text *Black Rage* and spoke to the impact that slavery, discrimination, and racism has had on the psyche of African Americans. Clinicians have subsequently expanded on this theory stating that past racist and insensitive ideas and behaviors of psychologists have caused "Cultural Mistrust" which makes potential clients doubtful that therapists would be capable and/or willing to render effective therapeutic treatment (Whaley, 2001). In addition, a 2016 study conducted by Kugelmass found that Black middle-class individuals were considerably less likely to be offered an appointment and working class individuals were three times less likely to receive an appointment.

Couples who are able to access services that are culturally responsive, trauma informed, empowering, and facilitated by clinicians who understand their past and current issues are better served than those couples that have to fit the mode of an ideal therapy client. This mode is historically described by Schofield (1964) as YAVIS, young, attractive, verbal, intelligent, and successful, traits more often attributed to white women. Clinicians who deny or minimize the historical trauma and continued impact of systemic racism, oppression, and implicit bias on their African American clients are not only ineffectual but harmful to the healing process and should under no circumstances attempt to serve these couples.

7.1 Racist Experiences of Black Couples in the United States

During every period of Black existence in the United States, systemic racism and disregard of the Black family unit have negatively impacted

African American couples (Gaskin et al., 2004). During enslavement, Black marriages were not legally recognized because the enslaved were considered the property of their white enslavers. Although informal marriages were pursued, the relationships were consistently undermined so that white enslavers could rape, breed, and sell women as they desired (Franke, 1999). Following the era of legalized slavery, Black Codes were created to maintain free labor lost from its abolishment. These "laws" restricted freedom and when broken, led to Black males being placed in forced work situations. Former enslaved Africans who chose to work less than they had while enslaved to focus more time on family were considered vagrants, which was determined to be unlawful and grounds for the punishment of forced labor, thus removing Black men from the home. During this time the Freedmen's Bureau, established to "help" former slaves, designated Black husbands as heads of households, when previously an egalitarianism system had been practiced. This caused new friction in households by imposing a white construct on Black families that still exists today (Giddings, 2014).

The current generation of African American marriages has been impacted by early welfare laws, high unemployment, and mass incarceration. In all three instances, men have either been prohibited from being in the home, unable to financially contribute to the home, or removed from the home, all causing lasting damage to women and children and destabilization of relationships. Systemic issues that start early in life, including miseducation, generations of missing fathers, and geographic disempowerment also contribute to issues in adult relationships. These frequent occurrences support DeGruy's (2017) framework of PTSS, in that many of the current issues in Black relationships can be linked to the aforementioned issues that are rooted in Black displacement to America, issues that have now been passed down through generations with little significant acknowledgment, help, or intervention. This historical context must be considered by therapists because couples will often present with what the author refers to as *veiled shackles*. These unconscious blocks in relationships, and subsequently therapy, may be hidden but the impact is far reaching. Veiled shackles can be further hidden because of time passed, success, education, and charismatic personalities. Years of unacknowledged, unrecognized, and untreated trauma has an impact on the ability to form healthy relationships. Therapists must be aware of the deeply embedded issues and adaptions that individuals have made in order to survive generations of psychological and physical trauma.

7.2   Post-Traumatic Slave Syndrome

DeGruy (2017) defined PTSS as the condition that exists when a population has experienced multigenerational trauma resulting from centuries of slavery and continues to experience oppression and institutionalized racism presently. Added to this condition is a belief (real or imagined) that the benefits of society in which they live are not accessible to them.

DeGruy (2017) indicated that the presence of PTSS and the attitudes and behaviors therein are counter to the skills needed to build and nurture healthy marriages and relationships. She explained

> A Black couple bears the same burdens as any couple bears: finding gainful employment to support themselves; establishing a strong base from which to raise healthy children; carving out time to escape life's daily hassles and rekindle tender bonds of affection; time to simply do life in the best possible way. However, they have some additional baggage given to them by family long gone-old, dirty, and heavy baggage that needs to be repaired or discarded. (p. 136)

She further indicated that although every African American has been impacted by PTSS, all individuals respond to trauma differently and there are many patterns and degrees of behavior that can manifest. Her explanatory theory focuses on the three categories that are most pervasive: vacant esteem, ever-present anger, and racist socialization (DeGruy, 2017).

According to DeGruy, *vacant esteem* is the act of minimizing your worth as it is minimized in society, community, and/or family. Examples of societal constructs that lead to vacant esteem include poorly funded schools, inadequate social services, discriminatory policies, unjust laws, and negative media portrayals. Community may serve as a microsystem of society by establishing norms that do not support equity or reinforce stereotypes that are misaligned with the uniqueness of the individuals within. Families, who have their own long-standing trauma, may inadvertently raise children to conform to the society and community in which they were born. When society, community, and family present a negative and/or limited identity that feels confining, vacant esteem can result. This esteem not only impacts how one views him or herself, it effects how they view other African Americans as well, especially their romantic partners (DeGruy, 2017).

DeGruy (2017) explained *ever-present anger* as "a well spring of anger that lies just below the surface of many African Americans, and it doesn't take much for it to emerge and be expressed" (p. 112). This anger is often a result of years of societal abuse, blocked goals, fears, frustrations, and the expectation of survival under oppressive conditions. Slavery, systemic racism, Jim Crow, present- day police brutality, Trumpism, and overall white supremacy are the most angry and violent processes that have existed in the United States. According to DeGruy, any group of people living under such harsh conditions would eventually learn the ways modeled by their captors over the last 400 years. Anger and violence have been the American way; however, when it manifests in African Americans it is scorned, criticized, and often times, viciously punished. Because the true orchestrators of oppression and frustration are out of reach, partners may become the unintentional targets of this fury, just because they are present (DeGruy, 2017).

Lastly, *racist socialization* is theorized as the adoption of the attitudes, values, and views of white superiority. People, things, and ideas associated with European Americans are taught and thought to be better, more intelligent, and overall, more desirable. From the inception of the slave trade, African Americans were taught to see Black characteristics, religion, vernacular, and people as inferior and not to be valued. In addition, white standards including beauty, material success, and denial of the significance of Black history, have been adopted by many African Americans in an attempt to assimilate to the dominant culture. Racist socialization, akin to the idea of internalized racism in the literature, is further demonstrated by African Americans who glamorize violence, lack of education, sexual irresponsibility, substance abuse, and the deprecation of themselves and other African Americans (DeGruy, 2017).

7.3   Hope in the Struggle

Despite systemic racism, veiled shackles, and the multilayered traumas that African Americans have faced in this country, one-third of African American adults are married (Cohn et al., 2011) and many others indicate that they desire to be married (Bent-Goodley, 2014). This demonstrates that Black love is miraculous and real but generational adaptions to structural racism have resulted in some attitudes and behaviors that undermine the strength and health of Black relationships.

Effective therapeutic interventions must acknowledge systemic challenges as well as the impact that these challenges have had on clients. Whereas not all African Americans have been negatively impacted to the same degree, the denial of systemic racism and PTSS by clinicians is detrimental to clients and may lead to incomplete assessments and inadequate treatment. In addition, clinicians must recognize the importance of cultural mores, spirituality, family and community; encourage individual and collective functioning; and acknowledging the critical ways that people are interdependent (Bent-Goodley et al., 2017). Lastly, couples should be empowered with tools and interventions that they can use independently, outside of therapy, in order to establish new, healthier patterns of behavior and relationship. These therapeutic elements utilized by culturally responsive, trauma informed therapists are critical to facilitate greater therapeutic success and minimize harm.

7.4 Gottman Method Couples Therapy Overview

The Gottman Method, developed by John and Julie Gottman, was based on more than forty years of research with thousands of couples (Gottman & Silver, 2015). The primary goals of the Gottman Method are to focus on emotion, skill building for managing conflict, the development of new skills for enhancing friendship, and helping the couple to create a system of shared meaning together (Gottman & Gottman, 2016). To achieve these goals, the Gottman Method begins with a comprehensive assessment. To begin, a thorough assessment of the couple is completed using a computerized "Relationship Checkup" tool, along with joint and individual in-depth oral interviews. During the oral interview the couple also engages in a ten-minute conflict discussion that is used to recognize communication patterns and difficulties. Following the assessment, the couple is presented with a synopsis that identifies their strengths and challenges based on the Sound Relationship House Theory, the Gottman's integrative approach to couple therapy. This three-part assessment is used to form a projected duration of therapy and the Gottman Interventions to be used within the couple's treatment plan.

Gottman-trained therapists have at their disposal a plethora of therapeutic interventions designed to strengthen relationships through friendship, conflict management, and creation of shared meaning. All of these interventions strengthen the various levels of the Sound Relationship House and result in more fulfilling, positive interactions. The foundational exercises include the Gottman-Rappaport, Dreams within Conflict, Self-Soothing, Compromise, and Aftermath of a Fight or Regrettable Incident, each of which is discussed later in the chapter.

7.5 Use of the Gottman Method with Black Couples Impacted by PTSS

Being trauma informed means couples therapists will recognize, understand, and address the impact and persistence of trauma in the lives of the

African American couples they see (Levenson, 2017). Funding, time, and interest have often not been dedicated to the explicit study of Black couples; therefore clinicians often have to adjust broader research and methods to effectively serve this population. Although the Gottman Method has not focused specifically on the current and historical traumas, oppression, systemic racism, and importance of the extended families in the lives of Black couples, no evidence-based couples therapy method has. In developing their Sound Relationship House theory and their therapeutic interventions, however, general trauma, triggers, the importance of learning new behaviors, empowerment, and storytelling have been incorporated. Many of their interventions can be enhanced if skilled therapists are the facilitators and special consideration is given to the impact of PTSS and the family and societal culture that exist within African Americans.

7.5.1 Considerations for Gottman Assessment with African American Couples Impacted by PTSS

There are thirteen standard Gottman "Oral History" interview questions, ten of which are asked at the discretion of the therapist. Only one of the optional questions inquires about their parent's marriage/relationship, and none focus on extended family, community, culture, impact of racism/oppression, or childhood/current trauma. Therapists working with African American couples should include these questions as standard practice when working for a thorough assessment. DeGruy encourages couples to create a "virtual village" with a network of individuals who can support the relationship – individuals who are trusted and respected regardless of their familial relationship. This village is present to provide support, advice, and guidance. During the assessment phase the therapist should inquire about the village's input during the dating stage and early stages of the relationship. Healthy village involvement can serve as a strength when difficulties arise. The quality of the village becomes very important and in the early stages of therapy couples should be encouraged to evaluate these relationships. Additionally, asking about the relationships "cheerleaders and haters" and detailed information pertaining to both is extremely valuable. In addition, the enhanced relationship checkup has an optional demographic section that asks questions related to income levels that clinicians might consider asking couples to skip as this information may be off-putting to African American couples who are forming a relationship with a new therapist. Clinicians must be aware of the aforementioned Cultural Mistrust (Whaley, 2001) in that clients are often suspicious of the intentions of helpers as well as how they are being judged. These questions are also aligned with Western concepts of worth and wealth and can shade the therapeutic lens of therapy and activate implicit bias.

7.5.2 The Sound Relationship House and Post-Traumatic Slave Syndrome

Gottman's method is based on a structural framework for partnership that he calls the Sound Relationship House (Gottman & Gottman, 2016). This house has seven components that build upon each other as well as two pillars that support the relationship structure. The assessment and interventions are incorporated into this house.

7.5.2.1 Love Maps

This level is the first of the three friendship foundational levels and it focuses on how well a couple knows each other's inner psychological world including their worries, stresses, joys, and dreams. This level also indicates how well a couple knows and is responsive to each other's triggers, pain, and past traumas.

Couples who have demonstrated strengths in the assessment of their Love Maps know and understand themselves and their partner's racial socialization including the impact that assimilation and acculturation have had on their lives, positive and negative experiences with the majority culture, and experiences with colorism – the judgment of individuals based on the shade of their skin. They will be in regular communication with their partner, allowing them to vent often, and keeping abreast of the external stressors, including those of racism and oppression.

Couples challenged in this area will likely not be in consistent, healthy communication with each other and may even demonstrate the Chameleon Effect – becoming what their partner wants them to be, detaching from who they really are (Gottman & Gottman, 2017)-related to DeGruy's (2017) concept of Vacant Esteem. Lack of knowledge of each other's world and inner workings will lead to greater emotional distance, which can be disconnecting when isolation already exists due to structural racism and/or PTSS-related family of origin dysfunction.

In addition, a couple impacted by PTSS likely has difficulty understanding their own true selves, which makes it extremely difficult to know and understand their partner. The client may be displaying his or her representative and how they want to be viewed, either from a prosocial or antisocial lens, which may make it difficult to truly know who they really are. An antisocial persona may be displayed as a protective factor and an overly prosocial persona may be demonstrated because the partner may have great disdain for themselves and their perceived inadequacies and have been taught that they must always demonstrate social compliance in order to be liked and accepted by others. The PTSS-impacted individual may be so cut off from their own feelings that their triggers and comforts may be unrecognizable to themselves.

7.5.2.1.1 Examples of PTSS Issues That May Appear Related to Love Maps Vacant Esteem. Rayshard has had difficulty achieving financial success as expected by society and sees himself as having no worth. He devalues himself and feels unworthy of being known or recognizing his other qualities.

Ever-Present Anger. Marcus lost his football scholarship and was kicked out of college because of false exam cheating accusations. He later married and began having children and never obtained his degree. Although he is brilliant, without out a degree he has never been able to achieve the career success that he once dreamed of. Anger may be the emotion that is in the forefront to his partner, while fear and sadness may remain hidden and unknown, not allowing true triggers to be understood.

Racist Socialization. Aura has been conditioned to idolize white people and has learned to assimilate to their perceived attributes. Her view of herself and her African American partner is through the lens of inferiority and she is often degrading herself and him.

7.5.2.2 Fondness and Admiration

The next level of the Sound Relationship House focuses on affection and respect and is achieved by shifting focus on what the partner is doing wrong to what they are doing right. Couples who demonstrate a strength in this area will create a culture of appreciation (Gottman & Gottman, 2017) in which they make it a regular practice to find the positive in their partner and verbalize their appreciation for the relationship.

Couples who are challenged in this area may vilify their partner as the enemy, when the true enemy is out of reach, making consistent shows of fondness and admiration difficult. They may struggle with accepting fondness and admiration and see it as not genuine, especially when the world around them tells them that they are no good. They may block out loving words because it is in direct conflict with what they have been taught to think about themselves by society. They may also feel the need to maintain their own emotional distance and their invisibility (Gottman & Gottman, 2017).

7.5.2.2.1   Examples of PTSS Issues That May Appear Related to Fondness and Admiration
Vacant Esteem. Stephon sees himself as having no worth so he distrusts his partner's expressions of fondness and admiration.

Ever-Present Anger. Botham's displaced anger has turned into emotional abuse which has made it difficult for Michelle to feel fondness or admiration.

Racist Socialization. Philando's value system is based on what is admirable in white couples and Western society standards. He sees the strength of Janisha as unattractive and masculine while viewing the vulnerability and meekness of Bob's white wife as more desirable and feminine.

7.5.2.3   Turning Toward
The third level of the Sound Relationship House focuses on the couple's emotional connection. According to Gottman's theory, individuals make small bids to their partners in order to connect. One can decide to either turn toward these bids (respond positively), turn away (ignore), or turn against (reject). When partners turn toward each other, Gottman says that they have built their "Emotional Bank Account," which they can then pull from when challenging times arise (Gottman & Silver, 2015). African American couples who demonstrate this area as a strength see themselves and their partner as lovable, are confident in their ability to fill their partner's love bank, and recognize the source of their anger, without wrongly targeting their partner. They focus on the small things that occur on a daily basis that strengthen their relationship and utilize the relationship as a protective factor against a harsh society.

For a couple challenged in this area, the vulnerability of making an emotional bid that is not accepted may invoke fears of rejection and ridicule based on past experiences. Partners may be ill equipped to recognize the bid and their high defense level or suspicion may cause them to automatically turn against. Bids for emotional connection may also be minimized because of the ever threat of harm, equating to loss of one's partner. Reducing intimacy may be thought to reduce the experience of future hurt. Loss has been present since arrival in the United States and has manifested by being sold (through slavery or imprisonment), killed, or dying prematurely from a preventable disease.

7.5.2.3.1   Examples of PTSS Issues That May Appear Related to Turning Toward
Vacant Esteem. Eric does not see himself as having the tools or

ability to fill Gabriella's Emotional Bank Account. He does not feel worth being turned toward.

Ever-Present Anger. Tanisha's bids are often rejected by Akai because of his anger that lingers from outside situations and clouds his ability to see her efforts and desire to connect with him. She has now stopped making bids.

Racist Socialization. Alexia makes bids for emotional connection but becomes complacent in needing to be turned toward because she assumes she is not worthy of connection because of disparaging remarks that have been made about her skin color in past relationships.

7.5.2.4 Positive Sentiment Override

The first three levels of the Sound Relationship House are referred to as the friendship levels. If these levels are solid, positive affect will be present, even in times of conflict. Couples who demonstrate strengths in this area will be more likely to repair when missteps occur and have the tools necessary to build and maintain authentic friendships despite the challenges they face.

For couples challenged in this area, by the time they are at an age to be partnered, their experiences with trauma, disappointment, and injustice make it extremely difficult to have a Positive Sentiment about life, much less their partner. When Negative Sentiment Override exists, signals, whether neutral or positive, are automatically seen as negative. Their lens may be clouded in that no matter how much they attempt to see the glass as half full, their life experiences have reflected emptiness. They are not just seeing life as hypothetically negative, they are assured that negative experiences and events are a daily occurrence.

7.5.2.4.1 Examples of PTSS Issues that May Appear Related to Positive Sentiment Override Vacant Esteem. Mya sees herself as worthless, so her view of her life and relationship is negative in general.

Ever-Present Anger. Miriam's adverse experiences in childhood and repeated blocked goals result in anger, which leads to an override of negative sentiments.

Racist Socialization. Tamir has been shown throughout his life that that Black love, Black life, and Black existence are all negative. He has found it impossible to have a positive sentiment override in the midst of 400 years of this disparagement being ingrained.

7.5.2.5   *Managing Conflict*

In order to manage conflict (according to Gottman, resolution of conflict is not the goal) the therapist helps the couple identify core issues and communication failures that trigger escalation. Gottman places conflict into two categories, resolvable and perpetual, which could lead to gridlock. Positive dialogue is taught and practiced throughout sessions. In theory there needs to be a 5–1 positive-to-negative ratio of affect, which means that for every negative exchange, five positives need to occur (Gottman & Silver, 2015). Couples who demonstrate strengths in this area often come into the relationship with the ability to compromise, self-soothe, and understand their own triggers.

PTSS impacted couples who are challenged in this area may have had models of ineffective conflict management that have been passed down through generations have difficulty embodying new modes. Strict discipline techniques are often used as a protective method, to control children's behaviors to lessen the risk of harsher punishments from whites in power that could include harassment, brutality, or death (Patton, 2017). DeGruy (2017) further explains that many parents have downgraded the positive characteristics of their children, starting during slavery as a protective factor so that they would not be seen as desirable, financially, sexually, or industrially, by white enslavers, a practice that unconsciously continues today. Relatedly, even in adulthood, individuals may have adapted to receiving and giving these criticisms and need additional assistance in breaking these patterns.

Childhood trauma also manifests because of neighborhood violence, poverty, substance abuse of family members, fatherlessness, and illness. The more traumatic one's childhood is, the more triggers are transferred into adulthood and pulled within relationships. Children may be taught that they have to fight to get what they want and too much discussion may be seen as manipulation, often times in racist and dysfunctional school settings. Being raised by traumatized parents, raised by prior traumatized generations often leads to more trauma and maladaptive problem solving. Because independent opinions and intelligence have not historically been valued by Whites, the attempt to demonstrate these qualities in school or in the workplace, have been discouraged and this adjustment may be made within relationships as well.

One major tenet of conflict management is the ability to self-soothe, which is made much more difficult by constant trauma and an inability to "quiet one's mind." Conflict at home may be downplayed or not addressed, because the conflict outside of the home requires an enormous amount of energy to sustain.

7.5.2.5.1 Examples of PTSS Issues that May Appear Related to Conflict Management

Vacant Esteem. Mannie believes that his ability to win physical and verbal fights is equated to his manhood, so he vows to never lose, even in his marriage.

Ever-Present Anger. LaTanya has been the paralegal for a law firm and is berated on a daily basis. The job pays well, and she sees herself with no other prospects because of how well her bosses are connected. Her anger is hidden during the workday but at home she utilizes all four of the Horsemen of the Apocalypse when dealing with her husband.

Racist Socialization. Shelly does not feel the right to advocate for herself and express her needs so she just accepts behaviors from her husband, even though his behaviors bother her and could likely be corrected

7.5.2.6 Making Life Dreams Come True

On this level, the focus is on both knowing one's partner's dream and working to help them make it come true. Couples who demonstrate this as a strength let their dreams be known so that their partner can help in the realization of these dreams. They talk openly and honestly about their dreams, values, aspirations, needs, and convictions.

Couples for whom this presents as a challenge may not have been able to dream or have their dream realized. One may have been taught to focus on only what one can see and manifest now and not look too far into the future. Day-to-day survival often becomes more critical than future planning. Dreams coming true may be seen as the foundation of fairy tales and white privilege. It is also a possibility that their dreams ae in opposition which create gridlock. At the heart of all gridlocked conflicts are unmet, unrealized dreams or longings.

7.5.2.6.1 Examples of PTSS Issues that May Appear Related to Making Life Dreams Come True

Vacant Esteem. Antwon was raised to focus on the here and now and told that his dreams have no worth or purpose; he does not dream and often criticizes his partner when she shares her dreams.

Ever-Present Anger. Demontre has worked extremely hard to become a supervisor at his job, he's been passed over repeatedly. His anger will not allow him to dream and his embarrassment will not allow him to let his dreams be known.

Racist Socialization. Sharmel was 21 before she saw even a Black Disney Princess; aside from her uncle who won the lottery for $5,000, she's never personally known anyone whose dream has come true. She does not believe in dreaming. Dreams are fairy tales that are created and realized only by white people.

7.5.2.7 Create Shared Meaning

On the top level of the house, couples explore their shared meaning, which may include shared thoughts about legacy, spirituality, service to others, and purpose. Couples that demonstrate this area as a strength, build their life together, recognizing how they prioritize their resources, time, and energy shapes this shared meaning system. The formal and informal rituals that they implement in the relationship and in their families also further explore culture, roles, symbols, and family of origin. Discrepancies and common ground between partners in life meaning are also investigated.

Couples challenged on this level may have a distorted sense of purpose and meaning because they have received messages that their life does not matter. The meaning of life and the decisions regarding how to raise children may be influenced by perceived limits placed by society and it may be difficult for couples to come to a consensus on what rituals, goals, roles, and symbols actually matter.

7.5.2.7.1 Examples of PTSS Issues That May Appear Related to Create Shared Meaning

Vacant Esteem. Shelly focuses on how things look in her marriage as opposed to how things really are and what meaning exists. She has been conditioned to be superficial and not to focus too deeply on things with meaning, because those things always seemed transient in her youth.

Ever-Present Anger. Alton hates the materialism of Christmas and the way that they go broke every year buying extravagant presents for the family. He feels forced to do this because the majority culture requires it. He and his wife have verbal altercations throughout the holiday season.

Racist Socialization. Shareese has been acculturated to view European-based religious systems as the only ones that have meaning ,which causes great friction when Terrence wants the family to explore the African religion of Yoruba.

7.5.2.8 Trust and Commitment

The Sound Relationship House is held up by two pillars, Trust and Commitment. Trust is focused on how confident one is in the notion that their partner has their back. This means trusting that their partner is making decisions, in relationships, money, career, etc., that consider both of their needs and wants. Commitment is the partner's beliefs and actions that indicate that they are in the relationship for a lifetime and are dedicated to celebrating the good times and working through the bad. Couples that demonstrate a strength in this area allow themselves to be vulnerable and do not compare them to others, real or imagined (Gottman & Gottman, 2016).

Couples with PTSS symptoms may be challenged by never seeing examples of commitment and being taught that people are untrustworthy. The aforementioned attacks on the Black family and historical constructs that remove Black husbands and fathers from the home leave models few and far between.

7.5.2.8.1   Examples of PTSS Issues That May Appear Related to Trust and Commitment   Vacant Esteem. Sandra does not know her worth and makes decisions that are not in the best interest of herself, much less her partner, Jonathan. Because of her poor decisions, he has difficulty trusting her and loses hope in the longevity of the relationship.

Ever-Present Anger. Walter's frustration and fear have manifested in a lingering anger that is often misdirected toward his wife, making him suspicious of her actions, often believing that she will betray him as he feels that life has.

Racist Socialization. Atatiana married Marqueese three years ago; however, her commitment has waned because she no longer believes that he is "good enough" for her because of his inability to provide the lifestyle that her coworkers' husbands provide.

7.6   Four Horsemen of the Apocalypse

Gottman and Gottman (2016) indicate that there are four mistakes in communication that are so lethal, they refer to them as the Four Horsemen of the Apocalypse: Criticism, Defensiveness, Contempt, and Stonewalling. When utilized, these weapons of destruction tear down the house and can become strong predictors of divorce.

Criticism is a direct attack on your partner's character versus making a legitimate complaint about their behavior that is impacting you negatively. The antidote to Criticism is a Soften Start-Up. Whereas a harsh start-up typically leads to further difficulty and an unproductive end, a softened start-up states a partner's feelings, trigger, and need. A harsh start-up regarding a partner not answering his phone would be "you are so shady, you must be doing something wrong, you never answer my calls when you leave the house." However, a softened start-up would be "I feel anxious, when you sometimes don't answer the phone. I need for you to answer the phone or send a quick text to strengthen our communication." Research indicates that criticism is most used by women.

Contempt is like criticism's big, bad brother. When a partner uses contempt, not only are they being critical, they are also expressing an air of superiority in intelligence, common sense, or morality. A contemptuous comment would be, "your junk is everywhere, you are so triflin', I guess that's just how you were raised." This comment is not only a character attack, it implies that the contemptuous partner was raised better by their parents, because they do not engage in such "trifliness." The antidote to contempt is to describe your own feelings and needs. the Gottmans indicate that contempt is the most dangerous of all of the Four Horsemen and the biggest indicator for divorce.

Defensiveness is described by the Gottmans as a tactic used to not accept feedback given by their partner. Defensiveness manifests in two ways, as an aggressive pushback in that they may blame the partner for doing similar things or as a victim in which they may whine and accuse the partner of "picking on" them when they are doing the best they can. The antidote to defensiveness is accepting responsibility for your partner's complaint, even if you are only able to own a small piece of what is being accused. By attempting to put yourself in your partner's shoes you try to see the issue as they do versus denying all of their feelings and perceptions regarding your behavior and/or actions.

Stonewalling, the last of the Four Horsemen, is often seen as being present in a conflict in body, but having your mind removed. This often happens when a partner gets flooded, a physiological response to stress that prevents you from processing information and communicating in an effective way. Couples who become flooded are encouraged to call a time out and resume the conversation after a twenty-minute to twenty-four-hour break during which both partners spend time self-soothing, a concept that we will dive deeper into when presenting the Gottman interventions. Research indicates that Stonewalling is most used by men; however, women who have been abused or traumatized in any way will experience physiological flooding at the same rate as men.

Gottman and Gottman's (2016) research indicates that even couples who have been using these lethal weapons for years can learn to recognize them and offer their antidotes instead.

7.7 Gottman Foundational Interventions

7.7.1   Gottman Rapoport

The Gottman Rapoport is often one of the first exercises that clinicians will use with clients when they are teaching couples to connect and understand each other. Partners take turns being the listener and the speaker and are instructed not to argue or persuade, but instead just explain their thoughts and feelings about their position on the issue. The "speaker" states their feelings, along with their needs, and is encouraged not to blame or criticize and to recognize that there is a longing that underlies every complaint. The "listener" is encouraged to focus in on their partner's world and hear their pain. They ask open-ended questions to better understand their partner's perspective. During this process they take notes so that they can summarize that they have heard what their partner has said, and later validate and express empathy for their partner's feelings and perception. Both the listening and speaking roles may be difficult for couples impacted by PTSS because of the vulnerability required to share one's heart and to completely shift from their own pain and trauma to focus on their partner's distress. According to Gottman and Gottman's (2017) *Treating Affairs and Trauma* manual, clinicians must be aware of the retriggering and difficulties in completing the exercise in order to tune into clues of deeper trauma. This clinical awareness may lead to gateways toward healing.

7.7.2   Dreams within Conflict

Dreams Within Conflict is used to assist clients in working through a gridlocked or perpetual problem by helping them understand underlying dreams, history, beliefs, and/or values behind their position on the issue. The goal here is not to solve the issue, but to reframe conflicts to be seen as life dreams in opposition. The clinician must be sensitive to the speaker not wanting to talk about historical traumas and recognize the tremendous opportunity for them to be heard and their story to be validated. The couple takes turns talking about their feelings and beliefs and asking six questions that the Gottman Method have found to be effective in exploring the dream. During their turn, the partner is given a sample list of dreams to help identify their ideal dream and then asked about their deeper purpose or goal. The therapist can also encourage the listener to ask questions that delve deeper into relevant values, history, emotions and symbolic meaning in this intervention.

7.7.3   *Self-Soothing*

For the couple impacted by PTSS, self-soothing may be hard to achieve not only because it may not have been modeled or permitted if complex (trauma inflicted by caregivers) or chronic trauma was present in childhood. In conflict, not only is there an emotional reaction, there is also a physiological reaction, which is seen when someone becomes flooded and is most obviously detected when heartbeats exceed 100 per minute. Individuals impacted by PTSS have often normalized flooding and feel that they should just push through it. When feeling tense, couples are encouraged to take a time-out and self-soothe so that they can avoid becoming overwhelmed and engaging in destructive communication. During this process the couple spends time calming themselves through breathing, self-care, relaxation, and healthy distraction. This may present a challenge, however, if taking a break for self-care is seen as a sign of weakness and an inability to handle life and relationship stress.

7.7.4   *Compromise*

The Compromise exercise encourages couples to identify their core needs within a conflict, followed by areas in which they are most flexible so that they can communicate and share in order to find common goals and reach a temporary compromise. The understanding is that everyone is willing to sacrifice something so that they can both make a gain. According to Gottman and Gottman's (2017) *Treating Affairs and Trauma* manual, when the trauma is brought to light, couples may be in a better place to understand what their partner needs, including understanding why their core needs are so important. A traumatized partner may feel safer and become less rigid in their needs. In couples impacted by PTSS, clinicians must be mindful that both partners have likely been traumatized and may not be able to hear or respond to their partner's need or recognize their own. This blockage may need to be more fully processed to determine if there are creative solutions or if the relationship cannot be continued because the intensity of trauma and the rigidity that has followed makes compromise impossible. This exercise should be used only after a Gottman Rapoport or Dreams Within

Conflict so that a meaningful conversation can be held regarding the conflict before a compromise is attempted.

7.7.5   Aftermath of a Fight or a Regrettable Incident

The Aftermath of a Fight or a Regrettable incident is utilized following an episode that is antirelationship and hurtful. The Gottman Method recognizes the role that past incidents, often from childhood, trigger reactions and worsen even the most minute conflict. There are five steps to the exercise and couples are guided through steps that begin with the feelings they experienced during the incident to constructive plans that will prevent a reoccurrence in the future. Couples are asked to discuss the incident without reliving it, remaining calm and emotionally distant from the fight. The Gottmans warn that while going through this exercise, traumatized couples may report feelings that appear disproportional to the incident that has occurred. This is a signal that time must be devoted to processing and connecting their feelings to past occurrences. They are asked to think about how they felt and "review the video tape of their mind" to another time in their past that they have felt a similar way during their childhood or teenage years. Often traumatized individuals make deals with themselves that they will never allow themselves to experience negative feelings or experiences from childhood again, and once feelings return, their anger and frustration toward their partner is intensified for making them renege on their promise. Once each partner is able to recognize these triggers and underlying traumas in the other, healing and efforts to avoid retriggering can begin.

7.8   Couple Conceptualization: Breonna and Trayvon

7.8.1   Brief History

Breonna (age thirty-five) and Trayvon (thirty-eight) have been married for six years and have no children. She recently earned a master's degree and works in the development office of a large predominantly white institution (PWI), while he has his PhD and works as a clinical researcher. Both were born in the South and are considered success stories in their respective families and communities. Trayvon's father was largely absent from the home, as his grandfather had been absent before him. Breonna was raised in a two-parent family but indicates that no emotional support was offered and she and her siblings were simply expected to focus on school, be active in church, and not cause any "problems" for their parents, who both worked extensive hours.

7.8.1.1   Reasons for Seeking Therapy

During their third year of marriage Breonna was laid off from work and, unable to find another job locally, she moved to a city four hours away. While there, Breonna realized that she enjoyed not having the responsibility of a marriage and began to make new friends, reconnect with old friends and enjoy focusing solely on her own needs and wants. Although she denied having an affair, she indicated that she was interested in a divorce, but changed her mind once they were reunited. Trayvon was deeply impacted by her words and actions and no longer trusted her commitment to their union. Breonna now feels that he has emotionally detached from her and because he began spending more time with "the guys" and being what they both refer to as "selfish." They both have tired of their constant arguing and contempt and were seeking help to make a definitive decision regarding their relationship. To complicate matters, Breonna now desperately wants to have a child and Trayvon is not interested.

7.8.1.2   Systemic Racism Impacts

Trayvon entered into his relationship with a commitment to do better by his wife than his father did by their family. Although he had not seen an example of a healthy relationship, he pledged as a child to never cheat, divorce, or be cruel to his wife. Breonna also sought a different relationship from her parents, viewing them as cold, unaffectionate, and mundane. She dreamed of family vacations, date nights, and a single-family home, versus the tightly budgeted apartment lifestyle she grew up in. Both Trayvon and Breonna believed that their parents' poverty were attributed to systemic racism and not their intelligence or drive to change their financial situation.

Breonna and Trayvon were resentful that they were initially not able to obtain jobs in the same state. Breonna was often told that she was overqualified, but the upper-level positions were also unobtainable. They both spoke of the difficulties they faced in school at PWIs and now, in their careers. In both cases, they were the only African Americans in their respective offices and the scrutiny and micro-aggressions that each faced were well documented in yearly reviews.

The couple were also deeply impacted by the witnessing of nationwide police brutality that occurred throughout their marriage and the divisive presidency of Donald Trump. They both reported that the level of government-sanctioned racism that they have witnessed was reminiscent of what their parents and grandparents recounted from their experiences in the south throughout the 1950s and 1960s, but nothing they imagined occurring during their lifetimes. Trayvon often spoke of feeling hopeless because no matter what amount of education he achieved, the reality of being a Black man and being made to feel inferior had taken its toll over the past few years. He also felt powerless to protect Breonna from racism at her job and the aftereffects of a promotion she was denied. Breonna was scared of the possibility that Trayvon would be stopped by the police or harassed by their white neighbors. In addition, the murder of Ahmaud Arbery was especially impactful in that Trayvon often jogged to ward off his risk for diabetes. Trayvon stopped his daily jogs around their neighborhood and was resigned to run on the treadmill in their basement, which was not optimal and ultimately not maintained. Trayvon was also deeply impacted by the shooting of Jacob Blake and reported feeling more and more like his life did not matter and, with the political climate of the country, that things would never get better. Conflict also ensued because of Trayvon's admission that he was hesitant to have children because of the social climate and fear of raising children in this society. Breonna was concerned that her "biological clock" was ticking and she desperately wanted to be a mother. She had an abortion during college because of the stigma and lack of support she would likely receive as an African American teenaged mother. She now felt as if she was being punished. Although she had similar fears regarding raising a child in an oppressive society, she wondered if her limited finances and Trayvon's distrust of her were fueling his position on child-rearing with her.

7.8.1.3 Post-Traumatic Slave Syndrome Impacts

7.8.1.3.1 *Vacant Esteem*   Trayvon had always been motivated to achieve financial and material success because he felt that would be the only way to earn respect from white men and the attention of women. Without a sizable income, Trayvon believes that he has no worth and, in his words, would be view as "mediocre," similar to how he perceived most Black men as being viewed.

Breonna's worth has always been connected with her looks and her physique. She has always received compliments and she believes that her mother was always invested in how she physically presented, more so than her emotional well-being. In high school and college she became promiscuous after being cheated on by her high school sweetheart. She began to use sex for material gain, believing that her desire for a monogamous relationship could not be fulfilled. During her period of "pseudo-singlehood" she questioned if she loved Trayvon for his personality or his material stability. Trayvon's preference to hang out with his friends and unwillingness to have children with her reinforced her feelings of not being enough.

7.8.1.3.2   Ever-Present Anger   Because of his frustration with society as a whole and because his marriage had not turned out to be the haven of love, affection, and escape that he had always dreamed about, Trayvon was plagued by ever-present anger.

Breonna is angry that she has been objectified by men and, at times, welcomed this attention. She now is hypervigilant to anything she perceives as attention from the opposite sex and has "cursed out" men at work, gym, and at church for paying her compliments or "staring" at her for too long.

7.8.1.3.3   Racist Socialization   Trayvon was deeply impacted by colorism as a dark-skinned boy and now man, and often wondered if his lighter skinned wife was really attracted to him or was with him only because he was financially stable and faithful. When she called him a disparaging name related to his color during an argument last year, feelings of inferiority swept over him and he had difficulty forgiving her or forgetting her comment. He often felt like he was not enough in outside spaces, and because of her earlier suggestion of a divorce, he also felt like he was not enough inside of his home. In addition, he had secretly resolved to not procreate, because he feared that his child would carry his features and dark skin color.

Breonna's frustration had recently been exacerbated because she had always believed and been treated as a "prize" because of her "fair" skin, straight hair, and European features. The rejection that she had been experiencing from Trayvon was foreign to her and she had assumed that he would have gotten over it as soon as she apologized.

7.8.2   Gottman Connect Relationship Analysis

According to the Gottman Institute, the Enhanced Gottman Relationship Checkup was developed from over forty years of scientific research by John and Julie Gottman and encompasses evidence-based information on why relationships succeed or fail. The questionnaires are completed individually and utilize 337 questions to access the strengths and challenges of the relationship over five categories: Friendship and Intimacy, Trust and Safety, Conflict Management, Shared Meaning, and Individual Areas of Concern.

7.8.2.1 Friendship and Intimacy

Breonna and Trayvon's strengths included that they felt well known by their partner and had a friendship in which they both turned toward each other's bids for emotional connection. The relationship was challenged in that they were both dissatisfied with the current level of passion, romance, and sexually intimacy. Breonna felt sexually rejected and unloved by Trayvon. Their issues led to the reason that most relationships fail, emotional disengagement and loneliness (Gottman & Silver, 2015).

7.8.2.2 Trust and Safety

Breonna and Trayvon's strengths included that they felt security and peace in their home and they both valued the expression and exploration of their emotions. They were challenged by their ability to trust each other and the fact that although Breonna now felt committed to the relationship, Trayvon did not.

7.8.2.3 Conflict Management

Breonna and Trayvon's strengths included that they both felt comfortable accepting each other's influence, demonstrating flexibility and consideration to avoid power struggles. Their challenges included being gridlocked on reoccurring problems, becoming easily flooded, utilizing the Four Horsemen, and beginning most of their conflict discussions with criticism and blaming.

7.8.2.4 Shared Meaning

Shared Meaning is a strength of Breonna and Trayvon's relationship in that they have created rituals to connect and ways to support each other's roles and goals. The challenge is that they may not be clear on how they symbolize the underlying meanings of pieces of their marriage including home, money, and love. According to the Gottman's the way they view these symbols together influences how connected they feel in their sense of shared life purpose.

7.8.2.5   Individual Areas of Concern

A strength for this couple is that there are no major individual concerns that were captured by this assessment. The challenge for Breonna and Trayvon is that the traumas often experienced in individuals impacted by PTSS, including the impact of systemic racism, instability in their families of origin, parental coping and parenting styles, and perception of self, are not assessed by the instrument but should always processed in the individual portion of the interview.

7.8.3   Brief Summary of Treatment Plan and Outcome

In the couple's initial assessment session, the couple was asked to introduce their partner to the therapist sharing information, both factual, assumed, and perceived, regarding their partner's family of origin structure, gender roles, and lessons about dating, love, and marriage. This activity served as a way of breaking the ice to therapy and the "introduced" partner had an opportunity to confirm or correct information shared. During this exercise, which exemplifies how therapists are encouraged to use their own style in clinical tools and fit the Gottman Method within, the clinician was able to assess for ease of communication, connection, love maps, early traumas, and how each partner conceptualizes their partner's upbringing and family impact. Following this exercise, the full Gottman Oral History interview was conducted, which included thirteen open-ended questions that yielded information regarding both the history and the philosophy of the relationship. At the end of this interview additional questions regarding the "cheerleaders and haters" of the relationship, strengths and deficits that they brought into the relationship, and the prior traumas that have negatively impacted the way that they related to each other were asked. This foundational knowledge was a key to the awareness of the external and internal impacts that play a role in their daily lives together. Breonna and Trayvon presented as lighthearted and well connected throughout, both congratulating the other on how well they did with their introductions. They described dating and their decisions to marry as seamless, but both described feeling inadequate shortly thereafter, realizing that they were ill equipped to meet their partner's needs because they were unsure of how to meet their own.

Following the first joint session, the couple each had individual sessions where trauma, individual reasons for seeking couple therapy, individual mental health concerns, their personal commitment and goals for therapy were discussed in depth.

In the intervention stage, both the Gottman Rapoport and the Dreams Within Conflict were utilized to help Breonna and Trayvon voice their varying needs to each other. Breonna's needs often centered around love and appreciation, whereas his needs centered around affirmation and the necessity of trust. They were also taught to utilize the Stress Reducing Conversation, in which they both had an uninterrupted time to share the stresses and frustrations of their day, outside of the relationship, so that they could stay connected and protect their relationship from the stress caused from work, society, and extended family.

Because ongoing conflict and flooding were an issue, the couple was also given tools to manage both including practicing Gentle Start-Ups, Avoiding the Four Horsemen, and Self-Soothing. These exercises led the couple to be more mindful, and although awkward at first, they both reported utilizing these tools to have more meaningful interactions while caring for themselves and each other. The Aftermath of a Fight tool was also used extensively so that they could each process these reoccurring incidents and connect them with past traumas so that they can be more authentically discussed and acknowledged, versus focusing on the less significant issues that were repeatedly being brought to the forefront. This exercise was used to also speak to issues of skin color and Breonna was able to better understand how triggering and cutting her insult truly was.

Toward the end of therapy, extended time was spent on the Art of Compromise exercise in which Breonna and Trayvon were able to determine their core needs and those in which they were more flexible. The most significant compromise that they were able to work through surrounded the issue of sex and time devoted to physical intimacy. Because of an abuse history, and the meaning associated with sex from their family of origins' religious affiliation, work had to be done to help them understand and be sensitive to each other's positions, and not serve as triggers. Here, they were able to also discuss their hopes and fears regarding child-rearing and ultimately decided to procreate.

7.9   Conclusion/Implications for Therapists

Degruy's PTSS theory clearly summarizes the long-standing history of trauma and retraumatization for most African Americans in the United States. Although these traumatizations are internalized in varying ways, couples work requires awareness and processing so that any veiled shackles present in the relationship can be processed and addressed. Although specific theories, research, and methods created to strengthen Black love are extremely limited, the Gottman Method utilizes critical pieces that are necessary to the work of healing and healthy relationships. The Gottman Method emphasizes a need to empower the couple and give them the tools that they need to strengthen their relationship. The Gottmans have also based a portion of their theory on the role trauma plays in conflict and the ability to communicate, expanding that work in 2017 with their workshop and manual focused on treating affairs and trauma. An extensive assessment in which the therapist gets to know the client through joint and individual interviews and a research-based questionnaire, makes sure the couple feels seen and better known before the work begins, which is a critical piece necessary before therapy with couples impacted by PTSS begins. It is clear that no matter how many critical pieces a therapeutic method has, the most critical element of therapeutic care for African American couples is having a therapist who understands the impact of slavery, oppression, and systemic racism on the couple. This therapist must take the time to do a thorough assessment so that not only they can better understand the couple, but so that the couple can better understand themselves and each other.

Discussion Questions

1. What strategies can a therapist use to counter the *Cultural Mistrust* Black clients might hold for mental health professionals?
2. Describe the relationship between *Post-Traumatic Slave Syndrome (PTSS)* and *Veiled Shackles*?
3. How might a therapist introduce the concept of the Four Horsemen of the Apocalypse to a couple where PTSS and veiled shackles are present?
4. Describe the dangers of having a therapist who does not understand the impact of slavery, oppression, and systemic racism poses to a Black couple seeking therapy.

REFERENCES

Bent-Goodley, T. (2014). In circle: A healthy relationship, domestic violence, and HIV intervention for African American couples. *Journal of Human Behavior in the Social Environment, 24*, 105–114.

Bent-Goodley, T., Fairfax, C. N., & Carlton-LaNey, I. (2017). The significance of African-centered social work for social work practice. *Journal of Human Behavior in the Social Environment, 27*, 1–6.

Cohn, D., Passel, J. S., Wang, W., & Livingston, G. (2011, December 14). *Barely half of U.S. adults are married – A record low*. Pew Research Center. https://www.pewresearch.org/social-trends/2011/12/14/barely-half-of-u-s-adults-are-married-a-record-low/

Davis, R. G., Ressler, K. J., Schwartz, A. C., Stephens, K. J., & Bradley, R. G. (2008). Treatment barriers for low-income, urban African Americans with undiagnosed posttraumatic stress disorder. *Journal of Traumatic Stress, 21*(2), 218–222. https://doi.org/10.1002/jts.20313

DeGruy, J. A. (2017). *Post Traumatic Slave Syndrome: American's legacy of enduring injury and healing* (rev. ed.). Joy DeGruy Publications Inc.

Franke, K. M. (1999). Becoming a citizen: Reconstruction era regulations of African American marriages. *Yale Journal of Law and the Humanities, 11*, 251–309.

Gaskin, D. J., Headen, A. E., Jr., & White-Means, S. I. (2004). Racial disparities in health and wealth: The effects of slavery and past discrimination. *Review of Black Political Economy, 32*(3–4), 95–110. https://doi.org/10.1007/s12114-005-1007-9

Giddings, P. J. (2014) *When and where I enter*. HarperCollins e-Books.

Gottman, J. M., & Gottman, J. S. (2016). *Level 1 clinical training: Gottman Method couples therapy, bridging the couple chasm*. Gottman Institute.

(2017). *Treating affairs and trauma*. Gottman Institute.

Gottman, J. M., & Silver, N. (2015). *The seven principles for making marriage work*. Harmony Books.

Grier, W. H., & Cobbs, P. M. (1968). *Black rage*. Basic Books.

Guthrie, R. V. (2004). *Even the rat was white: A historical view of psychology* (2nd ed.). Pearson Education.

Kugelmass, H. (2016). "Sorry, I'm not accepting new patients": An audit study of access to mental health care. *Journal of Health and Social Behavior, 57*(2), 168–183.

Levenson, J. (2017, January 1). Trauma-informed social work practice. *Social Work, 62*(2), 105–113.

Mikle, K. S., & Gilbert, D. J. (2019). A systemic review of culturally relevant marriage and couple relationship education programs for African-American couples. *Journal of Ethnic & Cultural Diversity in Social Work, 28*(1), 50–75.

National Healthy Marriage Resource Center. (n.d.). *Supporting an African American healthy marriage initiative*. Retrieved October 15, 2022, from http://www.healthymarriageinfo.org/resource-detail/supporting-an-african-american-healthy-marriage-initiative/

Patton, S. (2017). *Spare the kids: Why whupping children won't save Black America*. Beacon Press.

Schofield, W. (1964). *Psychotherapy: The purchase of friendship*. Prentice-Hall.

Whaley, A. L. (2001). Cultural mistrust: An important psychological construct for diagnosis and treatment of African Americans. *Professional Psychology: Research and Practice, 32*(6), 555–562.

CHAPTER 8

Transcending the Binary: A Narrative Therapy Approach to Work with Black Trans Men Navigating Gender Transition with Romantic Partners

Moe A. Brown

8.1 Introduction

Despite the growing visibility of Black transgender identities in culture and in academic discourse surrounding mental health, there still remains a large deficit in theories and models that are sensitive to the nuances of intersectionality as these nuances surface for Black transgender men and their romantic partners. This chapter addresses the challenges that often arise for Black transgender men and their families, summarizes major narrative therapy concepts, and explores the adaption of Narrative Therapy for use in work with Black transgender men and their romantic partners. A case example will serve as an education tool to illustrate Narrative Therapy with Black transgender men and their romantic partners.

8.2 The Gender Spectrum

Before understanding how to navigate couples therapy with Black transgender men and their partners, it is important to have a strong comprehension of gender and other facets of identity that often coalesce at the intersection of gender identity. Prior to the 1970s, the pervasive theories about gender and sex asserted that gender was a given byproduct of biological sex. Biological *sex* is characterized as biological characteristics that are often rooted in DNA, presentation of genitalia, and reproductive organs. Humans are assigned male or female at birth based on these biologically expressed features. Even in the case of *intersex* people, those who are born with ambiguous genitalia and/or DNA that are a combination of both male and female, historically they are given a binary male or female sex determination at birth (Lev, 2004). After the feminist constructivist movements of the 1970s, psychologists have come to understand gender as *socially constructed* and very different from biologically determined characteristics. West and Zimmerman (1987) suggest that *gender identity* is a socially constructed articulation of societal roles related to masculinity and femininity, that the path to each articulation of masculine and feminine varies across cultures, and that these articulations have little to do with biological sex. Lev (2004) further expounds that gender identity is a person's internal sense of being masculine or feminine and their own sense of roles they would like to perform in society. While gender identity, for many people, often aligns with the typical roles expected from their biological sex assigned at birth, meaning they are *cisgender*, sometimes people's internal sense of masculinity and/or femininity differs greatly from the biological sex they were assigned at birth and the performances typically expected of that sex, meaning they are *transgender* (Bischof et al., 2016, p. 40).

Gender identity is not determined solely based on other social factors while it is inherently related to and impacted by other social identities. For this reason, it is important to continue to further separate gender identity from biological sex. While traditional articulations of transgender identities have often been placed in the binary context of transitioning from male-to-female or female-to-male, these binary markers are in fact, rooted in a framework that centers biological sex and not gender because the terms *female* and *male* are in fact sex categories whereas *masculine* and *feminine* are gender categories. For our work, we urge therapists to view transitioning as both an individualistic and relational process that looks differently across couples (Boe et al., 2019). For example, according to Boe et al., some may choose a social transition (e.g., use of different name and pronouns), a medical transition (e.g., hormone replacement therapy), or surgical procedures (e.g., hysterectomy, double mastectomy, phalloplasty), a combination of some or all of these categories, and some may decide not to transition at all.

This distinction is an important one as it supports the emergent literature that gender, like sexuality, and sexual orientation, is on a spectrum rather than a traditional binary. The importance of acknowledging and understanding the gender spectrum is crucial to the work of counselors as we work to dismantle structures that marginalize and make invisible, those who do not easily fit binary categories. The spectrum view of gender provides the framework to support gender identities at the intersection of other identities (i.e., race) as culture heavily influences gender identity and other aspects of gender like gender presentation or gender expression. Cultural influences like race, socioeconomic status, and religion create so much variation in gender identity and expression that a binary view of gender would intentionally exclude anyone who is not in the majority or in the dominant group. This has been historically true as transgender identities have quite often been invisible in the binary view of cisgender identity. As this chapter progresses and narrative therapy is further explained, it is important to release any rigid structures or binaries around identity as narrative approaches to identity are fluid. These approaches promote flexibility while creating space for evolution over time rather than a static or fixed self-identity.

To further understand gender, it is important to deconstruct gender a bit more than sex and gender identity. While gender identity is one's internal sense of being masculine or feminine and one can exist anywhere along that continuum, the performance of that internal sense of gender is impacted by other variables. *Gender expression* is defined as the outward manifestation of internal gender identity, through clothing, hairstyle, mannerisms, and other characteristics (Burnes et al., 2010). Gender expression, is essentially how someone performs their internal sense of masculinity or femininity via external manifestations. Gender expression is different than *gender presentation*, which is defined by how other people experience and perceive a person's gender. This experience is often based in their own cultural and personal understandings of gender. Gender presentation is essentially how other people "read"someone's gender. For this reason, people can often misgender transgender people based on their own assumptions about gender presentation. It is important to be aware of gender presentation as distinctly separate from gender identity and expression as we work with populations of people who are often being oppressed via dominant cultural institutions and practices that exclude and marginalize transgender people. For individuals who seek the alignment of their gender identity, expression, and presentation, transitioning becomes an integral process of their alignment. *Transitioning* is the process that an individual undergoes to feel aligned in their gender identity, gender presentation, gender expression, gender role, and sometimes their physical body. One individual's process of alignment looks different from another person's process and the details of that process are deeply personal and unique to them. It will be important for a clinician to explore with each client individually what their process of alignment looks like and to never make assumptions about their process. This is imperative and essential to the therapeutic process as well as the alliance between the therapist and the client.

Figure 8.1 depicts the common assumptions made by clinicians about client demographic information when meeting a couple for the first time. The assumption is often that if a person is assigned male at birth then they

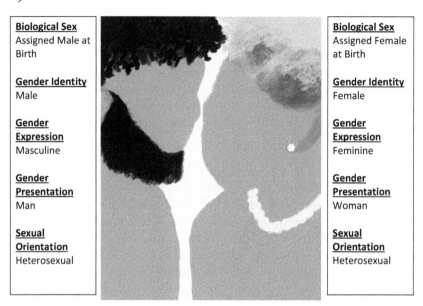

Biological Sex Assigned Male at Birth		Biological Sex Assigned Female at Birth
Gender Identity Male		Gender Identity Female
Gender Expression Masculine		Gender Expression Feminine
Gender Presentation Man		Gender Presentation Woman
Sexual Orientation Heterosexual		Sexual Orientation Heterosexual

Figure 8.1   Assumptions therapists typically make filling in demographic information for clients or when meeting new clients

must also have a masculine gender identity, masculine gender expression, masculine gender presentation, and they must also be heterosexual. The same could be said of how people would make assumptions about the identity of someone assigned the sex of female at birth. These are assumptions too risky to make as clinicians. Figure 8.2 depicts the identity of our case example clients, Mark and Tina. They each fall along the spectrum of identity at various points, each point exclusive of the previous category. In fact, moving away from assumptions is a major step in our work toward dismantling oppressive structures, not harming our clients in therapy, being more culturally sensitive, and helping our Black trans-masculine clients and their partners to explore the fullness of their narratives via narrative therapy in couples work.

8.3   Case Example

Mark (age twenty-eight) and Tina (twenty-seven) are in couples' therapy to help aid them in navigating Mark's gender transition and the impact on their relationship. They have been married for two years and in a relationship for seven years. They have one child together. They do not have any

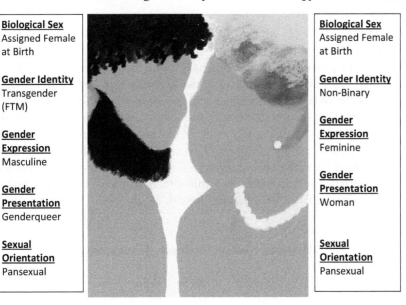

Biological Sex Assigned Female at Birth		Biological Sex Assigned Female at Birth
Gender Identity Transgender (FTM)		**Gender Identity** Non-Binary
Gender Expression Masculine		**Gender Expression** Feminine
Gender Presentation Genderqueer		**Gender Presentation** Woman
Sexual Orientation Pansexual		**Sexual Orientation** Pansexual

Figure 8.2   Identity categories that align with the case example couple, Mark and Tina

children from previous relationships. Both Mark and Tina are from traditional Christian backgrounds although they both consider themselves more spiritual than religious. They each want to work on integrating all the changes that are happening in their relationship so that they can enter parenthood together with more ease. They each report having trouble connecting romantically lately and want to explore how to reconnect romantically and emotionally.

8.3.1   Mark's Background

Mark is a Black, transgender, and pansexual man. He uses he/him pronouns. He grew up the youngest of six siblings, four brothers and one sister. Mark is originally from the Midwest. Mark has close relationships with family members and they are supportive of him. Mark has been taking testosterone for one year and underwent a bilateral mastectomy one year ago. Mark has changed his legal name and gender marker on all official documents. Mark has a master's degree and works as a writer. Prior to transitioning, Mark participated in gender processing groups and individual therapy to support him in processing the changes related to his transition. Mark had two significant relationships prior to meeting Tina.

8.3.2   Tina's Family

Tina identifies as Black, nonbinary, and pansexual. Tina uses she/her or they/them pronouns. Tina is originally from the southern region of the United States but currently lives in the Midwest with her partner, Mark. Tina is the oldest of five siblings and has close relationships with family members. Tina reports that family members have not always been openly affirming of her relationship with Mark and there have been several challenges with family members. Tina reports that family members attitudes toward her relationship impact her relationship with Mark. Tina has a master's degree and works as a midwife. Tina didn't have any serious relationships prior to her relationship with Mark.

8.4   Historical Issues for Black Transgender Men

8.4.1   Issues in Culture

According to Flores et al. (2016), 1.4 million adults in the United States identify as transgender. Considering underreporting and the lack of state and federal protections to prohibit discrimination on the grounds of transgender identity, which disincentivizes transgender visibility, we could assume that the overall transgender population in the United States is even larger than this number estimates. This bears significance because it offers us a tangible representation of just how many individuals would be impacted by gender affirming and celebratory therapy techniques just like the case example couple, Mark and Tina, who you will continue to learn about in this chapter. It is important to note that adults who identify as Black, Latino, or Hispanic or another race or ethnicity are more likely than white adults to identify as transgender (Flores et al., 2016). Adults who identify as transgender are more racially and ethnically diverse than the U.S. population overall (Flores et al., 2016). Keeping in mind that racial diversity is not an indicator of other socioeconomic factors, Flores et al. assert that broader racial and ethnic demographic patterns of U.S. residents are similar to the demographic patterns of adults who identify as transgender. This also bears great significance because this indicates that the socioeconomic disparities and other racial disparities that disproportionately disenfranchise cisgender people of color also are impacting transgender people of color at similar rates. In fact, transgender people of color are most heavily represented in states that do not have equitable transgender protections under the law. In fact, they are heavily represented in states where anti-transgender legislation is a common political practice. This offers insight into the impact of racial disparities on the transgender population and helps to characterize the ways in which transgender people of color are further marginalized than their white counterparts. Hence, this particular work with transgender men and their partners is immensely important.

8.4.2   Issues in Mental Health

There are various issues that arise as roadblocks to mental health services for Black transgender men. According to Herman et al. (2017), Transgender adults experience disparities in mental health, disability status, and access to prescription medicine. These disparities present challenges to help seeking for suicidality or other mental health concerns (Shipherd et al., 2010). These disparities are also present in the representation of Black transgender men in couple's therapy. Herman et al. (2017) indicate that compared to cisgender adults, transgender adults are more than three times more likely to have ever thought about suicide, nearly six times more likely to have ever attempted suicide, nearly four times more likely to have experienced serious psychological distress, and more than three times more likely to have emotions that interfere with their relationships, social life, ability to do chores, and work performance. Furthermore, these statistics are increased by lack of access to resources or being denied mental health or medicinal assistance, which transgender individuals are three times more likely to be denied overall. These statistics are compounded by a social landscape that works to systematically target transgender people and remove their protections under the law (Burnes et al., 2010). Negative attitudes toward Black transgender men in mass culture can deeply impact the individual experiences of Black transgender men. Stigma can have a lasting impact on the way the individual processes their gender transition, is able to come out to their family, or even whether they are accepted at work or social spaces – all facets of life that typically help support emotional and mental well-being.

8.4.3   Cultural Competency/Humility in the Therapy Room

There are large chasms in the body of knowledge that explores work with Black couples (DeVance Taliaferro et al., 2013). Furthermore, there is an overall lack of knowledge related to competency and sensitivity to the needs of Black transgender individuals and their romantic partners (Brown, 2010). There are still gaps in knowledge centered on competency with transgender clients that lead to transgender people experiencing microaggressions related to gender transition (Nadal et al., 2012). Subsequently, Black transgender individuals, with intersecting racial and gender minority identities, often face microaggressions in social contexts as well as inside of the therapy relationship due to this lack of cultural humility. Despite the growing visibility of Black transgender identities in culture and in academic discourse surrounding mental health, Black transgender men still represent an underserviced and underrepresented population in counseling.

With all the social obstacles that Black transgender men and their partners face in society, it is always important that allyship in the therapeutic alliance be present when working in this population (Burnes et al., 2010). An *ally* is a celebratory and affirming supporter of lesbian, gay, bisexual, transgender, queer, intersex, asexual, and all other identities (LGBTQIA+) within this community and in this context, an allied therapist would support racial, gender, sexual orientation, equity, and equality. This alliance is built through culturally sensitive, antiracist, gender-affirming, and celebratory practice (Kirk & Belovics, 2008). To work with Black transgender men and their partners, a therapist must not only be competent in work with one part of their clients' identities, but competent in care that supports their holistic identities. For instance, if a clinician is an expert in therapy approaches that are culturally sensitive to Black clients, the therapist will still need to enhance their competencies for working with the LGBTQIA+ population. If their main competencies rest in working with the LGBTQIA+ population but they lack cultural understanding of Black clients and the challenges they face in America, clinicians stand a great risk of not being sensitive to the intersectional needs of this population. Let's take a quick look at Figure 8.3, which offers some helpful ways to be a good ally to Black transgender men and their partners in therapy.

8.5   Narrative Therapy

Narrative and truth telling have been successful methods for analysis and tools for healing in the therapy room. Narrative Therapy, created by Michael White in partnership with David Epston in the late 1980s, offers a helpful model for structuring therapy work in an empowering way. Social workers and family therapists, Michael White from Australia and David Epston from New Zealand, developed Narrative Therapy in response to working with populations that were often degraded by society in the

Do	Don't
1. Ask general, open-ended questions.	1. Don't make assumptions based on client appearance.
2. Ask about the pronouns of clients.	
3. Please educate yourself on pronouns other than he/him/his or she/her/hers like they/them or ze/hir/hirs.	2. Do not assume gender, sexual orientation, race, religion, etc.
4. Ask clients what name they would like to be called if different from the legal name.	3. Don't assume that a romantic partnership only consists of two people.
5. Follow client cues about pronouns of individuals in their family/community.	4. Don't overgeneralize groups/populations of people.
6. Ask about different intersectional identities that clients hold.	5. Don't be judgmental.
7. Ask clients how they define their gender identity/sexual orientation.	6. Don't use body language that conveys openness or judgment.
8. Modify any handouts you give to clients to reflect clients' gender and sexual orientation.	7. Don't presume that all LGBT clients are the same.
9. Ex. Try not to provide an LGBTQIA+ couple with a premarital handout that only references "husband and wife."	8. Do not presume that all LGBT clients grew up in heterosexual households.
10. Be open and curious.	9. Don't think that one modality of therapy works for every client.
11. Understand the impact of culture on the presentation of symptoms.	10. Don't forget to do a social and cultural assessment.
12. Ask clients for feedback about services.	11. Don't underestimate transference and countertransference.
13. Explore what biases you come into the therapy room with.	
14. Stay up to date on terminology and essential updates in culture.	
15. Apologize and correct yourself if/when you make a mistake or misgender someone.	

What are some other "Dos" you think should be on this list?
What are some other "Don'ts" you think should be on this list?

Figure 8.3   Ways to be a good ally to Black transgender men and their partners in therapy

1970s. In their clinical work, they found their narrative techniques to be useful in empowering marginalized persons to invent solutions to their problems rather than internalizing their problems. Before exploring Narrative Therapy's application in work with Black transgender men and their partners, it is important to highlight and identify important concepts, techniques, and interventions for using Narrative Therapy with couples overall.

Narrative Therapy has become highly regarded in the field of family counseling as an effective method of treatment for a wide variety of systemic and intersectional issues. White and Epston (1990) state that Narrative Therapy is rooted in the idea that problems are created in social, cultural, and political frameworks. These socially constructed narratives then become the dominant narrative that guides individuals inside of the family context (White & Epston, 1990). Narrative Therapy offers a blueprint to help couples navigate challenges around personal problems, value systems, social context, and intersectional identities. Narrative therapy helps couples to externalize problems, deconstruct narratives, and reauthor stories. Kim et al. (2012) assert that it is through the remembering and reauthoring of stories that couples are able to understand the social context around their narratives while empowering them to reconstruct those narratives to strengthen their futures together. Narrative therapy also provides a framework to understand how these factors impact the stories clients construct about their lives and how those stories impact mental health as well as client perspectives of life challenges (Kim et al., 2012).

8.5.1   Tenets of Narrative Therapy

Let's take a closer look at Narrative Therapy and understand how the practice of narrative therapy is used clinically. Narrative Therapy works from a few essential premises. First, *clients are the experts of their lives.* It is imperative for clients to leave the therapy process more empowered than when they began. For this reason, clinicians work to remove assumptions from their therapeutic stance. Think back to Figure 8.1 and Figure 8.2. In therapy with Black transgender clients, it is extremely important to always allow clients the space to tell their own stories and through proper ally practice, remove any biases and assumptions that might enter the therapy room. Especially when working with populations that already experience oppression and prejudice, it is vital to the clinical work that therapists examine their own internalized heteronormative constructions. Another important premise of Narrative Therapy is that *there is no absolute truth and narratives are socially constructed.* This articulates the postconstructivist leanings of this work. Narratives are created in context and especially for couples; narratives are cocreated and are a product of social relationship. There is a saying: "there is your side, my side, and the truth." This maxim expresses that human narratives are subject to human experiences and human perspectives. It is important that therapists keep this in focus when conducting narrative work. Narrative therapists are not looking for absolutes or truths in therapy. Narrative Therapy questions can't be answered by "yes" or "no." Narrative therapy seeks to explore how clients arrived at the stories they hold about their lives and deconstruct those narratives so that those stories serve the vision of how clients want to live in the future. Narrative therapists are looking for space in the narrative to expand, adapt, or change enough so that the story continues to serve the clients and puts them in healed relationship with their own lives. Sometimes clients begin therapy with problem-centered narratives rooted in pain. A Narrative Therapy approach seeks to honor the pain and use it as a guidepost rather than a port. Moreover, the narrative approach uses the pain as a way to understand how the client got to where they are rather than determining that the pain is the reason for all the troubles. This approach allows clients to evolve as aspects of their lives change over time, in and out of social context. The last premise for us to note before exploring the methods of Narrative Therapy is that *Narrative Therapy is respectful and does not try to find blame.* This premise is crucial to narrative work. It is an act of real vulnerability for clients to share their stories with any clinician in the therapeutic context. The therapeutic stance of the clinician should always be respectful and sensitive to the client's vulnerability. Narrative Therapy is not an interrogative or solution focused approach to therapy. Therapists utilizing narrative work are asked to really listen mindfully to client's stories as they tell them because however the client tells their story is how they operate with that story in their day-to-day experience. How each client shares their narrative is likely, the perspective they experience the world from every day. For example, a therapist may know that a client's relationship with their mother seems dysfunctional but if the client reports that their relationship with their mother is perfect, a narrative therapist would seek to help them explore moments in their narrative where their relationship has proven dysfunctional but would never outrightly just say that the relationship is dysfunctional. More training on how to conduct narrative sessions will be offered, but the takeaway here is that the therapist is in the role of observer, listener, and holder of sacred vulnerable space.

8.5.2 Narrative Therapy Methods

There are several core methods that Narrative Therapy uses: telling the story, externalization of problems, identifying unique outcomes, deconstructing the narrative, and reauthoring the narrative. Telling the story is the first step in the narrative therapy process. Clients are asked to share with us how they view their life and the problems they face. In doing so, we allow space for the clients to tell us how they see their worlds and the context that they live in. Not only is this empowering for clients, who may not have ever had the space to share their voice or ever had someone listen empathically while they talk about subjects that might cause them shame, allowing them to tell the story offers the clinician an insightful look into the client's world while strengthening the therapeutic alliance. A strong therapeutic alliance is essential for this work.

Externalization of problems is a method of depathologizing the issues that clients face. So often, clients see their problems as self-inflicted or as a part of themselves. This stance is disempowering as it makes the client the problem and robs them of any power to find solutions. Through externalization of problems language, a safe space is created to see the problems as separate from the individual and therefore, creating space for the narrative to be separate from the individual as well. The externalization of problems is vital to the work as it makes room for the client to examine their narrative in the seat of co-author rather than victim and leaves room for the narrative to evolve with the client over time rather than setting up rigid and/or stagnant frameworks.

Identifying unique outcomes is the aspect of the therapy that narrative therapists will be keenly focused on while practicing this approach with clients. Identifying unique outcomes is the process of listening to the narrative as told by the client and looking out for counternarratives. The purpose of identifying unique outcomes is to highlight exceptions to the narrative that the client has constructed. These exceptions work as an entry point for altering the narrative. *Deconstructing the narrative* allows clinicians to take those unique outcomes and utilize them to better understand the origins of the existing narrative. Deconstructing the narrative is where therapists should strongly consider the influence of the larger society and dominant culture on the client's perspective. When deconstructing the narrative, therapists should also explore how the narrative came into being as well as discover if there are parts of the narrative that the client no longer needs or parts of the narrative that were formed by the influence of someone else. Deconstruction allows us to examine the narrative critically and in social context in order to put it back together by reauthoring.

Reauthoring or re-membering is the process of reorganizing the narrative so that the client's voice is centered in the story telling. Often, we ask clients to explore who and what have been the biggest influences on their narratives. Often when we explore these influencers, we find that so many external influences have been adding parts of the narrative over time and sometimes those external influencers carry much more weight in the authorship of the narrative. Framing the story within the larger societal context helps therapist and client to understand the influence of the larger systems at work. In the reauthoring and re-membering process, therapist and client are changing the influence of external forces on the narrative and giving authorship back to the client so that they feel empowered to decide for themselves what the narrative will be. Ultimately, it is the hope of the narrative therapist that through the Narrative Therapy process, the clients will have a life story that much better serves where they see themselves in the future as well as where they are in the present.

The reauthoring and integration of new narratives can be bolstered with the use of the *outsider witness* intervention, a practice involving inviting members of the client's community to witness the telling of the newly constructed narrative. There can be a literal witness or an imagined witness for this intervention. The clinician uses this intervention once clients have begun to identify unique outcomes and integrate new aspects of their narrative. Michael White's use of outsider witness would have consisted of asking key players who support the client or add to the narrative in a significant way to be present and witness the client's integration of their new narrative. The hope in this intervention is that the witnessing will continue to empower and affirm the emerging narrative.

8.6   Application of Narrative Therapy with Black Trans Men in Couples Therapy

Understanding the historical mistreatment of Black transgender individuals in the global society as well as in therapy, it is important to explore culturally sensitive ways to approach therapy with Black transgender men and their partners. Critical Race Theory, which emerged in the 1970s in response to the lack of adequate representation and understanding of race in dominant discourse about the law, offers counter storytelling as a fundamental method of analysis and as a tool for empowering people of color (DeVance Taliaferro et al., 2013). *Counter storytelling is* a means of telling a narrative that "aims to cast doubt on the validity of accepted premises or myths, especially ones held by the majority" (DeVance Taliaferro et al., 2013, p. 37). As a method, counter storytelling allows for marginalized individuals to tell their own stories, while as a means of analysis, counter stories are used to challenge the majority discourse (DeVance Taliaferro et al., 2013). The effectiveness of sharing narratives in racial justice work offers us meaningful insight into the power of narrative and truth-telling for clients who face oppression and marginalization. Furthermore, the narrative therapy approach offers these similar tools and methods for potential use in empowering Black transgender men and their romantic partners.

Existing research on Narrative Therapy, like the work of DeVance Taliaferro et al. (2013), and its effectiveness for use with couples has offered meaningful insights into how Narrative Therapy might be used in work with Black individuals in therapy. However, current research lacks a focus on Black transgender men in partnership specifically. Through the externalization of problems, deconstruction of narratives, and reauthoring of stories, Narrative Therapy is a useful and practical method for aiding Black transgender men and their romantic partners through challenges related to gender transition. In the following section, it is explained how Narrative Therapy might be applied to work with the case example couple, Mark and Tina.

8.6.1   Telling the Story

As a narrative therapist, your role is to invite your client into safe space and allow them to share their story. Narrative therapists want to make no assumptions about the clients and their challenges, and they want to listen carefully to how each client shares their story. Narrative Therapy questions are open ended and client centered. They are not solution focused, directional, and cannot be answered with a yes or no. The following is a snippet from a session between Mark and Tina and Therapist. Observe how the therapist creates space for Mark and Tina's story.

THERAPIST: What prompted your call this week to schedule another session? Tell me what happened.

MARK: I realized that Tina and I haven't been intimate for a while and every time we try to talk about it, it ends up with us arguing. I feel like she isn't attracted to me anymore because I'm transitioning, and I don't know what to do about it.

THERAPIST: Thank you for sharing, Mark. Tina, tell me what happened from your perspective. How does your viewpoint differ or mirror Mark's view?

TINA: We have not been as intimate as we were in the past. It does feel like a challenge, but I am not sure why. I know that it's been difficult to talk about with Mark and it's hard to get him to understand that he isn't the problem. I am the problem. I just lack an interest in intimacy overall. It's not Mark. I just don't know how to fix it.

THERAPIST: Thank you so much for sharing Tina. I know it took a lot of vulnerability for both of you to share what has been going on in your relationship. Let's go ahead and explore all of this some more.

Mark and Tina just expressed several things to the therapist about how they perceive their narrative. Mark deeply believes that their problems stem from his gender transition and he perceives that Tina is no longer attracted to him because of his changing appearance. Tina strongly believes that the issue regarding their intimacy rests inside of her as an individual. They each blame themselves for this issue they face and they are having a challenging time sorting out the details. Quite often, clients come to therapy believing strongly that the issue is a part of them, and often, the problem actually is that they are struggling to integrate something about themselves or their experience into the story they are telling about their relationship.

8.6.2   Externalization of Problems

Now that it is clear that Mark and Tina both view the problems regarding their challenges with intimacy as having to do with their own deficits, a narrative approach would encourage these clients to *externalize problems*. By externalizing the problem, the therapist could help them to deconstruct the challenges they are facing while depathologizing their view of themselves. This technique helps clients view their problems as separate from themselves and helps orient the clients toward exploring the impact of the problem on the relationship rather than seeing the relationship as the problem. The following is an example of how a therapist would help Mark and Tina to externalize the problems they identified.

THERAPIST: I appreciate you each sharing what has been going on for you. It sounds like you each agree that a lack of intimacy has been difficult to manage. Please share more with me about the impact of the lack of intimacy on your relationship.

TINA: Well, if I were a better spouse, Mark wouldn't be out here thinking that I am unattracted to him. I really want him to understand that I'm the issue here.

THERAPIST: I hear you. I hear that you really blame yourself for the challenges you are having. I want to offer you this small insight from one caring soul to another: you aren't the problem. The lack of intimacy is the problem and it is totally separate from who you are as person.

MARK: I agree! You aren't the issue, babe.

TINA: It's just so hard not to blame myself.

THERAPIST: I hear that the lack of intimacy keeps you blaming yourself. Is there anything else that the lack of intimacy stirs up for you?

MARK: It makes me feel like my partner isn't interested in me anymore because of my gender transition. It makes me worried that Tina doesn't like my body anymore since I have had top surgery.

TINA: It makes me feel inadequate and like I'm not being a good partner.

THERAPIST: It sounds like the lack of intimacy has been stirring up some self-doubt and self-criticism in each of you and we are all going to tackle this together.

Mark and Tina each began this work with a problem-centered narrative where they blamed themselves for the challenges they were facing. Mark placed blame on his gender transition for the lack of intimacy in their relationship. Taking the narrative approach, it is strongly encouraged to proceed with care and consideration for the external factors that would contribute to this kind of thinking for Mark and Tina. This would be called *deconstruction*, which is the process by which narrative therapists break down the narrative into smaller parts within the social context. Deconstruction helps therapist and clients explore the meaning behind the way the clients see the problem and where they derived their perspective.

MARK: When Tina and I first met, I was a woman and answering to a completely different name. I don't expect her to be able to just flip a switch on and stop being interested in women. So, I just feel like she has to always somewhere in the back of her head be thinking about how I used to look.

THERAPIST: What makes you feel so sure that she is thinking these things?

MARK: That's how people in the lesbian community can be. There is a lot of transphobia and shunning of masculinity.

THERAPIST: It sounds like you've experienced some prejudice in the social spaces you've been a part of. It sounds like there is a part of social culture you have experienced that holds negative attitudes toward transgender men. It sounds like these attitudes have had an impact on you.

MARK: Absolutely. I have heard people saying that all masculinity is toxic or that making a binary transition is participating in misogyny. I just don't want to be a part of a larger problem and I worry that Tina sees me this way too.

THERAPIST: It sounds like you got some negative messages and your social community has lacked affirmation and celebration of your identities in some regards.

MARK: Yeah, I guess they really have. I hadn't thought of it that way. Sometimes, I'm just so happy to have a community at all as a Black trans man that I may overlook the impact of these kinds of biases.

THERAPIST: It makes me curious if you worry that Tina has been impacted by these negative attitudes too. Let's get Tina to weigh in on her experience.

Mark was able to work with the therapist to explore where his thoughts come from regarding his partner's attraction to him. He identified that his struggles stem from rejection and negative attitudes he has faced in social community. This is a powerful intervention because it helps Mark to realize that this problem, which is separate from him, also is greatly influenced by his experiences in his social community. The social context surrounding the issues is often so important, especially when working with clients who experience oppression and marginalization of their identities. It's important to explore with clients how their identities are impacted by these external forces and deconstruct this impact prior to reauthoring.

8.6.3 Identifying Unique Outcomes

Another helpful intervention for use in narrative therapy is identifying unique outcomes. This exercise is not to simply poke holes in the client's narrative. Rather, this exercise is to help clients to explore the narrative more fully. Expanding the narrative from any rigid thinking or any narrow focus helps the clients to increase self-awareness and hold perspective in the future.

THERAPIST: Tina, I hear you saying that the lack of intimacy has been constantly impacting your relationship. Have there been any examples of moments where you were able to be intimate with one another? If so, what did you do differently?

TINA: Yes, we are intimate sometimes, I guess it's just not as often as we'd like. I guess we keep the lack of intimacy from impacting our relationship negatively by really trying to talk things through, coming up with fun new games to play together, or other ways to keep things interesting.

THERAPIST: Awesome, so I hear that when you really work together to tackle the lack of intimacy head-on, you all are successful. Does that feel intimate?

MARK: It certainly feels intimate to me. I love when we operate as a team, no matter what the outcome is.

TINA: Me too, Mark. I guess we have been really focused on one kind of intimacy; we really do have a wealth of emotional, spiritual, and mental intimacy. Those are aspects that I adore about our relationship.

MARK: Same here. I adore those things. And I adore you.

THERAPIST: Your reflection on intimacy is rather insightful. It highlights your strengths as a couple. When you work together, you both really enjoy the collaboration and all that collaboration builds the foundation for meaningful intimacy of all kinds.

Mark and Tina have done the hard work of identifying unique outcomes. In doing so, they were able to realize that intimacy comes in many different forms. The purpose of this exercise was to offer them a reflection of the potential for a new narrative about intimacy to emerge. Rather than the narrative they began with which was rooted in each of their perceived individual deficits, they now are identifying strengths as a couple that they will later use in collaborations with one another.

8.6.4 Reauthoring and Re-membering

Through the process of reauthoring and re-membering, we offer the clients an opportunity to explore how to reorganize their narrative so that their highest truth has the most prominent impact on the narrative, not outside forces. In our case example, Mark really was impacted by negative social attitudes and this affected his relationship to his gender transition and then to his partner. A narrative therapist would first help him deconstruct his narrative around his transition, explore the influence of these external forces, reorganize and prioritize his own voice in the narrative, and then help him to integrate unique outcomes and new potential for what the narrative could become. Keep in mind, Narrative Therapy is not a rigid process nor should it be used in pursuit of some absolute truth. The work with Mark and Tina is to help them leave room in the narrative for their relationship to continue evolving over time.

MARK: I hadn't realized just how deeply the social isolation, misgendering, and transphobia I experienced had impacted my self-esteem and in turn impacted our relationship.

TINA: I had no idea either. I also hadn't considered how those experiences had impacted me and how I was relearning my relationship to myself in relation to your transition.

THERAPIST: These are very valuable insights. It sounds like you both are acknowledging how external factors have played a role in oppressing your partnership. How does it feel to realize that in this moment?

MARK: It feels like an important realization. I don't want anyone else to prevent me from living my truth. I am who I am. I am certainly happy that we explored this.

TINA: Same. I want to commit to doing this work in collaboration with you, Mark. We don't need anyone else writing out story. That work is up to us.

MARK: I agree, 100 percent.

Mark and Tina, alongside their narrative therapist, have done some hard work to really explore their challenges resulting from a loss in intimacy. In subsequent sessions, they would work together to explore ways to enhance intimacy. The work of Narrative Therapy was to help them orient around their problems differently. If they had approached the work from where they began the session, assuming they each were the problem, they would have been working hard at "fixing themselves," which is a dead end. The reason that this session was successful was because they were able to see the problem in social context and separate the problem from themselves. This allowed them to collaborate and lean into finding solutions for enhancing intimacy rather than solutions for fixing what they originally thought were deficits in each other.

8.7   Chapter in Review

This chapter covered:

• Key terminology related to gender identity and its application to clinical practice with Black transgender men and their romantic partners

- Historical issues for Black transgender men in dominant culture and in mental health
- Key terminology related to narrative therapy and its application to clinical practice with Black transgender men and their romantic partners
- Narrative therapy interventions for working with Black transgender men and their romantic partners.

Discussion Questions

1. What biases or assumptions might you hold from your own social context that you may need to deconstruct before work with this population?
2. What narrative therapy interventions stand out to you?
3. Think about how you view problems now. Do you externalize them or do you often view them as part of yourself?
4. Are you an LGBTQIA+ ally? Have you taken any training to help you create safe space for working with Black transgender men and their partners?
5. If you were working with our case example couple Mark and Tina, what other narratives would you want to explore with them given the information you know about them?

REFERENCES

Bischof, G., Stone, C., Mustafa, M. M., & Wampuszyc, T. J. (2016). Couple relationships of transgender individuals and their partners: A 2017 update. *Michigan Family Review*, *20*(1), 37–47.

Boe, J. L., Bermúdez, J. M., Sharstrom, K. A., & Baldwin, D. R. (2019). Easing the transition: A critical narrative therapy approach to working with committed couples navigating gender transition. *Journal of Systemic Therapies*, *38*(1), 1–16.

Brown, N. R. (2010). The sexual relationships of sexual-minority women partnered with trans men: A qualitative study. *Archives of Sexual Behavior*, *39*(2), 561–572.

Burnes, T. R., Singh, A. A., Harper, A. J., Harper, B., Maxon-Kann, W., Pickering, D. L., & Hosea, J (2010). American Counseling Association: Competencies for counseling with transgender clients. *Journal of LGBT Issues in Counseling*, *4*(3–4), 135–159.

DeVance Taliaferro, J., Casstevens, W. J., & DeCuir Gunby, J. T. (2013). Working with African American clients using narrative therapy: An operational citizenship and critical race theory framework. *International Journal of Narrative Therapy & Community Work*, (1), 34–45.

Flores, A. R., Brown, T. N. T., & Herman, J. L. (2016). *Race and ethnicity of adults who identify as transgender in the United States.* Williams Institute, UCLA School of Law.

Herman, J. L., Wilson, B. D., & Becker, T. (2017). *Demographic and health characteristics of transgender adults in California: findings from the 2015–2016 California Health Interview Survey* (Policy brief no. 8). UCLA Center for Health Policy Research.

Kim, H., Prouty, A. M., & Roberson, P. N. (2012). Narrative therapy with intercultural couples: A case study. *Journal of Family Psychotherapy, 23*(4), 273–286.

Kirk, J., & Belovics, R. (2008), Understanding and counseling transgender clients. *Journal of Employment Counseling, 45,* 29–43.

Lev, A. I. (2004). *Transgender emergence: Therapeutic guidelines for working with gender-variant people and their families.* Haworth Clinical Practice Press.

Nadal, K. L., Skolnik, A., & Wong, Y. (2012). Interpersonal and systemic microaggressions toward transgender people: Implications for counseling. *Journal of LGBT Issues in Counseling, 6*(1), 55–82.

Shipherd, J. C., Green, K. E., & Abramovitz, S. (2010). Transgender clients: Identifying and minimizing barriers to mental health treatment. *Journal of Gay & Lesbian Mental Health, 14*(2), 94–108.

West, C., & Zimmerman, D. H. (1987). Doing gender. *Gender & Society, 1*(2), 125–151.

White, M., & Epston, D. (1990). *Narrative means to therapeutic ends.* Norton.

CHAPTER 9

Imago Therapy and the African American Couple

Beverley Boothe

9.1 Introduction

Imago Relationship Therapy was developed by Harville Hendrix to help couples work through conflict in their relationship. Hendrix's (1988) book *Getting the Love You Want: A Guide for Couples* and his accompanying workbook (1994) has sold numerous copies. Both the book and the workbook have successfully guided couples to work through their relational conflict skillfully. Numerous couples in the United States and worldwide have attended the two-day couple's workshop to learn about conflict resolution and strengthen their relationship. Many therapists have also attended the Imago Relationship twenty-one-day training to become a Certified Imago Relationship Therapist. The Imago Therapist is trained in understanding the unconscious self and how to help couples move to a conscious stage.

Imago Therapy incorporates various therapeutic approaches, including psychoanalysis, attachment theory, psychodynamic approaches, and gestalt therapy (Zielinski, 1999). A certified Imago Therapist's goal is to help the couple understand and learn techniques to consciously relate to each other. Hendrix outlines two unconscious stages of relating in a relationship that includes the Romantic and the Power Struggle Stage (Hendrix, 1988). He also outlines five essential principles in the conscious stage of Imago Relationship Therapy. According to Hendrix, they include re-imagining, re-romanticizing, restructuring, resolving, and re-visioning the couples' relationship. Healing occurs in the conscious stage. Each of these stages is discussed in more detail.

9.1.1 Benefits of Imago Therapy with African American Couples

Imago Relationship Therapy has been utilized with couples in seventeen countries in addition to the United States with over 2,000 certified Imago

213

clinicians. This type of therapy is useful in helping couples to improve communication and address conflict. Although no specific research has been completed on its effectiveness with African American couples, the principles of moving from an unconscious to a conscious way of relating as a couple are relevant to this population. African American couples are often unaware of how racism, childhood trauma, feelings of powerlessness, socioeconomic conditions, and other psychosocial factors affect how they relate as a couple. Imago Relationship Therapy enables the African American couple to look at their childhood story, increase awareness of the connections to their triggers in the relationship, and make a conscious decision to change their way of relating with their partner. Imago Relationship Therapy can also be adapted to use in church group settings because it can easily incorporate spirituality or a faith-based approach to support couples. Research shows that religion is vital to most African American families, and having a counseling approach that meets their spiritual needs is important (Taylor, 1988). Imago Therapy enables the therapist to consider African Americans' spiritual and other cultural needs in the individual counseling session and group settings.

9.1.2   *The State of Marriages in the United States*

Marriage rates continue to decline rapidly in our society. In the United States, marriage is regarded as a monogamous lifelong partnership; however, divorce rates continue to increase (Campbell & Wright, 2010). Research shows that divorce rates in the United States are approximately 40–50 percent (Emery, 2013). Emery states that finances, parenting issues, and emotional and psychological states of each individual contribute to divorce in couples. Studies also indicate that couples who experience marital distress have an increased risk of depression, anxiety, economic hardship, and long-term health concerns (Emery, 2013). With the high rates of divorce leading to the deterioration of families, there continues to be a need to provide supportive services to strengthen marriages. Despite the numerous premarital and marriage education programs that exist, there is a need to better understand how to help couples effectively work through their conflict and improve their communication skills.

Grief and other emotional and psychological distress are common emotions experienced by the individual or couple when they experience marital distress (Emery, 2013). Emotional and psychological distress is a state of emotional suffering associated with stressors, such as anxiety and depression, in which couples find it challenging to cope with daily life (Leeker &

Carlozzi, 2014). Numerous research studies have been conducted on Caucasian couples to examine interventions to address marital distress; however, research is scarce for African American couples and the interventions needed to help repair or strengthen their relationship.

9.1.3   The State of African American Marriages

African American culture is different from mainstream American culture because of external variables (Lavner et al., 2018). These variables include discrimination, disproportionate imprisonment rates, unequal socioeconomic levels, and imbalanced gender ratios, influencing the level of commitment given in a relationship (Lavner et al., 2018). In the first half of the twentieth century, most African Americans married and rarely divorced (Allen & Olson, 2001). However, these patterns have changed, and research shows that African Americans tend to marry later and divorce earlier than other races (Chambers & Kravitz, 2011). They also have the lowest rate of never been married compared to other ethnic groups. (Chambers & Kravitz, 2011). Studies show that regardless of educational level and socioeconomic background, African Americans report lower marital quality, which influences their decision to contemplate getting divorced (Burdette et al., 2012). Some of the factors affecting the decrease in marriage in African American marriages are the decrease of available men for African American women, the inability of many African American men to provide for the family financially, and sometimes the lack of desire for couples to marry (Chambers & Kravitz, 2011).

   All marriages have strengths and challenges. Marital strength involves the couple learning techniques to address crises when they arise in their relationship (Chaney, 2014). African American couples experience unique strengths and challenges in their relationship (Chaney, 2014). Despite the decline of African American marriage rates, research shows that they continue to see marriage positively (Chaney, 2014). Their marriage expectations include commitment, love, trust, covenant, partnership, and friendship (Marks et al., 2008). Research also shows that role sharing, division of household labor, strong kinship bonds, and strong religious orientation are protective factors for African Americans (Vaterlaus et al., 2017)

9.1.4   Spirituality and the Black Couple

Many African American couples have a strong religious orientation and incorporate it into their daily lives. Studies indicate that religion has been a buffer in African American marriages because it improves marital interaction and contributes to lower stress levels in couples (Phillips et al., 2012). Historically, the Black church has played a significant role in African Americans' lives and is central to the Black community (Collins & Perry, 2015). African Americans will often seek help from the Black church when they are making significant family decisions (Collins & Perry, 2015). Perry (2013) found that more religious Black men reported more favorable attitudes toward marriage than other, less religious Black men. In the Black community, marriage involves entering a covenant with the spouse and with God and spirituality is seen as a strength in African American marriages (Vaterlaus et al., 2017). When the couple feels close to God and active in their religious community, it can increase their commitment level to their spouse because they are accountable to their religious community. With the high divorce rate, there is a need to support African American couples through marriage enrichment programs that are culturally sensitive and incorporate their core value system (Hurt et al., 2012).

9.1.5   The Impact of Slavery and Racial Discrimination on the African American Couple

The impact of slavery has had a profound effect on the African American family. It has left deep emotional and psychological scars; however, it has also caused resilience in the African American family (Wilkins et al., 2013). Clinicians must understand how slavery and other historical traumas have impacted African Americans to provide more effective treatment that considers diversity concerns from a theoretical and clinical perspective (Wilkins et al., 2013). Studies show that African Americans are reluctant to seek mental health services due to the 400-year history of being seen as inferior to other races (Wilkins et al., 2013). When counseling is sought, clinicians often lack cultural sensitivity to meet this population's needs due to the lack of understanding of how slavery and racial discrimination inform African Americans' presenting problems. The effects of slavery have impacted African Americans for multiple generations. There is limited clinical literature available to help clinicians understand the techniques needed to better support the African American family and strengthen the couples' relationship.

More than other ethnic groups, African American families are impacted by financial strain and poverty, contributing to racial discrimination (Clavél et al., 2017). When couples experience financial strain, this can damage their relationship, primarily if the strain is attributed to both individuals in the relationship. Racial discrimination is another stressor that exists on an institutional level. African American couples are unable to control the changing presentation of racial discrimination. Therefore, their response as a couple may be to protect their loved ones from being victimized. Research studies show that African American couples take on a supportive role with their partner due to being mistreated in society (Clavél et al., 2017). Clavél et al. (2017) states that there is evidence that racial discrimination promotes bonding within the same cultural group. Couples have more awareness of the partners' vulnerabilities and an increased desire to protect them from harm (Clavél et al., 2017).

9.1.6 Childhood Wounds and African Americans

Couples are more likely to have a stronger, healthier relationship with their partner when their childhood experiences are positive. Research indicates that family or origin experiences contribute to the success of an intimate partner relationship. Supportive experiences in the childhood home will enhance the couple's relationship (Simons et al., 2014). Negative experiences and childhood trauma can contribute to attachment issues in the couple relationship. Studies indicate that identifying social competencies experienced in childhood, such as warm parenting or hostile parenting, can explain how to better support couples in establishing a healthy romantic relationship (Simons et al., 2014). Imago Therapy enables the African American couple to examine their childhood experiences and determine how they impact their current relationship. They learn to identify their emotional wounds and their partners' wounds from childhood and work to support each other in their healing.

9.1.7 Communication and the African American Couple

Effective communication is a foundation for a healthy marital relationship. Research shows that African Americans desire to have open, honest, and frequent communication in their marriage. Vaterlaus et al. (2017) state that African American couples who had high expectations for open communication, relationship goals, and acquired skills could strengthen their relationship. Studies reveal that the following factors helped to sustain marriages: when African American couples agree in their faith and religion; have open, honest, and frequent communication; and respect differences or individuality and relationships (Vaterlaus et al., 2017).

9.2   Introduction to Imago Theory

The term Imago is a Latin word for "image." It is a relational approach to therapy that focuses on working through unresolved childhood conflicts as they surface in our intimate adult relationship. Hendrix (1988) explains that this image is "a composite picture of the people who influenced you most strongly at an early age. This may be the mother, father, siblings, or close relative. Hendrix states that a part of the brain called the amygdala records everything about them, including their physical features and experiences. Scientist report that people have hidden information stored in their brain from childhood that is forgotten. The most vivid memory recorded are often formed from caretakers early in life and the most deeply engraved interactions are usually the most wounding experiences (Hendrix, 1988).

Hendrix (1988) expressed that although we are born whole with the full potential to thrive, we experience pleasure and pain in childhood and learn to adapt through these experiences. According to Hendrix, positive and negative childhood experiences are imprinted in the brain because they feel the most pleasure or the most threatening, and they leave deep wounds. During childhood, the experience of unmet needs creates feelings of pain and often maladaptive ways to work through the conflict. Hendrix further states that people learn to adapt to survive, contributing to our basic needs being unfilled. He states that since human beings desire to experience wholeness, working through childhood wounds in the context of an intimate relationship will enable couples to fulfill their potential and work toward restoring their wholeness (Hendrix, 1988).

9.2.1   The Effectiveness of Imago Therapy with African American Couples

Although Imago Therapy was developed in the 1980s, many people are not familiar with this type of therapy. While some research exists, more is needed to examine the effectiveness of Imago theory in helping couples resolve conflict. Even less research on its effectiveness with African American couples exists. Few studies have examined Imago Therapy's weekend workshop. Heller (1999) conducted a research study with sixty participants six weeks after the workshop and determined that both men and women felt there were improvements in their marital satisfaction, communication, commitment, conflict, and insight into one's family of origin. The study also determined that improvements in the couples' relationship continued three months after the workshop, except for issues with commitment (Heller, 1999).

A study was conducted examining Imago education with African American couples to determine if they improved communication, increased understanding of self and the partner, increased understanding of childhood wounding for self and partner, and the need for increased Imago education (Martin & Bielawski, 2011). The study determined that participants did report increased communication and insight into themselves and their partners. There was more awareness of the importance of being more understanding and empathic to their partner's needs. There is an increased understanding of how childhood experiences, particularly childhood wounds, lead to self and relational healing (Martin & Bielawski, 2011). The Imago therapy process gives African American couples an opportunity to learn more about how past childhood and psychosocial experiences impact their ability to thrive in their relationship. It also gives them the tools to learn how to resolve conflict more effectively. Imago Therapy provides the tools to move from an unconscious way of relating to a conscious one.

9.3   The Unconscious Self

9.3.1   Childhood Wounds

Hendrix expands on Erik Erikson's theory of childhood development to describe the impact on the couple's relationship. He describes the importance of the child being able to attach, explore, experience a sense of identity, and become competent as they grow. Hendrix believes that even though we may grow up in a nurturing home environment, we may still experience invisible scars, which leads to childhood wounds due to our never-ending cycle of needs.

Hendrix (1988) states that we were born whole, and babies experience oneness inside their mothers' wombs. This type of existence comes to an end when babies are born; however, there is a desire to feel oneness again. According to Hendrix, there is a desire for attachment and to experience physical and spiritual union as it was in the womb. Hendrix states that as children grow, they need to feel connected to their caretakers. When children have painful experiences, they will feel disconnected from others, which leads to problems in their romantic relationship. Hendrix also states that although adults can take care of their physical needs, people unconsciously desire someone to take care of them and return to that emotional safety they experienced in the womb.

Hendrix states that childhood wounds occur when children are not nurtured and protected to grow and feel secure. He indicates that we receive messages from our parents and caretakers about how we should be, and negative messages affect how children perceive themselves. Hendrix explains that children may have feelings of insecurity and rejection when negative messages are received from caregivers and society. This is seen when children are forbidden to express their feelings, especially if they are angry and throw temper tantrums. Children then learn to repress their feelings and live according to their caretakers' expectations of them, states Hendrix. They also learn to create a "false self" to protect themselves from further hurt. Imago theory states that children learn to find their adaptive character traits and continue these traits into their adult relationship to protect themselves from hurt and pain. Hendrix states that adults learn to disown the negative traits because they are too painful to acknowledge in order for adults to maintain a positive self-image.

Due to racial discrimination, poverty, single-parent households, and other stressors in African American families, many couples are impacted by childhood wounds they carry into their intimate relationship. They learn how to protect themselves in their intimate relationship because they may feel unprotected in their family of origin and in a society that does not protect them (Lavner et al., 2018). Imago Therapy enables them to examine these childhood wounds and become aware of how their family of origin, community, and society have impacted them and their relational dynamic. Understanding their childhood wounds enables the African American couple to find new adaptive traits when they experience triggers in their couple's relationship. They begin to recognize each other's wounds from childhood and support each other in their healing journey.

9.3.2   Stages of the Relationship Cycle

9.3.2.1   Romantic Love Stage

Hendrix (1988) states that we are drawn to partners who have positive and negative traits of our parents or caretakers. He claims that people are drawn to a partner in the areas in which they are emotionally shut down. They are drawn to them unconsciously to finish unmet needs in childhood fueled by the desire to reach their potential. Initially, the person sees and is drawn to only their partner's positive traits versus the negative traits during a relationship's "romantic stage." The romantic stage is euphoric and short term due to oxytocin or "feel good" chemicals being experienced. The romantic stage gives the couple a glimpse of what it is like to love fully and what it is like to feel whole and fulfilled. Unfortunately, this stage does not last forever. Kuula et al. (2020) state that research indicates that "romantic love or infatuation is an overwhelming passion toward one person, whereas attachment is a more stable emotional bond." This romantic stage can last up to seventeen months of a relationship (Kuula et al., 2020, p. 3). Imago Therapy helps African American couples understand that this stage does not last forever, and moving to a conscious way of loving makes relationships endure.

9.3.2.2   Power Struggle Stage

Hendrix (1988) highlights that the power struggle stage occurs when we select partners who match our Imago. These partners represent the best and worst traits of the people who have been most significant to us with the unconscious desire to heal our childhood wounds. People unconsciously feel that their partner will meet their unmet childhood desires of being nurtured and loved consistently in order to feel whole. When they are unable to provide this to each other, it changes the dynamic of the relationship. When conflict occurs, the couple may experience triggers because they realize that their partner is not meeting their needs due to their own unmet childhood needs. The "flight-fight" responses are often experienced during the couple's conflict. According to Hendrix, the current responses are based on the earlier responses adapted in childhood when the pain was experienced. He further states that the power struggle stage involves disillusionment, frustration, and anger. Couples learn that their partner cannot make them feel whole but can help them heal their childhood wounds. Imago Therapy helps the couple move from an unconscious way of functioning to a conscious way of dealing with relationship conflict. Most couples end their relationship during the power struggle phase, according to Hendrix. Helping African American couples work through their power struggles using Imago Therapy will help reduce divorces in this population.

9.3.2.3   Minimizer and Maximizer

Hendrix's Imago Therapy utilizes the terms maximizer and minimizer to describe how couples relate to each other. Maximizers tend to externalize or expand their affect, and minimizers tend to internalize and diminish their emotions (Zielinski, 1999). The maximizer tends to pursue their spouse. The spouse, who is the minimizer, tends to be the distancer in the relationship. Hendrix expressed that maximizers tend to marry minimizers. The maximizer must learn to contain their emotions and allow their minimizer spouse to be more expressive and pursue them in the relationship. This will enable the couple to improve how they relate to each other.

Research has indicated that women, more often, tend to be the pursuer and men tend to be the distancer in the relationship because women are often raised to be expressive and dependent and men to be independent and nonverbal (Betchen, 2005). Betchen states that a woman's ability to connect, empathize, and bond is partially impacted by hormones such as estrogen, progesterone, and prolactin. Also, he states that males have higher testosterone levels and exhibit more aggressive behavior, are less empathic, and more task oriented than women. Betchen (2005) further indicated that factors that impact the pursuer-distancer role include changes in social, cultural norms, gender equality, and familial influences that may change this dynamic. He stated that gender equality had impacted intimate relationships because women can distance emotionally from men, and there is more power struggle for control in the relationship (Betchen, 2005).

Traditional roles indicated by researchers may not be relevant for African American couples since they are impacted by racial discrimination. Studies show that over 80 percent of African American couples express being treated unfairly due to their race (Lavner et al., 2018). They often experience economic hardship and psychological distress due to racial stressors (Lavner et al., 2018). African American women had to step into a provider role due to being single mothers often caused by racial discrimination. African American men have been denied access to resources to take care of the family due to institutional racism (Clavél et al., 2017). Familial and societal influences have significantly impacted African American couples in how they relate to each other. Imago Therapy helps the African American couple learn to become more conscious of their maximizer-minimizer or pursuer-distancer roles and change maladaptive behaviors to healthy ways of communicating to enhance the relationship and increase connection.

9.4   The Conscious Self

According to Hendrix's theory, when couples move to a conscious way of relating, they become aware of their own unfulfilled needs from childhood and their unconscious desires in relating to their partner. They can identify their triggers and how they unconsciously adapt to protect themselves due to these triggers. Couples learn the importance of being intentional in working through conflict in their relationship. Further, Hendrix (1988) states that when couples have a conscious relationship, they see conflict as a way to grow versus a negative experience to avoid. The conscious relationship involves recommitment, doing the work, an awakening, and ultimately real love. Couples learn to move to a conscious stage of relating through the Couples Dialogue, the Parent–Child Dialogue, and the Behavior Change Request Dialogue. Experiencing these dialogues bring insight and increase knowledge of oneself and the partner.

9.4.1   Recommitment

Hendrix (1988) states that a recommitment to the relationship involves being aware of one's own unfulfilled needs from childhood and deciding to move toward a conscious view of self and way of relating. He further explains that each of the couples will need to become more aware of their adaptive coping style when they experience conflict and pain when triggered by their partner. There must be a conscious decision to create safety for their partner and a desire to heal their relationship. Couples learn how to process and release feelings of childhood hurts and release hurt in their relationship. The couple develops a plan to grow the relationship and recommit to making the couple's relationship healthy again. Since research shows that African American couples have the highest divorce rates in the United States, helping them get to conscious relating will contribute to a committed couples' relationship.

9.4.2   Doing the Work

Hendrix (1988) claims that when couples decide to "Do the Work" to get through their power struggle phase, conscious healing begins. There is a decision to make their relationship strong and focus on learning techniques to better understand their partner. When couples learn to close exits, then feelings of anger begin to reduce. Closing exits mean that couples choose to communicate their feelings versus acting it out with negative behaviors. Couples learn to express their feelings effectively by using the couples' dialogue by mirroring, expressing empathy, and learning how to validate one another. They also learn to express feelings of appreciation and caring behaviors to their partners. Helping African American couples learn the Imago Couples Dialogue and becoming intentional to care for their partner will strengthen their relationship and cause their relationship to thrive.

9.4.3   Awakening

Hendrix's (1988) Imago theory states that during the awakening phase, the couple is more aware of their unfulfilled childhood needs carried into their adult relationship. They become aware of their triggers and what triggers their partner. The couple also learns the importance of closing exits in their relationship and finding opportunities to communicate to resolve conflict. The couple begins to see their relationship as a new and exciting journey. They learn to release old hurts and old patterns of relating to each other that are ineffective. There is a conscious decision to work on the relationship intentionally.

The awakening process includes five steps. They include re-imaging their partner as a wounded child who requires healing; re-romanticizing the relationship by expressions of caring behaviors, surprises, and appreciation to their partner; restructuring their frustrations by requesting an appointment with their partner to have an intentional dialogue; resolving conflict by working together; and re-visioning their relationship by developing a joint vision and goals for connection. When African Americans become awakened to how societal injustices have contributed to the couples' breakdown, they will become intentional in learning and utilizing the necessary tools to repair and strengthen their relationship. Imago Therapy is an effective tool used to identify childhood wounding and learning techniques to promote healthy relationships.

9.4.4   Real Love

Hendrix (1988) indicates that couples commit to keeping each other safe in the relationship when they move from the romantic phase to "real love." They feel safe and experience joy in their relationship. Hendrix states that a couple establishes a vision for their relationship and sets goals to maintain a relationship that will continue to grow. They learn that conflict naturally happens in a relationship, and it provides opportunities to experience growth, primarily when the Imago techniques are utilized. The couple learns the importance of committing to deepen their love for one another and see their partner as their greatest gift. African American couples can learn the importance of developing a vision of what they want their marriage to look like. Even if they have had no previous couples as role models, they can imagine a relationship that moves beyond infatuation to long-lasting ones.

9.4.5   Caring Behaviors and Surprises

Hendrix (1988) states that engaging in caring behaviors and giving surprises is important to sustain the couples' relationship. When the couples engage in caring behaviors, they will list the type of behaviors they received in the past, the present, and the caring behaviors they wish to receive in the future. The couple will initiate a dialogue with the sender saying, "I feel loved or cared for when you . . .." The receiver will mirror. The couple will identify their secret desires and be specific about their needs. Communicating secret desires brings about vulnerability. These desires can be words of affirmation, gifts, or activities that are desired. Hendrix also expressed the need for couples to surprise each other with the things their partner identifies as important to them. The couple must have a sense of safety to share their deepest desires hoping that their partner can meet these desires. Helping African Americans express their desires to their partner will encourage giving and receiving in their relationship and feelings of belonging.

9.5   The Imago Dialogue Process

Using the Imago Couples Dialogue is central to Imago education. There are different types of dialogues. The Parent–Child Dialogue helps the couple to work on healing their childhood wounds. The Couples Dialogue enables the couple to work on the frustrations they are experiencing in their relationship. The Behavior Change Request Dialogue gives couples the opportunity to request change from their partner to reduce their frustration. Each of these dialogues is discussed in more detail.

9.5.1   Parent–Child Dialogue

According to Hendrix (1988), the Parent–Child Dialogue allows each person in the relationship to express the pain and hurt they experienced in their childhood with their significant caregiver(s). Each person can describe the pain they experienced in their childhood to their partner using the present tense. The sender of the information can describe a childhood hurt experienced at a particular age, and the partner who is the receiver assumes the parent role and mirrors back their partner's childhood experience. The receiver asks the sender to describe their worst frustration and hurt experience with their caretaker during the dialogue. The receiver will also ask the sender what is needed in order to heal. When the receiver ends the

Parent–Child Dialogue, the receiver will then ask their partner what can be done in the partner relationship for healing to occur. The couple is then allowed to help heal each other's childhood wounds using this dialogue.

Hendrix (1988) delineates that the Parent–Child Dialogue process utilizes sender and receiver roles. The dialogue states, "I am your mother or father. What is it like living with me?" The sender will describe the experience in the present tense using the age that the wounding may have occurred. The receiver will mirror back and encourage the sender to provide more information. Once the sender is complete, the receiver will summarize and ask the sender to describe the worst feelings experienced with their mother or father. At the end of the summary, the receiver will de-role and let the sender know that they are not back to be their spouse and ask the question, "What can I do to help you heal?" This dialogue is important to African American couples because of the pain they may continue to carry into their intimate relationship due to the childhood trauma that they may have experienced through the impact of slavery and racial discrimination. Using this dialogue enables them to increase their vulnerability, release their pain, and increase the attachment with their partner.

9.5.2   Understanding the Imago Couples Dialogue

When the couple is consciously relating, they learn to communicate differently. They begin to learn and use the Imago Couples Dialogue to express their feelings. The Couples Dialogue includes Mirroring, Validation, and Empathy. Using the Couples Dialogue will enable the couple to address feelings of frustration. During the dialogue, each person will work through their various frustrations using the steps of mirroring, validation, and empathy. The Couples Dialogue helps the couple address their conflict safely and in a healthy manner. Shuper (2019) states that mirroring the partner's messages will avoid defensive reactions and improved communication in the relationship. Shuper (2019) indicates that when the partner's words and feelings are mirrored, it facilitates a close and empathic connection because it ensures that the couples listen and empathize with their partner's feelings. Mirroring, validation, and empathy are included in all the dialogues used in Imago theory.

9.5.2.1   Mirroring

Hendrix (1988) explains that mirroring involves an active listening process, and it allows the partner to reflect the content that is being communicated accurately. Hendrix further explains that mirroring can include paraphrasing, which conveys what the partner is saying but reflecting one's own words. Word-for-word mirroring reflects the partner's words, which gives the message that one can suspend one's thoughts and feelings to focus on the partner, according to Hendrix. A sender communicates the message, and the receiver mirrors back the message that is communicated. The couple is also encouraged to sit facing each other to provide eye contact. An example of mirroring given by the sender is, "I feel frustrated when you spend more time on your phone than talking with me." The receiver will say, "I heard you say that you are frustrated when I spend more time on my phone than I do speaking with you." When the couple hears their words repeated, they feel that their spouse is listening to them, which increases connection (Shuper, 2019). Since mirroring increases feelings of connection, using this technique in African American couples' counseling will strengthen their ability to have increased attachment in their relationship.

9.5.2.2 Validation

The validation portion of Hendrix's Couples Dialogue informs the partner that the information that is being mirrored "makes sense." It lets the partner know that their thoughts and feelings being experienced are valid because the couple can see their partners' perspective. Couples often struggle with validation because they feel like they have to agree with their partner's feelings. However, Hendrix (1988) reminds the reader that there are two points of view in a relationship, and each person is entitled to their truth. According to Hendrix, the couple learns to listen to their partner's view and learn to validate their experience to increase trust and connection. An example of validation is when the sender has communicated a frustration, and the receiver validates the sender by stating, "What makes sense about what I just heard is . . ..". The receiver takes the time to let the sender know that the frustration that they have experienced makes sense. African American couples have not been validated throughout history due to discrimination. Their contributions to society have often been overlooked, which has impacted the family structure. There is a need for African American couples to learn how to validate each other to feel that their thoughts and feelings are heard.

9.5.2.3 Empathy

According to Hendrix (1988), empathy in the dialogue helps the couple become more cognizant of their partner's feelings. Each person can reflect on what is being communicated and imagine what the experience must be like for their partner. Hendrix states that this process encourages the couple to move beyond their feelings of separateness and see their relationship as a partnership. Couples begin to reflect on their partner's feelings and empathize with their partner's hurt and pain. In this dialogue process, the sender will express their frustration, and the receiver of the frustration may say, "I imagine you might be feeling …" to provide empathy to the partner. Learning to empathize will help the African American couple move beyond their hurt and pain and see their partner's hurt and pain. This encourages emotional, physical, and spiritual oneness in the couple.

9.5.3   Behavior Change Request

The Behavior Change Request Dialogue's premise is to help couples work through their frustrations by requesting their spouse to meet their hidden desires (Hendrix, 1988). To engage in the Behavior Change Request Dialogue, the sender will request an appointment, and the receiver will grant the request as soon as possible. Couples use the Imago Couples Dialogue by learning how to mirror, validate, and empathize with their partner's frustration. Hendrix states that the sender will express, "I feel frustrated when …." The receiver will mirror back, "When this happens, I feel …." The receiver mirrors, "How it makes me behave is …." The receiver mirrors, "What hurts the most is …." The receiver mirrors, "These feelings remind me of my childhood experience of …." The receiver summarizes the dialogue and asks, "Did I get that right?" The receiver validates the information makes sense and asks, "The receiver will ask what is it that you desire of me?" The sender's responsibility is to state a global desire to be mirrored by the receiver. The receiver asks, "What is it that you desire of me?" The sender will express three specific requests to their partner. The Behavior Change Request must be completed as a SMART goal. It must be specific, measurable, attainable, relevant, and time limited, according to Hendrix. The couples will commit to giving their partner one of the Behavior Change Requests and will tell their partner how giving them this gift will help them grow and heal their partner's childhood wounds.

9.6   The Practice of Imago Therapy

9.6.1   Case Study Example

James and Susan are both African Americans who have been married for seven years. They have two children, ages five and two. The couple requested counseling because they were struggling with their connection. They expressed that they have very little time to connect and felt overwhelmed with caring for their children and working full time. James is a business owner, and Susan works for the government. James felt that Susan was more concerned with taking care of the kids and too tired to connect emotionally and sexually. Susan felt that James was more focused on his work than spending time with the family. The couple often found themselves in conflict and struggled to communicate effectively to work through them. Susan expressed that James does not share his feelings when he is upset, which contributed to her yelling at him. James felt that he could not open up and share his feelings with Susan due to her volatile emotional outburst.

James was raised in a family of five children with a single mother. James expressed that his father was close by and contributed to the family after the divorce; however, he was not emotionally present. Susan expressed that she was raised in a two-parent household with two siblings. She expressed that her parents argued repeatedly, and she was often fearful that the situation would become physical. The couple was afraid that they would not change their communication patterns and salvage their relationship. They decided that they wanted to try couples' therapy for the first time to repair their family.

9.6.2   The Assessment Process

The therapist completed an evaluation session with James and Susan together. Obtaining a thorough family history enabled the therapists to understand each of the couple's backgrounds to support them better. Conducting a biopsychosocial history allowed the therapist to better understand the culture, medical history, family or origin, psychological background, faith, and financial concerns. Also, the therapist reviewed the concerns that brought them into therapy and their desired goals. When the therapist obtained a thorough understanding of the couple, a plan was formulated to support them in repairing the relationship. Once the biopsychosocial history was discussed with the couple, the therapist explained the plan for therapy and delineated how Imago Therapy would support the couple to resolve their conflict. The couple was allowed to commit to the process.

9.6.3   Beginning the Imago Therapy Process

The couple agreed to commit to the therapy process; therefore, the therapist taught the couple about the Imago dialogue process. They were also taught about the importance of mirroring using the Appreciation Dialogue. The Appreciation Dialogue enabled them to identify positive qualities in their partner despite the frustrations they were experiencing. Even though the couple may be in a difficult place in their marriage, helping them see the positive gave them hope.

9.6.3.1   Couples Dialogue

The therapist worked with James and Susan for twelve sessions following the evaluation session. Susan was more eager to participate in couples counseling than James. Both expressed that they were committed to doing the work to improve their marriage. The therapist engaged the couple in the Couples Dialogue and the Behavior Change Request Dialogue to address various frustrations in their relationship. Susan expressed her frustration with James due to his long work hours and lack of focus on the family. She did not feel she was a priority to him. Susan complained to James about this behavior, but nothing seemed to change. Out of frustration, she resorted to yelling to get him to listen. She felt overwhelmed with work and managing the children on her own.

James expressed his concern about Susan's anger. He expressed that he was trying to provide for the family, and it was not easy to manage the business and spend more time with the family. James also expressed that it was more peaceful at work than at home. He expressed frustration with Susan's nagging behavior so he ignored her when she complained. He also stated that he was feeling very alone because Susan withdrew affection when she was angry.

The couple was able to identify their childhood wounds during the twelve sessions of Imago Therapy. Susan learned that James represented her father, who was present in the home but absent emotionally from the family. She expressed that she felt unwanted by him growing up and tried to get his attention by excelling in her school work and taking care of her younger siblings. Susan expressed that no matter how hard she tried, she just could not get noticed by him. She expressed resorting to yelling to get James to pay attention to her. James reminded her of her father because, like her father, he had very little time for her and the family.

James realized that his childhood wound related to unintentional neglect due to being raised by a single mother who worked two jobs to take care of the family. He was responsible for five of his siblings, and it was difficult for him to get his needs met. James expressed that he had very little time to be a "kid." He also expressed that due to his mother being so busy and stressed, she had very little time to show him affection. He resented his father for not being a support to the family. Susan reminded him of his mother because her attention focused on the children and not meeting his needs. The couple was able to use the Parent–Child Dialogue to help them heal their childhood wounds.

The childhood experiences of Susan and James are common experiences of the African American community. Since African Americans are more likely to be impacted by economic disenfranchisement, poverty, oppression, and racial discrimination than other racial groups, this negatively affects their family system (Clavél et al., 2017). Many African American families are not aware that these discriminatory experiences in their community contribute to childhood wounds that they bring into their relationships. Even when couples remain together, African American families' social, economic, and psychological stressors can destabilize the family system. Many African American couples may not understand that these experiences in childhood create emotional wounds that impact their couples' relationships. James and Susan recognized their childhood wounds and their need to help each other heal through Imago Therapy.

The couple learned how to create a safe space for each other to share their frustrations. They learned different couples' dialogue techniques to effectively address childhood experiences and work through conflicts in their relationship. The couple used the Behavior Change Request Dialogue to change the patterns that were ineffective in their relationship. Susan requested that James set aside two evenings and a Saturday to spend with the family and resume date nights once per month. James requested that Susan set aside time to acknowledge him with a warm greeting when he arrived home from work and that she set aside time once a week to resume sexual intimacy. Both agreed to work on giving each other what they desired, and they saw improvements.

James and Susan were able to understand better their triggers and the triggers of each other. They became very intentional in applying what they learned in therapy to strengthen their relationship. They used the Couples Dialogue when they had conflicts at home. They were able to establish a vision for their relationship and identified goals to operationalize their vision. They practiced giving caring behaviors and surprises to each other. James and Susan committed to keeping each other safe and closing exits to grow in their connection. Since they were intentional in using the Couples Dialogue to address conflict in their relationship, they were ready to move toward concluding weekly couples' therapy sessions.

9.7 Conclusion

Imago Relationship Therapy is a useful form of therapy for all couples, including African American couples. It enables couples to work through conflict by learning effective communication tools through the Imago dialogue process. Couples learn the importance of moving from an unconscious to a conscious way of relating in their relationship. They learn to see each other's childhood wounds and commit to helping each other heal. This is a focus on finding strengths in the relationship and helping couples to envision and commit to learning new healthy ways of relating. This approach builds on African American couples' strength and encourages them to deepen their commitment to one another.

Discussion Questions

1. How might the relational approach of Imago Therapy be used to strengthen African American marriages?
2. How might the sociocultural history of Black people in the United States impact their unconscious relational behaviors?
3. Why is it important for therapists to be aware of their own childhood wounds when working with couples?
4. How does Imago Therapy differ from your usual way of conceptualizing couple discord?

REFERENCES

Allen, W. D., & Olson, D. H. (2001). Five types of African-American marriages. *Journal of Marital and Family Therapy, 27*(3), 301–314. https://doi.org/10.1111/j.1752-0606.2001.tb00326.x

Betchen, S. J. (2005). *Intrusive partners – elusive mates: The pursuer-distancer dynamic in couples.* Taylor & Francis Group.

Burdette, A., Haynes, S., & Ellison, C. (2012). Religion, race/ethnicity, and perceived barriers to marriage among working-age adults. *Sociology of Religion, 73*(4), 429–451. http://www.jstor.org/stable/41818898

Campbell, K., & Wright, D. W. (2010). Marriage today: Exploring the incongruence between Americans' beliefs and practices. *Journal of Comparative Family Studies, 41*(3), 329–345.

Chambers, A. L., & Kravitz, A. (2011). Understanding the disproportionately low marriage rate among African Americans: An amalgam of sociological and psychological constraints. *Family Relations, 60*, 648–660. https://doi.org/10.1111/j.1741-3729.2011.00673.x

Chaney, C. (2014). Perceptions of emotional closeness, commitment, and relationship stability among African American couples. *Marriage & Family Review*, *50*(2), 129–153. https://doi.org/10.1080/01494929.2010.543037

Clavél, F., Cutrona, C., & Russell, D. (2017). United and divided by stress: How stressors differentially influence social support in African American couples over time. *Society for Personality and Social Psychology*, *43*(7), 1050–1064. https://doi.org/10.1177/0146167217704195

Collins, W. L., & Perry, A. R. (2015). Black men's perspectives on the role of the black church in healthy relationship promotion and family stability. *Social Work and Christianity*, *42*(4), 430–448.

Emery, R. E. (2013). *Cultural sociology of divorce: An encyclopedia.* Sage Publications.

Heller, B. C. (1999). *An evaluation of imago relationship therapy through its use in the getting the love you want workshop: A quantitative/qualitative assessment* (Order No. 9955251) [Doctoral dissertation, Saybrook Graduate School and Research Center]. ProQuest Dissertations & Theses Global; ProQuest One Academic. https://www.proquest.com/openview/a07080825aa93965682ef d79ee797495/1?pq-origsite=gscholar&cbl=18750&diss=y

Hendrix, H. (1988). *Getting the love you want: A guide for couples.* Henry Holt and Company.

(1994). *Getting the love you want: A couples workshop manual.* Institute for Imago Relationship Therapy.

Hurt, T. R., Beach, S. R. H., Stokes, L. A., Bush, P. L., Sheats, K. J., & Robinson, S. G. (2012). Engaging African American men in empirically based marriage enrichment programs: Lessons from two focus groups on the ProSAAM project. *Cultural Diversity and Ethnic Minority Psychology*, *18*(3), 312–315. https://doi.org/10.1037/a0028697

Kuula, L., Partonen, T., & Pesonen, A. (2020). Emotions relating to romantic love – Further disruptors of adolescent sleep. *Sleep Health*, *6*(2), 159–165. https://doi.org/10.1016/j.sleh.2020.01.006

Lavner, J. A., Barton, A. W., Bryant, C. M., & Beach, S. R. H. (2018). Racial discrimination and relationship functioning among African American couples. *Journal of Family Psychology*, *32*(5), 686–691. https://doi.org/10.1037/ famo000415

Leeker, O., & Carlozzi, A. (2014). Effects of sex, sexual orientation, infidelity expectations, and love on distress related to emotional and sexual infidelity. *Journal of Marital and Family Therapy*, *40*(1), 68–91. https://doi.org/10 .1111/j.1752-0606.2012.00331.x

Marks, L. D., Hopkins, K. Chaney, C., Monroe, P. A., Nesteruk, O., & Sasser, D. D. (2008). Together we are strong: A qualitative study of happy, enduring African American marriages. *Family Relations*, *57*, 172–185.

Martin, T. L., & Bielawski, D. M. (2011). What is the African American's experience following imago education? *Journal of Humanistic Psychology*, *51*(2), 216–228. https://doi.org/10.1177/0022167809352379

Perry, A. (2013). African American men's attitudes toward marriage. *Journal of Black Studies*, *44*, 182–202.

Phillips, T., Wilmoth, J., & Marks, L. (2012). Challenges and conflicts ... strengths and supports: A study of enduring African American marriages. *Journal of Black Studies, 43*(8), 936–952. http://www.jstor.org/stable/23414682

Shuper, E. (2019). Embodying the couple relationship: Kinesthetic empathy and somatic mirroring in couples therapy. *Journal of Couple & Relationship Therapy, 18*(2), 126–147. https://doi.org/10.1080/15332691.2018.1481801

Simons, L. G., Simons, R. L., Landor, A. M., Bryant, C. M., & Beach, S. R. H. (2014). Factors linking childhood experiences to adult romantic relationships among African Americans. *Journal of Family Psychology, 28*(3), 368–379. https://doi.org/10.1037/a0036393

Taylor, R. (1988). Structural determinants of religious participation among Black Americans. *Review of Religious Research, 30*, 114–125.

Vaterlaus, J. M., Skogrand, L., Chaney, C., & Gahagan, K. (2017). Marital expectations in strong African American marriages. *Family Process, 56*, 883–899. https://doi.org/10.1111/famp.12263

Wilkins, E., Whiting, J., Watson, M., Russon, J., & Moncrief, A. (2013). Residual effects of slavery: What clinicians need to know. *Contemporary Family Therapy: An International Journal, 35*(1), 14–28. https://doi.org/10.1007/s10591-012-9219-1

Zielinski, J. J. (1999). Discovering imago relationship therapy. *Psychotherapy: Theory, Research, Practice, Training, 36*(1), 91–101.

African American Narratives of Trauma: An EMDR Approach to Tapping into the Strengths of Black Love

Alice Shepard & Katherine McKay

There is no fear in love. But perfect love drives out fear.
1 John 4:18 (New International Version)

Romantic love is anything but perfect, but even with our limitations as humans, love holds the promise to transcend pain, heal our hearts, and inspire hope. However, incidents of trauma uniquely test the strengths of love. Trauma is an abrupt and devastating event that overwhelms our physical, emotional, and mental coping capacity. It can rattle our souls, shatter our beliefs, and destroy our relationships. Trauma has far-reaching effects. It disrupts one's ability to regulate their emotional state for years to come (Herman, 2015). Unfortunately, the impact of trauma on Black relationships often goes unaddressed in traditional couples counseling.

In a national behavioral health survey (National Epidemiologic Survey on Alcohol and Related Conditions [NESARC]), over 71 percent of Americans reported at least one exposure to a traumatic event. For African Americans, the prevalence of trauma is even greater (76.4 percent) (Roberts et al., 2011). For example, African Americans experience increased assault victimization (Roberts et al., 2011) and intimate partner violence (Smith et al., 2018). The ubiquity of trauma, combined with continuing societal, racial oppression, creates added layers of stress for African Americans and their loved ones. Therefore, couples counselors have a real opportunity to improve the health and wellbeing of Black communities through the effective treatment of unprocessed trauma in Black romantic relationships.

Eye Movement Desensitization Reprocessing (EMDR) is an essential tool for couples therapists seeking guidance in working with trauma. Francine Shapiro developed the EMDR approach in 1987, and it continues to gain popularity (Shapiro, 2002). EMDR is an evidence-based intervention shown to improve the therapeutic process and outcome.

The EMDR method is highly structured and thorough. It supplies a strategy for how to identify repressed memories and unlink them from feelings of victimization. Therapists create a holding space to delve into clients' shut-off aspects of themselves. This work can alleviate clients' shame and guilt and renew their connection to themselves and others. This chapter details how therapists can incorporate EMDR within a racially informed couples therapy framework. Hypothetical examples illustrate key concepts to portray the potential range of issues encountered in working with Black couples. The authors aim to improve the understanding and accessibility of EMDR and to promote its use. Black couples deserve access to culturally sensitive clinicians who have expertise in treating trauma.

10.1   Trauma in Black Couples

Couples counselors are in a unique position to heal both individual and shared trauma for Black clients. When working with Black couples, it is essential to thoughtfully assess if one or both members have experienced a form of trauma. Much of the literature dichotomizes trauma into either "big T" or "little t" (Shapiro & Forrest, 2016). Big T traumas include events that threaten one's physical integrity or in which a person believes their life or someone else's life is in danger (Shapiro & Forest, 2016). Feelings of terror often mark big T traumas. An example of a big T trauma event is the Black father witnessing the murder of his son.

In contrast, "little t" traumas are often covert daily and relational injuries that leave the individual feeling rejected, isolated, or ashamed (Shapiro & Forest, 2016). An example of a "little t" trauma is the Black woman who experiences isolation and microaggressions at work because she is the only person of color in her department. "Microaggressions are often linchpin memories that reinforce negative beliefs. Targeting these memories (in trauma processing) typically benefits clients" (Nickerson, 2016, p. 36). To varying degrees, both Big T and little t experiences negatively impact intrapsychic and interpersonal functioning. Therefore, couples therapists are encouraged to gain insight into the aggregated effect of multiple types of traumas.

EMDR is highly effective in uprooting trauma (Shapiro, 2002, 2014). The EMDR approach is especially beneficial to Black men in couples who may underreport incidents of victimization and assault (Motley & Banks, 2018). The guided processes of EMDR are structured to alleviate long-repressed feelings of anger and isolation and to create emotional intimacy, compassion, and trust. Through EMDR, Black couples can recognize the pernicious ways past trauma impacts their relationship and dismantle their communication and connection blocks. EMDR offers the possibility for Black couples to rebuild emotional intimacy, compassion, and trust by identifying and directly addressing trauma.

10.2   Neglect

It is imperative to highlight neglect as a form of trauma. Neglect is the most common form of child maltreatment (Children's Bureau, 2020). Clinically the impact of neglect can sometimes be overlooked as a salient factor in psychological and relational distress (Perry et al., 2002). However, studies show that neglect, like other forms of trauma, impacts a child's sense of safety. Those subjected to neglect struggle to form healthy romantic relationships later in life (Perry et al., 2002). "Indeed, neglect in early stages of life may lead to severe, chronic, and irreversible damage" (p. 194). The legacy of neglect may show up relationally for couples in their difficulty in both receiving and expressing empathy or their beliefs about parenting or emotional closeness.

A higher incidence of substance use, divorce, and rates of incarceration in the Black community combined with disproportionately high poverty leads to a greater likelihood of childhood neglect for Black children (Jonson-Reid et al., 2013). Even the culturally acceptable practice within the Black community of sending one's child to live with close friends and relatives can elicit feelings of neglect. As a result, Black clients may downplay or not include the history of early-life neglect in their self-report. During intake, clinicians are encouraged to assess for both adult and childhood trauma and be alert to occurrences of neglect. To help Black couples, providers need to gain additional training in listening for, assessing, and working with a range of traumas.

10.3   Racial Trauma

Racial trauma is a significant part of the American Black experience. It can occur as a direct attack or by witnessing harm done to another (Helms et al., 2010). The murder of George Floyd in May 2020 brought international attention to violence against Blacks and the racial trauma they experience. Floyd's killing and the media attention that followed inflicted large-scale vicarious racial trauma. Racial trauma increases stress, insecurity, fear, and adverse health outcomes (Carter, 2007). Early in life,

Blacks learn how to interact with racist societal forces. Instructions on navigating racist acts are part of intergenerational narratives in Black families (Guillory, 2021). Guillory calls on couples therapists to have humility and educate themselves about racism to better inform their work with Black clients. "Black romantic love relationships have been and continue to be negatively impacted" by racist societal systems (Guillory, 2021, p. 11).

10.4   Using EMDR to Treat Trauma

Culturally competent therapists need to be appropriately trained in the treatment of trauma. Therapists should be grounded in the knowledge that trauma behaviors are often unconscious, maladaptive strategies driven by the survival instinct, and are often attempts to cope, control, or gain mastery. The trauma survival actions can take the form of shutdown, control, reaction/alarm, or avoidance behaviors (Lancaster et al., 2016). Trauma control behaviors are typified by the Army veteran who walks point nightly, checking his doors and windows multiple times while his children sleep. Classic avoidance behaviors may take the form of a sexual assault survivor who recoils at her partner's touch, both physically and emotionally cutting off any avenue to sexual intimacy. Not all therapeutic approaches are alike. There are only a few evidence-based treatments that address trauma-related behaviors. EMDR is one of only a handful of trauma interventions that have been shown to be effective (World Health Organization [WHO], 2013).

EMDR, developed by Francine Shapiro (1995), is a research-validated treatment for trauma that has been approved for the treatment of Post-Traumatic Stress Disorder (PTSD) by several international bodies, including the Department of Defense, Department of Veterans Affairs, and the American Psychiatric Association (Trauma Recovery/HAP, 2020; Ursano et al., 2004). EMDR and trauma-focused cognitive behavioral therapy (CBT) are the only two trauma treatments recommended by the WHO (2013). WHO stated that "Like CBT with a trauma focus, EMDR aims to reduce subjective distress and strengthen adaptive cognitions related to the traumatic event. Unlike CBT with a trauma focus, EMDR does not involve (a) detailed descriptions of the event, (b) direct challenging of beliefs, (c) extended exposure, or (d) homework" (WHO, 2013, p. 1). Furthermore, EMDR has been shown to be applicable across cultures and effective in not just the treatment of trauma and PTSD but depression, anxiety, and other forms of psychopathology as well (Wilson et al., 2018).

At the foundation of EMDR is what Shapiro (1995) coined as the Adaptive Information Processing (AIP) model. "The AIP model views the human brain as a physical mechanism that translates perception into stored memories. These memories become the basis of knowledge that guides future activity. Memories are composed of complicated neural networks that impact perception, response tendencies, attitudes, self-concept, and personality traits" (Nickerson, 2016, p. 19). For Black survivors who struggle with PTSD or other trauma-related psychopathology, the AIP posits that unresolved memories result in trauma images, sensations, beliefs, or emotions that dominate the survivors' perceptions and behaviors. To use a hypothetical example, when John, a Black man in his late forties, sees his partner's face contorted with anger, he becomes frozen as his heart races, his throat tightens, and images of his father's fists flash through his mind along with the negative cognition of "I'm powerless," his trauma is alive. Although it has been three decades since his abuse, in those moments, his brain cannot distinguish the difference between the past and present. The past now disrupts his ability to navigate conflicts with his wife.

Central to EMDR is the premise that unresolved trauma memories are stored in one's neural pathways in a different way when compared to other memories, specifically emotionally neutral or positive events. These unresolved memories, because they are not "filed away" in a manner that either makes sense to the brain or ensures safety, continue to have the power to interfere with the survivor's functioning. Intrusive thoughts, memories, or dreams are some ways the memory may present, but the intrusion may also result in the form of an explosive, aggressive response to the slightest hint of a threat.

These behavioral responses, along with body sensations, visual images, and cognitions, are all part of the AIP. When applying an EMDR approach to couples therapy with Black Americans, the cognitions or narratives are often the easiest to access. Within the AIP framework of EMDR, the impact of the clients' trauma experiences can be accessed through their narratives. We all have narratives, which are stories our brains use to organize and make sense of our world. These narratives are framed by experiences both individual and collective; they are the stories shared not just within one's family, but within communities and inter-generationally. This can include historical narratives of one's own ancestors as well as the entire culture. Narratives are often grouped into three categories: view of self, view of others, and view of the world, which can include the perception of larger systems like governments, spiritual forces, or other entities bigger or more encompassing than any specific person. Narratives help individuals navigate through the world, establishing a template regarding what to expect and how to respond to life events.

From an EMDR perspective, narratives are identified as cognitions. A traumatic experience has the potential to challenge and radically shift one's cognitions. The trauma experience does not fit within the framework of what is expected and has the potential to shatter one's sense of self and the world. When confronted with trauma, the brain is faced with two urgent tasks: how to organize one's world and how to keep safe. Here is where the trauma becomes organized within the AIP. The brain's processing system takes over. Narratives are used to organize and make sense of the horrific experience and figure out how, with this newly recognized threat, one can attain safety. The brain starts scanning for all the past narratives that may apply, filtering through what fits. Like a ticker tape machine, the scripts start rapidly moving. The brain takes into account the cognitions that have governed one's life thus far and evaluates how to integrate this new experience. For example, a female survivor of sexual assault now must incorporate her rape within her narrative about the world. "So, if 'good things happen to good people,' what does this now mean about me?" From this automatic process, trauma cognitions are born. The examination of trauma narratives is an essential component of treating Black couples. The trauma survivor who now has to integrate her assault within the narrative that "good things happen to good people," now is left with the negative cognition of "I must have done something wrong. I am bad." Within EMDR treatment, this negative cognition is targeted as part of the trauma reprocessing.

For Black trauma survivors, the trauma cognition can be further complicated by historical and cultural narratives. For descendants of the African diaspora, these narratives can hold special meaning and power when spoken by the descendants of enslaved peoples. The narratives can be positive, retelling the stories of resilience in the face of the slave trade and the legacy of systemic oppression. They can also be negative, as seen in the co-opted and twisted images used to dehumanize, criminalize, and degrade the Black race. When working with a Black trauma survivor, it is imperative to assess not just the trauma narratives of the client's present victimization, but also the cultural and historical narratives they may have learned.

10.5   Culturally Competent Application of EMDR with Black Couples: From Consultation to Treatment

When working with African American couples, it is important to incorporate a culturally sensitive lens to assess trauma as well as understand racial and cultural factors as they shape narratives and the clients' identities. A failure to do so can be discriminatory and detrimental to the couple. Therapists who adopt a "culture-blind" approach without acknowledging the impact that systemic racism has on their perceptions and their clients often unknowingly engage in invalidating and harmful behaviors and perpetuate the psychological injuries inherent in racism (Ridley, 2005). This can further exacerbate the trauma response. An example of the importance of assessing for racial factors can be seen in the example of a Black couple who presents in therapy due to conflicts regarding the wife's controlling behaviors. Contributing factors of the wife's distress may be missed if the therapist fails to assess through a culturally relevant lens. For example, a woman's anger and demands for explanation when her husband is late to return home may be exacerbated by fears of him being profiled by the police. The need to assess directly for trauma history as well as the relevance of the couple's racial and cultural identity cannot be overstated.

EMDR is a culturally adaptive therapeutic approach. Whether it is the recent trauma of a Black couple who had a car accident, or the Black family whose house was destroyed in a natural disaster, or a young Black man describing his experience with police violence, adjustments are made to ensure that the therapeutic needs of the client are met. EMDR has been applied across the globe within various cultures and has been shown to be effective, even when cultural or language differences exist between therapist and clients (Nickerson, 2016). Through the Trauma Recovery, EMDR Humanitarian Assistance Programs (Trauma Recovery/HAP), there has been a global effort to provide trauma therapy and train EMDR therapists in culturally marginalized or underserved populations worldwide. "Not only can EMDR standard treatment be adapted to different cultures, but it can be used to specifically treat the overall effects of culturally based trauma" (Nickerson, 2016, p. 11).

For Black couples with a trauma history, utilizing EMDR can be an effective conjoint treatment. "The aim of integrating EMDR into couple therapy is to repair attachment wounds while providing a tangible experience of availability, empathy, and the promise of reliability" (Moses, 2007, p. 115). Availability, emotional engagement, and reliability are foundational to all healthy relationships and facilitate trust. Whether in a romantic relationship or in a psychotherapeutic setting, for Black trauma survivors, the presence of trust and safety is required for healing. Let's examine some of the factors that contribute to the creation of a safe therapeutic space when utilizing EMDR with Black couples who have a trauma history.

In order to create a safe, trusting alliance with the couple, the therapist strives to convey knowledge and empathy, patience and confidence, transparency and authenticity. In its practice, EMDR relies on these pillars in the creation of a sacred therapeutic space. In the earliest stage of therapy, in fact even before the first session during the initial contact, providing basic education about trauma, making sense of the survivors' symptoms in light of trauma's impact, and informing the couple about the expected course of treatment help to set the foundation for a successful therapy. This is done in a collaborative and attuned manner, paying close attention to the couple's experiences. In the initial phone consultation, it is beneficial to set the parameters of treatment and establish a balanced alliance. Speaking to both partners and sharing with them the pacing of treatment, outlining the process and purpose of the planned approach, and giving them the opportunity to ask questions and share their goals for the couple's work, assists in setting a base for a safe therapeutic space. The phone consultation gives the first opportunity to educate and assist the traumatized couple to organize and make meaning of their psychological responses, which up to this point have often left them feeling alone, chaotic, and "crazy."

During the phone consultation, the therapist should be mindful of the factors to consider in determining if the timing is appropriate for the couple to engage in treatment using EMDR. Treatment may not be appropriate if there are questions regarding either partner's commitment to the relationship, the presence of active infidelity, or significant addiction. Treatment may not be safe if there is current violence between the couple. The therapist must assess the risk of escalation in interpersonal violence (IPV) (physical, financial, sexual) and determine if the treatment will exacerbate IPV. Assessment of each partner's level of trauma distress is also crucial to determine if individual treatment is a necessary precursor to couples work. If one partner has severe PTSD or psychopathology, it may be necessary to first focus on that individual's stability by referring to an individual EMDR therapist, or if deemed manageable within the couple's framework, arrange the order of trauma processing to begin with a lengthier stabilization in the preparation phase (discussed in detail later). The decision to engage in EMDR couples treatment must be evaluated based on each partner's level of distress, including dissociation and issues related to risk of suicide or self-harm. Some deescalation of the couple conflict cycle as well as stabilization and grounding are also essential prior to engaging in conjoint sessions with EMDR, as emotional tolerance and other nuances related to the couple dynamic can impact trauma processing in the couple setting. This requires the EMDR therapist to be alert and attuned to the couple and their individual needs (Moses, 2007). These factors, especially monitoring the risk of interpersonal violence within the relationship and risk of suicide or self-harm, should be evaluated at the beginning and throughout the course of therapy.

If the consultation reveals that the couple is appropriate for EMDR couples therapy, then the therapist can evaluate if the standard protocol needs to be altered. EMDR allows for the adaptation of the standard protocol to meet clients' cultural or relevant trauma needs (Nickerson, 2016). The EMDR standard protocol consists of distinct phases that guide the therapist and organize the treatment (Shapiro, 1995). This eight-phase protocol can be applied to treat traumatized couples. This model will be used to demonstrate applicability of EMDR to couples therapy with African Americans.

10.6   The EMDR Protocol (Eight Phases)

Working with traumatized clients requires specialized training. The information contained in this chapter is used for descriptive purposes and is not intended to replace formal EMDR training or supervision. In the following section, the eight phases of the EMDR treatment protocol will be described in detail to show the full arc of the treatment process.

Phase One of the EMDR protocol is to obtain client history and devise a treatment plan. The culturally sensitive couples therapist will once again assess the level of commitment to the relationship, and any risks for self-harm or interpersonal violence within the relationship. In addition, the couple's relational history as well as a deliberate assessment of trauma and cultural experiences should be conducted. A thorough and culturally attuned assessment of the couple's history to include trauma provides the information necessary to plan and apply the treatment. The use of structured assessments as part of the intake process can be very helpful. However, there is no substitute for sitting with the clients and hearing directly from them about their lives. The culturally competent EMDR couples therapist is attentive to trauma and cultural experiences and asks direct questions about both areas. Gaining the clients' permission to talk about cultural and trauma experiences contributes to creating therapeutic safety. In line with being transparent and empathetic to create a trusting and safe space, the therapist should also be deliberate in stating the plan and purpose of the assessment. Letting the couple know that during the intake process they will be seen jointly or independently and that the goal is to get to know them better by learning about their family of origin and earlier relationships, will help the therapist understand how these experiences shape the clients' narratives about themselves and expectations in relationships.

Use of a cultural genogram (Nickerson, 2016) with special attention to trauma may be a good option in gaining insight regarding the personal, familial, and cultural experiences of Black couples. A culturally sensitive trauma-informed genogram includes not just asking about the family tree, but gaining information about relatives' experiences with trauma, family narratives regarding racism, any messages about seeking therapy, gender expectations, and coping. It means inquiring about the lessons learned from their parents' relationship, and sensitive and direct questions about child abuse and adult trauma. Examples of these questions include:

1. Sometimes as children, we have experiences that leave us feeling scared or uncomfortable. These experiences can impact the way we see ourselves or our relationships. Is it okay for me to ask you some questions about things that may have occurred when you were a child?
2. Sometimes people have the experience of being exposed to situations that leave them feeling uncomfortable sexually. Is it okay for me to ask you some questions about this?

Asking permission and gauging the comfort level of both partners is especially important in building alliance and trust while treating Black couples. Once a thorough trauma history is conducted, it is then possible to determine the trauma targets that will be included in the treatment as well as organizing the order of trauma processing. This is done in collaboration with the couple, being alert to the issues that are most important to them. When both partners have a trauma history, in addition to assessing the level of distress and ordering trauma processing, it will be necessary to assess if both partners have the capacity to be present for the other partner's processing without being activated. If not, strategies for managing the risk of activation for the non-processing partner will be necessary.

Phase Two is preparation. The focus is on setting the framework for the therapy by educating the clients about trauma, the process and purpose of the intervention, creating emotional regulation resources, and setting reasonable expectations about the treatment (Menon & Jayan, 2010). It is in this phase that the couple is first introduced to bilateral stimulation (BLS) to create or strengthen resources. BLS is integral to EMDR. When initially designed by Shapiro (1995), BLS was limited to eye movements, but has now evolved to include any sensory input that accesses the left and right hemisphere of the brain (audio played through left and right head-phones, tapping on shoulders or knees, jumping from left to right foot). EMDR theorizes that, similar to what occurs in the Rapid Eye Movement portion of sleep, BLS assists the brain in clearing out the debris and organizing memories in useful ways.

Using BLS to equip the client in building emotional safety and tolerance is key in the treatment of trauma from an EMDR perspective. It ensures that the client is not psychologically overwhelmed or is left feeling revicti-mized during trauma processing. The resources that can be beneficial to install during the preparation phase include the original Calm Place intervention (Shapiro, 1995) or other resources that allow the client to feel capable and safe. In addition to Calm Place, several EMDR resources have been devised over the past twenty-five years (Luber, 2009) and like the treatment in general, they can be adapted to meet the cultural and individual needs of the clients. When treating Black couples, tapping in to any positive narratives about the strength of their ancestors or power of survival can activate the cultural resilience of African Americans. Spiritual or positive family relationships can also be invoked as a resource. If both partners are not actively engaged in processing, it can be helpful to have the non-processing partner utilize the "Container" resource and other grounding resources while the clinician is conducting reprocessing. For couples who view their relationship as a secure, sacred bond, installing the feeling of being loved and accepted as a resource can be strengthening for both the relationship and each partner. If the relationship is not yet a safe space, once deescalation and a stronger bond is created through therapy, installation of the relationship as a resource may be possible.

Phase Three of EMDR treatment is called the assessment phase. It is not the same as gaining a history, instead it is where the clinician focuses in on what specific target will be addressed in the session. This is specific to each session as the therapist focuses the clients on the memory they wish to target. The client's AIP is accessed by getting data regarding their emotions, body sensations, trauma cognitions (both negative and posi-tive), and validity of the positive cognition. Once this occurs in Phase

One, the target is selected in this phase to begin working through the trauma memory.

Phase Four consists of applying BLS to desensitize the trauma memory. This phase is focused on reprocessing the trauma(s). BLS is applied to the target memory. When working with Black couples, if both partners have traumas that need reprocessing, the clinician should have a clear plan regarding the order of processing as well as if joint or individual processing is necessary. Since the client does not need to verbalize the trauma details while processing, EMDR allows for partners to be guided through processing their separate traumas while in the same session with an adapted protocol (Luber, 2009). When assisting Black couples to heal from racial trauma, there are unique factors to consider. The clinician should determine if there is an overlap with the clients' view of self or negative views of the world and if these are linked with any negative messages related to racial trauma (Nickerson, 2016).

If it is not needed or appropriate for both partners to be present during processing, as mentioned earlier, a separate session can be held; or if the couple wants the non-processing partner to attend, it can be useful to utilize containing resources with the non-processing partner to avoid activating them during their partner's processing. Organize couples sessions to ensure enough time for one relationship partner to process a specific trauma memory and enough emotional space for the other relationship partner to make sense of the experience. In working with Black couples, the clinician will need to address the impact of the specific trauma on the relationship and ideally assist the couple in creating a shared understanding and a new narrative with the now-integrated trauma.

BLS is used again in Phase Five to install and strengthen positive cognitions. Strengths of the relationship and the emotional support of the non-processing partner may be integrated into the survivor's positive cognitions. Phase Six is focused on processing any lingering physical distress that may be related to the trauma, and BLS is once again used to strengthen positive sensations. Phase Seven allows for the closure of the session and educating the clients regarding what to expect in the days following processing. Phase Eight is the final phase and is focused on the reevaluation phase in which a review of the processing and checking for additional target memories are conducted. Typically, not all eight phases will occur in a single session, and appropriate pacing with attunement to the couple, individually and as a unit, is paramount during treatment.

10.7   Cultural Competency and Attitude, Skills, and Knowledge

Throughout therapy with Black couples, the EMDR therapist must be emotionally and culturally attuned in a consistent and predictable manner, regardless of the phase of treatment. Nickerson (2016) proposes a culturally competent model to apply EMDR, by utilizing the framework of *ASK – Attitude, Skills,* and *Knowledge* – in order to work with "cultural humility." "Cultural humility entails suspending one's own culture-centric views when entering the world of a client" (Nickerson, 2016, p. 6). Clinicians who are able to demonstrate an attitude of humility and personal awareness when working with clients from diverse backgrounds show their openness to learn and in return earn patients' trust (Nickerson, 2016).

The *Attitude* required for clinicians to be competent begins with being humble and curious about their own culture and that of the couple. The culturally competent EMDR therapist engages in self-reflection, seeking to gain insight into their beliefs, attitudes, and blind spots, while being open and respectful of the couple's racial and ethnic experience. This allows for a curious approach to learn about the couple's culture from an inside-outside perspective. The therapist educates themselves with an outside lens on the general diversity of the Black couple, and remains open by engaging in dialogue with the clients to learn about their specific cultural experiences in order to understand the clients' perspective.

The *Skills* utilized by the culturally competent EMDR clinician are grounded in a model based on attunement to the client's individual and cultural experience, a collaborative approach that requires a partnership versus an up-down power hierarchy and allows for adaptation of the eight-phase protocol to meet the couple's needs. "EMDR clinicians can employ culturally informed modifications to other aspects of the eight-phase approach as long as these modifications remain consistent with the adaptive information processing model (AIP)" (Nickerson, 2016, p. 9).

Knowledge is the third factor that Nickerson (2016) proposes as a filter for applying EMDR in a culturally competent manner. "Culturally competent knowledge refers to having an understanding of the importance of culture in general as well as an understanding about specific cultural realities of any particular client" (Nickerson, 2016, p. 9). This requires clinicians not just to have an understanding of the culture of the client in general terms, using a checklist or profiling to see the Black couple, but instead requires an active engagement with the couple to determine how the clients may adhere to or differ from the cultural norms of their group. When working with a Black World War II Marine and his wife who was born in the South, the culturally competent EMDR clinician may actively seek out information about the history of segregation and discrimination and invite the couple to share how they navigated these realities. Asking questions to gain insight regarding their narratives creates trust and safety and facilitates a successful treatment. The therapist's curiosity about the couple's racial and cultural experiences can yield rich data. Learning that the veteran was one of the first Black Marines to integrate this branch of the military and the impact this has had on his narrative of self and the world will be an important component in processing this veteran's combat trauma. "EMDR clinicians can appreciate that adverse and traumatic experiences of stigmatization and discrimination become physically stored memories that may remain 'frozen' and isolated from other memory networks. When activated either consciously or unconsciously, these unre-solved memories affect perception, feelings, and behavior" (Nickerson, 2016, p. 19).

Central to EMDR is the premise that unresolved trauma memories are stored in our neural pathways in a very different way in comparison to other memories, specifically emotionally neutral or positive events. These unresolved memories, because they are not "filed away" in a manner that makes sense to the brain, continue to have the power to invade and interfere with the survivor's functioning. Intrusive thoughts, memories, or dreams are some ways the memory may present, but this intrusion also occurs with trauma-linked behaviors. These trauma behaviors are driven by the survival instinct and are often attempts to cope, control, or gain mastery. Trauma survival responses can take the form of shutdown, control, reactionary/alarm, or avoidance behaviors. An example of trauma-controlled behaviors is the Black Army veteran who served three tours in Iraq and in spite of his wife's requests for him go to sleep, walks "point" nightly, checking his doors and windows multiple times while his children sleep. Classic avoidance behaviors may take the form of an African American sexual assault survivor who recoils at her partner's touch, both physically and emotionally cutting off any avenue to sexual intimacy. Reactive or alarm behaviors may take the form of an explosive, aggressive response to the slightest hint of a threat. This is seen in a twenty-five-year-old Black man who, after witnessing over two decades of neighborhood violence, exists in the world with a kind of "hair trigger," living by the motto that "the best defense is a preemptive offense." The shut-down and walled-off African American husband, stone-faced as he literally escapes to his internal "cave," seemingly unresponsive to the protests of his wife, is perhaps the most misunderstood trauma survivor.

Although they may experience significant trauma and emotional distress, Black Americans are less likely to seek treatment for PTSD and other mental health issues than white Americans (Roberts et al., 2011). The barriers for African Americans seeking treatment and disclosing trauma and neglect are well documented (Conner et al., 2010; Motley & Banks, 2018). The obstacles range from lack of access to mental health professionals, cultural taboos regarding not "airing dirty laundry," lack of support, shame, cultural stigma of mental health care, lack of concrete resources like childcare or health insurance, and mistrust of the "system" based on fear of police and other governmental agencies (Motley & Banks, 2018). In addition, many clients may not realize the impact of their past experiences on their present functioning. Many Black Americans have adopted the narrative that suffering is a "part of being Black" and may minimize their present struggles by comparing them to the historical oppression Blacks have endured. It is crucial that clinicians who work with Black couples be aware of higher incidences, and lower reporting of latent trauma (Alegría et al., 2013; Motley & Banks, 2018) and incorporate that understanding into the couple's treatment.

The EMDR model presented in this chapter offers a culturally sensitive and effective treatment of traumatized Black couples. Ethical utilization of EMDR with Black couples requires appropriate training and supervision. Clinicians are highly encouraged to pursue formal training through Eye Movement Desensitization Reprocessing International Association (EMDRIA, https://www.emdria.org/page/21).

10.8 Summary

"The human response to psychological trauma is one of the most important public health problems in the world. Traumatic events such as family and social violence, rapes and assaults, disasters, wars, accidents and predatory violence confront people with such horror and threat that it may temporarily or permanently alter their capacity to cope, their biological threat perception, and their concepts of themselves" (van der Kolk, 2000, p. 7). This, coupled with a history of racial victimization and continued oppression and injustice, increases the cumulative effect of trauma for Black Americans. Black people have endured atrocities on historical, societal, and interpersonal levels. Whether it is sexualized violence or racial injustice, the legacy of trauma on intrapersonal and interpersonal functioning affects the emotional wellbeing of Black relationships.

"Racial and ethnic minorities are at high risk for developing post-traumatic stress disorder (PTSD) after experiencing a traumatic event and are less likely to receive evidence-based treatment for their symptoms" (Dixon et al., 2016, p. 107). Recognizing the high rates of trauma as well as the disparity in receiving mental health treatment, this chapter explored the impact of trauma on Black romantic relationships and introduced the application of Eye Movement Desensitization Reprocessing Therapy (EMDR) to treat Black couples. EMDR therapy has been successfully utilized to treat trauma survivors from "culturally marginalized or under resourced populations throughout the world" (Nickerson, 2016, p. xx). Counselors have an important role in bringing to light the prevalence of trauma and using EMDR to heal relationships and strengthen Black love.

Discussion Questions

1. How do trauma experiences differ for African Americans compared to other racial groups in the United States?
2. Describe how experiences of socially induced trauma might impact intimate relationships.
3. Discuss the importance of a culturally sensitive trauma-informed genogram when working with Black couples.
4. How might the framework of ASK (Attitude, Skills, and Knowledge) be integrated into your work with Black couples?

REFERENCES

Alegría, M., Fortuna, L. R., Lin, J. Y., Norris, L. F., Gao, S., Takeuchi, D. T., Jackson, J. S., Shrout, P. E., & Valentine, A. (2013). Prevalence, risk, and correlates of posttraumatic stress disorder across ethnic and racial minority groups in the US. *Medical Care*, *51*(12), 1114–1123. https://doi.org/10.1097/MLR.0000000000000007

Carter, R. T. (2007). Racism and psychological and emotional injury: Recognizing and assessing race-based traumatic stress. *The Counseling Psychologist*, *35*(1), 13–105.

Children's Bureau. (2020). *Child maltreatment 2018*. U.S. Department of Health & Human Services, Administration for Children and Families, Administration on Children, Youth and Families. https://www.acf.hhs.gov/cb/report/child-maltreatment-2020

Conner, K. O., Copeland, V. C., Grote, N. K., Rosen, D., Albert, S., McMurray, M. L., Reynolds, C. F., Brown, C., & Koeske, G. (2010). Barriers to treatment and culturally endorsed coping strategies among depressed African-American older adults. *Aging and Mental Health, 14*(8), 971–983.

Dixon, L. E., Ahles, E., & Marques, L. (2016). Treating posttraumatic stress disorder in diverse settings: Recent advances and challenges for the future. *Current Psychiatry Reports, 18*(12), 108. https://doi.org/10.1007/s11920-016-0748-4

Guillory, P. (2021). *Emotionally focused therapy with African American couples: Love heals*. Routledge.

Helms, J. E., Nicolas, G., & Green, C. E. (2010). Racism and ethnoviolence as trauma: Enhancing professional training. *Traumatology, 16*(4), 53–62. https://doi.org/10.1177/1534765610389595

Herman, J. (2015). *Trauma and recovery: The aftermath of violence – from domestic abuse to political terror*. Basic Books.

Jonson-Reid, M., Drake, B., & Zhou, P. (2013). Neglect subtypes, race, and poverty: Individual, family, and service characteristics. *Child Maltreatment, 18*(1), 30–41.

Lancaster, C. L., Teeters, J. B., Gros, D. F., & Back, S. E. (2016). Posttraumatic stress disorder: Overview of evidence-based assessment and treatment. *Journal of Clinical Medicine, 5*(11), 105. https://doi.org/10.3390/jcm5110105

Luber, M. (Ed.). (2009). *Eye movement desensitization and reprocessing (EMDR) scripted protocols: Basics and special situations*. Springer.

Menon, S. B., & Jayan, C. (2010). Eye movement desensitization and reprocessing: A conceptual framework. *Indian Journal of Psychological Medicine, 32*(2), 136–140. https://doi.org/10.4103/0253-7176.78512

Moses, M. D. (2007). Enhancing attachments: Conjoint couple therapy. In F. Shapiro, F. W. Kaslow, & L. Maxfield (Eds.), *Handbook of EMDR and family therapy processes* (pp. 146–166). Wiley.

Motley, R., & Banks, A. (2018). Black males, trauma, and mental health service use: A systematic review. *Perspectives on Social Work (Houston), 14*(1), 4–19.

Nickerson, M. (Ed.). (2016). *Cultural competence and healing culturally based trauma with EMDR therapy: Innovative strategies and protocols*. Springer.

Perry, B. D., Colwell, K., & Schick, S. (2002). Neglect in childhood. In D. Levinson (Ed.), *Encyclopedia of crime and punishment: Vol. 1* (pp. 192–196). Sage.

Ridley, C. R. (2005). *Overcoming unintentional racism in counseling and therapy: A practitioner's guide to intentional intervention* (2nd ed.). Sage.

Roberts, A. L., Gilman, S. E., Breslau, J., Breslau, N., & Koenen, K. C. (2011). Race/ethnic differences in exposure to traumatic events, development of post-traumatic stress disorder, and treatment-seeking for post-traumatic stress disorder in the United States. *Psychological Medicine, 41*(1), 71–83. https://doi.org/10.1017/S0033291710000401

Shapiro, F. (1995). *Eye Movement Desensitization and Reprocessing: Basic principles, protocols, and procedures*. Guilford Press.

(2002). EMDR 12 years after its introduction: Past and future research. *Journal of Clinical Psychology*, *58*(1), 1–22.

(2014). The role of eye movement desensitization and reprocessing (EMDR) therapy in medicine: Addressing the psychological and physical symptoms stemming from adverse life experiences. *Permanente Journal*, *18*(1), 71–77. https://doi.org/10.7812/tpp/13-098

Shapiro, F., & Forrest, M. S. (2016). *EMDR: The breakthrough therapy for overcoming anxiety, stress, and trauma*. Basic Books.

Smith, S. G., Zhang, X., Basile, K. C., Merrick, M. T., Wang, J., Kresnow, M. J., & Chen, J. (2018). *The national intimate partner and sexual violence survey: 2015 data brief – updated release*. National Center for Injury Prevention and Control, Centers for Disease Control and Prevention.

Trauma Recovery/Humanitarian Assistance Programs. (2020). *Research findings*. www.emdrhap.org/content/about/research-findings/

Ursano, R. J., Bell, C., Eth, S., Friedman, M., Norwood, A., Pfefferbaum, B., Pynoos, J., D., Zatzick, D. F., Benedek, D. M., McIntyre, J. S., Charles, S. C., Altshuler, K., Cook, I., Cross, C. D., Mellman, L., Moench, L. A., Norquist, G., Twemlow, S. W., Woods, S., Yager, J., & Steering Committee on Practice Guidelines (2004). Practice guideline for the treatment of patients with acute stress disorder and posttraumatic stress disorder. *American Journal of Psychiatry*, *161*(11 Suppl.), 3–31.

van der Kolk B. (2000). Posttraumatic stress disorder and the nature of trauma. *Dialogues in Clinical Neuroscience*, *2*(1), 7–22.

Wilson, G., Farrell, D., Barron, I., Hutchins, J., Whybrow, D., & Kiernan, M. D. (2018). The use of Eye-Movement Desensitization Reprocessing (EMDR) therapy in treating post-traumatic stress disorder – A systematic narrative review. *Frontiers in Psychology*, *9*, 923. https://doi.org/10.3389/fpsyg.2018.00923

World Health Organization (2013). *Guidelines for the management of conditions that are specifically related to stress*. WHO.

PART IV

Sex and Intimacy

Sexual Intimacy in Black Heterosexual Couple Relationships: Challenges and Opportunities toward Relational Intimacy

Danielle Y. Drake & Daktari Shari R. Hicks

11.1 Introduction

There is a lack of research exploring the factors contributing to interference between heterosexual Black women and men creating and preserving healthy sexual intimacy in couple relationships. Sexual intimacy in couple relationships in the Black community have been under siege since the arrival of enslaved Africans into the United States (Baca-Zinn et al., 2015; Kelly et al., 2013; Winek, 2010). With little control over their bodies and the day-to-day activities of their relationships, Black couples have developed, to varying degrees of success, unique relationship configurations that reflect resilience in the face of racism, discrimination, and other social ecological factors (Baca-Zinn et al., 2015). Beyond these issues, specific barriers related to Black sexual intimacy in couple relationships include (a) the degree of flexibility in gender roles between Black men and women, (b) economic stress, (c) exposure to early childhood trauma and violence, and (d) fidelity and sexual problems (Gillum, 2007).

This chapter explores (a) sociopolitical factors historically affecting sexual intimacy among Black couples, (b) the role of gender and sex, (c) power in sexually intimate relationships and sexuality and intimacy among Black heterosexual men and women respectively, and (d) creative interventions for addressing sexual intimacy with Black couples toward increased communication and relationality. It must also be stated that the relationship configurations discussed in this chapter are presented from a cis-heterosexual stance, a perspective that reflects the historical lens of much of the research done on Black couples and the authors' area of focus for this paper. This discussion is limited to configurations where (a) a couple is discussed, rather than addressing polyamorous relationships; and (b) both members of the couple dynamic identify as Black, rather than interracial couples. The topics explored in this chapter highlight the ways in which a focus on culturally specific factors can promote resilience in sexual intimacy among Black heterosexual couples toward viewing their relationships as emotionally supportive and culturally congruent, with the emphasis of these aspects as acts of social justice.

11.2 Sociopolitical Factors Historically Affecting Sexual Intimacy among Black Couples

The history of enslavement among people of African descent affects every aspect of life for contemporary Black people, including perspectives of sexuality and intimacy among these individuals in couple relationships. Chattel enslavement denied Black people the ability to have agency over their own bodies, hence affecting their relational intimacy and sexual behaviors (Crook et al., 2009). Furthermore, women's sexuality and access to sexual intimacy, and Black women's access specifically, have been historically blurred by secrecy and shame (Rouse-Arnett & Dilworth, 2006). Through biogenetic, physiological, behavioral, psychical, spiritual, psychological, cultural, and societal mechanisms, historical trauma legacies (Danieli, 1998) and residual behaviors have often been passed down intergenerationally to impact current relational patterns between Black women and men in couple relationships (Crook et al., 2009).

Black men have also been historically depicted as having extreme sexual prowess, virility, and extraordinary genitals (Wyatt et al., 1976). As such, during enslavement, African men were often used to impregnate African women for breeding more chattel property. Again, it is noted that African men did not hold agency over their bodies and intimate experiences.

Since the beginnings of their experiences in the United States, Black people have been subject to sexual exploitation, placing Black sexual intimacy within the realm of a sociopolitical act. In addition to bearing the weight of enslaved ancestors' unresolved historical trauma, much of which has been transgenerationally transmitted, contemporary Black couples grapple with inescapable daily encounters of oppression and marginalization. Black couples still navigate the effects of slavery and postemancipation discrimination in the form of structural racism, which encompasses large-scale systems such as education, economics, law, and media (Kelly et al., 2013). Data show that these social ecological factors weigh heavily on Black people individually and also disproportionately affect Black couples and their relationship dynamics (Kelly et al., 2013; LaTaillade, 2006; Wilkins et al., 2013). Factors such as high rates of incarceration among Black men, lower levels of education of Black men (compared to Black women), unemployment, underemployment, and insecure employment, each of which is created by chronic systemic oppression and racism, come to bear in determining the viability and success of couples in the Black community. Research additionally demonstrates that Black men who have stable employment are twice as likely to marry as those who do not (Pinderhughes, 2002).

11.2.1   *The Role of Gender and Sex*

Issues of gender and sex are also connected to social ecological factors. Research regarding gender relations among Black couples often views the structure of female-headed households as deviant from traditional gender roles in society (Baca-Zinn et al., 2015). These gender role configurations harken back to the lack of control enslaved Africans had over their gendered and sexual experiences. Many Black men accept and understand manhood as being responsible/accountable to themselves and their families and being autonomous, free governing, and able to yield power, control, and authority over their lives (Hammond & Mattis, 2005). Black men have historically experienced a decreased ability to protect women from the hostilities of society in America beginning with the inability to protect their wives and children from rape during slavery (Pinderhughes, 2002). This diminished ability of Black men to physically protect Black women combined with a diminished economic capacity created a structure in which Black women have had to fend for themselves, work outside of the home, rely on female kinship networks, and thus create a sense of higher independence in general; owing to the "Strong Black Woman" stereotype (Baca-Zinn et al., 2015). This stereotype inherently pits Black men and women in a power struggle when contextualized through a Euro-American framework in which men are purported to be the stronger, more educated, economically secure, and head of household (Pinderhughes, 2002). One study found that Black men are more likely to grow up in a household with working mothers/wives and tend to be more open and receptive to their wives being in the labor force, which is also related to lived experiences of economic necessity (Blee & Tickamyer, 1995). Another study that analyzed data from two national surveys suggests that Black men are strong supporters of women's leadership in family life and gender equality (Harnois, 2014). In an earlier study utilizing data from two national surveys, Harnois (2010) found that Black men were as likely as Black women to accept core themes of the "Black women's standpoint," that being the intersectionality and interconnectedness of race, gender, inequality, and oppression. Yet, other research demonstrates Black men value traditional ideas of sex-role power distributions and male authority more than Black women, Euro-American men, or Euro-American women (Pinderhughes, 2002), further illustrating a potential clash in values within heterosexual Black couples.

11.2.1.2 Sexual Dysfunction among Blacks

Research addressing sexual dysfunction is a grossly understudied area within psychology, and specific to Black individuals and couples, studies, literature, and research relevant to sexual dysfunction are even more so devoid. Enslaved African/Black men, women, and children were incessantly exploited, routinely raped, and misused as super-breeders and reproducers to mass produce children of rape for capital gain (Leary, 2005). Fathers and mothers were forced to watch their young endure sexual abuse, assault, and molestation in their youth. Irrespective of age and gender, centuries of commercialized sexual exploitation have undoubtedly evoked feelings of powerlessness, helplessness, defenselessness, vulnerability, and mistrust. The enslaved were susceptible to the internalization of dysfunctional belief systems, distorted values, erroneous associations, and misunderstandings around the purpose, meaning, and significance of sexual intimacy/activity, childbearing, romantic relationships, family dynamics, and body ownership. These traumatizing and dehumanizing experiences are passed down through generations and culture (Leary, 2005). Thus, it is presumed that some level of residual sexual dysfunction linked to the sexual traumatization experienced throughout the Maafa (the middle passage, enslavement, and Jim Crow) may exist and impact Black relational and sexual intimacy, attitudes, values, beliefs, and practices in ways that we do not yet understand to what degree remains unknown, warranting a call for future and extensive research.

Research on Black sexual dysfunction is essential and vital to our understanding of healthy and optimal sexual functioning for Black couples. The sole research study found was conducted by Wyatt et al. (1976) and explored sexual and identity dysfunction as related to the myth of hypersexuality among Black people. Specifically, the study looked at what happens when sex in the relationship does not live up to the myth. Using sexual dysfunction therapy developed by Masters and Johnson, a Black couple was able to identify their culturally bound sexual beliefs, which led to the dysfunctional issues in the relationship.

11.2.2   Power in Sexually Intimate Relationships

Power in intimate relationships is an important factor to consider more broadly, but certainly comes to bear in Black sexually intimate relationships. Desire for emotional intimacy and/or physical arousal and passion are primary motives for involvement in sexual behavior (Seal et al., 2008). A qualitative narrative study with urban heterosexual couples regarding their first most physically arousing and most emotionally intimate sexual experiences found that physical arousal and passion were more predominant than emotional intimacy in first sexual experiences for both men and women, demonstrating men and women experience and enjoy physical arousal, without an emotional requirement, equally in the beginning of the relationship. Findings also suggest emotional intimacy and physical arousal were not mutually exclusive for both men and women, indicating these aspects of relationships are more intertwined than previously thought. Additionally, egalitarian interpersonal scripts were found to be increasingly normative, and initiation of sex becomes more mutual and bidirectional as the relationship becomes more committed.

For Black couples, more specifically, this study found that Black men reported greater adherence to traditional sexual scripts for their most physically arousing and emotionally intimate sexual experiences than did Black women (Seal et al., 2008). This information suggests Black men may desire more traditional roles and intimate partner relationship dynamics than Black women. This finding falls in line with what we know about the lack of power Black men often experience society at large. From this perspective, macro-level social justice work by all members of society, it seems would have the greatest impact on the success of Black couple relationships. Social justice efforts everywhere supporting a balance of power for Black men therefore would appear to support intimacy in Black couple relationships more specifically.

11.3   Sexuality and Intimacy among Black Heterosexual Men

Discussions regarding relational intimacy among Black heterosexual men are often laden with negative descriptions and propagation of unhealthy stereotypes. Rarely do these explorations highlight Black men as economic providers, emotionally engaged lovers, and supportive friends (Crook et al., 2009). These negative assumptions about Black men in intimate partner relationships often distort mental health practitioners' views regarding the intimacy desires of this population (Crook et al., 2009).

Some of the challenges specifically faced by Black men in developing sexually intimate relations include economic, value-based, and gender role conflict issues. Economic challenges, including unemployment, under-employment, and insecure employment, impact the intimacy goals of Black men. They often navigate depictions as being violent, criminal, libidinous, lazy, and lacking values, drive, and motivation to work, leading to descriptions of unmarriageability. These characterizations, while acknowledged to be legacies of racism and oppression, still impede relational intimacy among Black couples (Crook et al., 2009; Gillum, 2007).

The Black community has historically held matriarchal values, with women often being the head of the household and/or larger extended family. This runs opposite to the more dominant value of patriarchy propagated in the United States. Thus, Black men must often mediate their own, and Black women's, desires to be the more economically empowered "breadwinner," while recognizing a relational power imbalance of female-headed family systems in general within the Black cultural community context (Crook et al., 2009; Gillum, 2007).

Negative culturally bound masculine behaviors as an aspect of male gender role conflict (MGRC): MGRC is a psychological state in which socialized male gender roles have negative consequences stemming from rigid, sexist, or restrictive gender roles that result in restriction, devalua-tion, or violation of self or others (O'Neil, 2008). Negative messages surrounding masculinity suggest decreased definitions of success, fewer affectionate relationships between men and experiences of emotionality, and increased competitiveness, aggression, and homophobic perspectives. When Black men encounter traditional masculine ideals, they are some-times filtered through their ethnic-cultural experiences. As such, experi-ences as a "tough guy," "player," or adoption of a "Cool Pose," within a Black male context may predict decreased intimacy and emotional expres-sion in partner relationships for some (Crook et al., 2009). These percep-tions are, however, often mediated by age, education, and positive experience in intimate partner relationships. Black men who are older, have attained higher levels of education, and/or are in positive longstand-ing intimate relationships often have expanded perceptions of manhood that reflect the maturation processes involved in these life experiences (Blee & Tickamyer, 1995; Hunter & Davis, 1994; Hunter & Sellers, 1998). In a study conducted by Hunter and Davis (1994) Black men defined the components of manhood as consisting of having a sense of self-direction, family leadership and responsibility, spiritual groundedness, and connections to members of the community.

Furthermore, some of the opportunities for Black men to overcome sexual intimacy challenges in relationships include focusing on positive masculine characteristics, defying negative portrayals/stereotypes, and culture-based interventions. The reality is that a great many identify with positive characteristics associated with masculinity including the role of provider, protector and emotionally-engaged partner (Crook et al., 2009). Additionally, recognizing that African-centered perspectives of masculinity are bound by mastery rather than age provides a welcoming context for Black men to begin wherever they are in becoming the intimate partners they seek to be in sexually intimate relationships. More empowered conversations can include holistic explorations of sexual behaviors and sexual decision-making power and associations regarding ideas about masculinity, ethnic-cultural identity, sexual development throughout the lifespan, and the meanings they make among Black men (Crook et al., 2009).

11.4 Sexuality and Intimacy among Black Heterosexual Women

Black women have been stereotyped as motherly and nurturing, unattractive, matriarchs, sexual objects, and temptresses (Gillum, 2007). These stereotypic perceptions of Black women are often linked with characteristics such as chronic anger, depression, low self-esteem, adoption of a superwoman persona (which masks vulnerability), and difficulty creating and maintaining intimate interpersonal relationships. Mental health practitioners who adopt these beliefs about Black women may be influenced in their comfort level when working with this population, and by inaccurate beliefs about their sexuality (Gillum, 2007).

Some of the sexual intimacy challenges Black women navigate involve overcoming stereotypic representations and increased access to information about culturally empowered sexual intimacy. Research has demonstrated that a majority of men endorse stereotypic perspectives about Black women (Gillum, 2007). A study conducted by Gillum (2007) found that 48 percent of a male sample endorsed the Jezebel stereotype of Black women, and 71 percent of males in the sample endorsed the matriarch stereotype of Black women. Black women must also navigate the contemporary portrayal of the Jezebel stereotype in rap music and videos in which they are often portrayed as "freaks," "sluts," and "whores" (Rouse-Arnett & Dilworth, 2006), often suggesting disempowerment rather than a contemporary reclamation of sexual power and freedom.

In a study conducted by Rouse-Arnett and Dilworth (2006), access to high levels of good-quality sex education by caregivers was demonstrated to create barriers to intimacy among Black women. Furthermore, value judgments about self-worth as women and the merit of receiving protected care by trusted male caregiver figures were found to exacerbate the already tenuous grip many Black people hold regarding self-esteem and value as both women in general and Black women in particular. Moreover, restrictions on exploring sexuality only within the confines of a committed, socially endorsed relationship contribute to decreased sexual and intimacy satisfaction. Additionally, sexually intimate relationships among the Black women in this sample often became sexual through coercion rather than choice, suggesting a need for emerging adult women in this population to receive information on culturally empowering ways of advocating for the kind of sexual intimacy they desire.

While most Black men in the Black women stereotype study endorsed one or both of the stereotypic images, 94 percent of Black men also endorsed positive characteristics among Black women (Gillum, 2007). Additionally, warm, sensitive, and informative communication from caregivers about sexuality and intimacy is necessary (Rouse-Arnett & Dilworth, 2006). It is important to work with Black women in reconceptualizing their intimacy goals and perceptions from a more culturally empowered stance. African-centered relational ideals can be helpful in locating and defining worth through images drawn from the African and Black communities, as opposed to adopting the negative images emanating from the Euro-American sociocultural environment (Gillum, 2007). Emotional Emancipation Circles invite Black women to call out the lies told about them, to tell their truths, and to name their strengths, which allows Black women to be empowering, self-defining, and thriving (Grills, 2016).

11.5 Rationale for Culturally Congruent Creative Interventions

Black Americans' essential essence and core is African, that which is rooted in circularity, interconnectedness, collectivism, wholism, and "spiritness" (Nobles, 2015). Black people did not *only* inherit ancestral unresolved trauma. Notwithstanding bearing battle scars, Black people *also* inherited intergenerational life-affirming systems of knowing/being and legacies of healing, that is, culture, heritage, strength, survival, dynamism, vitality, resilience, and spiritual connectedness (Akbar, 1996; Ani, 1994a, 1994b; Billingsley, 1968; hooks, 1993; Kambon, 2004; Nobles, 1985; Richardson & Wade, 1999).

Black Americans acquired legacies of deep-rooted African spirituality and religion, which (a) are responsible for African Americans' survival, continued existence, and continued quest for liberation (Frame & Williams, 1996); (b) have been "important resource[s]" during and beyond slavery (Dunn & Dawes, 1999); and (c) continue to be used as coping strategies for loss, death, racism, trauma, violence, depression, etc. (Boyd-Franklin, 2010). African and African American religious and spiritual practices are versatile, multidimensional, and allow for connection, awareness, enlightenment, illumination, and healing through a variety of mediums, including but not limited to song, dance, drum, divination, storytelling, ritual, and prayer.

More than any other racial-ethnic group in the United States, Black people tend to resort to religion and spirituality to manage life problems and challenges (Lewis-Coles & Constantine, 2006). Given the unique sociopolitical narrative of the Black experience in America and in light of the relevance of religion and spirituality in the lives of most Black people, culturally congruent and deeply reflective interventions are warranted. Said interventions should restore Black contemporary and ancestral psychological, emotional, behavioral, social, and spiritual wellness through the process of liberating and illuminating the spirit (Nobles, 2013).

Creativity is associated with the act of creating new ideas or solutions and has been demonstrated to promote health and wellness, imbue openness and expressiveness, and pave the way for increased self-awareness (Drake, 2019). Black cultural aesthetics and expression have historically supported resistance and liberation strategies in the Black community through acts of flourish and adornment leading to an enhanced ability to self-define according to collective cultural values (Drake-Burnette et al., 2016). Language arts, dance, music, visual arts, food customs, and ritual are African-centered practices maintained by Black people in the United States, which have sustained and united the community (Durodoye & Coker, 2008; Parks, 2003). In working with Black couples in distress, turning toward creative practices that have historically sustained the Black community can assist couples in remembering and accessing familiar, culture-centered, strengths-based skill sets.

11.5.1   Creative Keys to Unlocking Sexual Intimacy in Black Couples

Nganga Fu-Kiau (2001) taught healing and therapy are mediums of art. ("Nganga" is a healer and powerful mediator between the visible and invisible/ancestral/spiritual realms in Kikongo culture [Fu-Kiau, 2001]). African-rooted (and Black) therapeutic and healing interventions "can take the form of debate, conversation, play, ritual, cooking party, dance, war game, trip, weaving, running, bathing or washing hands ceremony, working with clay (pottery), massage, meditation, singing, drumming, storytelling, laughter, play, touching, iconographical writing, inhalation, or hypnotism" (Fu-Kiau, 2001, p. 47). Healing invites creativity and must be grounded in mind, body, and most important, spirit. Intimacy requires the presence of spirit and cannot exist in absence of spirit. Somé (2000) offered, "Intimacy in general terms is a song of spirit inviting two people to come and share their spirit together" (p. 12). Black couples have been assaulted on every level imaginable and must dedicate time to attend to, and in many cases, repair their relationships and shared intimacy. We offer creative interventions to Black couples that celebrate, honor, acknowledge, and reflect their Blackness/Africanness and are steeped in their collective her/history, wisdom, narrative, memories, legacies, and DNA.

11.5.1.1   Swingin' with East Coast Swing Dance

Dance has served as a form of medicine for Africans and their descendants for thousands of years and invokes healing and restoration by synchronizing the mind, body, and spirit (Hicks, 2017). Through the medium of kinesthetic-affective expressivity, African and Black rooted dance has the power to invoke bodily integration, bliss, communion, connectivity, cathartic release, emotional expressivity, empathy, elation, tranquility, transition, transcendence, transformation, wholeness, and a healthy sense of self/community and commemorates life passages (Welsh, 2016). Hazzard-Gordon (1990) offered, "Social dancing links African-Americans to their African past more strongly than any other aspect of their culture" and functions as a resource for resisting systemic oppression and combating melancholy (p. 3). The first creative key/intervention for enhancing sexual intimacy we offer to Black heterosexual couples is East Coast Swing Dance.

In its most basic form, East Coast Swing Dance (*Swingin'*) is a collaborative pact for couples to voyage together via song and dance and consists of a cycle of movements completed and repeated in six counts. The first two counts make up the *rock-step*, a step backwards followed by a step forward, while steps three through six consist of *side-steps*, stepping and swaying from side to side. A brief release of the hand(s), called a *breakaway*, may be interjected to offer partners freedom for freestyling and improvisation, before ultimately returning to one another.

Each partner is invited to *assume* or *try on* a role, at least for the span of a song, and may choose to swap roles for the following song. Swingin' invites couples to explore alternative roles that they have shied away from or have not had access to due to preconceived notions of masculinity, femininity, and gender roles, and allows partners to cultivate, refine, reconceptualize, and redefine the roles they are accustomed to *leading* and/or *following*. Swingin' arouses *power play* and balancing of masculine and feminine energies to elicit innovation and harmony. Teach me how you love to be led. This is how I love to lead. Teach me how you love to follow. This is how I love to follow. These lessons of love, trust, self-disclosure, and consent through *leading* and *following* via dance can then be shifted, explored, and played within the privacy of couples' bedrooms.

The *rock-step* is significant for arousing intimacy for two reasons: (a) akin to the Adinkra notion of *sankofa*, we step backward before traveling forward to remember our past, our roots, our dreams, our memories, our experiences, and our stories that strengthen, empower, and prepare us for forward momentum, optimal tomorrows, and even children (African Heritage Collection, 2016) and (b) analogous to the idiom, "You can't see the forest for the trees," if we are too close or too near, we sometimes lose sight of the entire picture. In taking a step back, partners are able to get an enhanced perspective, more holistic view, and increased appreciation of their partner, their shared narrative, and their journey.

The *breakaway* creates a brief interval of distance in time and physical space between couples. In its essence, it is a quick act of separation before ultimately returning to closeness/togetherness. As an individual, each partner revels in her/his freedom and plays in time. As a unit, they energetically and kinesthetically communicate when the time is right to rejoin forces and unite as one. The *breakaway* allows couples to have sacred personal space to acknowledge their individual wants, needs, and desires. At the same time, the *breakaway* creates conditions for couples to map out sacred shared space to honor their commitment to each other. Couples must be mindful of not invading their partner's space by *stepping* on her/his toes.

Lastly, the *side-steps* are valuable because they arouse rhythm, romance, sensuality, seduction, and passion. I am dancing for me. I am dancing for you. You are dancing for me. You are dancing for you. We are dancing for we. Swingin' and swayin' back and forth together enraptures the couple into a sphere of harmony, a realm of togetherness, a spirit of synchronicity. When the unit feels in sync and harmonious, they feel safer and more open to exploring uncharted and undiscovered dimensions of romantic, relational, and sexual intimacy.

This is a mini-introduction to basic beginner East Coast Swing Dance, that is, Swingin'. Similar to Swingin', relationships traverse various stages: attraction, introduction, exploration, commitment, uncertainty, maturity, termination, and discovery. We invite Black heterosexual couples to seek a beginner swing dance class in your local area to access and tap into ancestral-spiritual-sexual power that may be beneficial and redefining in relationship.

11.5.1.2   Real Talk Pillow Talk

One of the challenges that most disrupts intimacy among Black couples are patterns of communication built over time that stifle authenticity, growth, and expansion. Couples come together at a particular point in their collective histories and often expect each other to stay the same way, though they are constantly being affected by their changing roles, relationships, environments, and events. Furthermore, for Black couples the daily realities of living in stressful and systemically oppressive environments can overshadow the need or ability to spend time cultivating conversations about intimacy that when unchecked can result in an unintended sense of disconnection. *Real Talk Pillow Talk* is an intervention designed to open communication through discussion prompts that require listening and creative engagement through the use of poetry and/or rap.

The couple is instructed to take turns asking questions of their partner specifically around themes of intimacy and sexuality. For example, in this activity Partner A may ask Partner B, "In what ways do you like to be touched?" Partner B will then have two to five minutes of uninterrupted time to respond. While Partner B is responding, Partner A is capturing with pen and paper words and phrases that seem meaningful, interesting, new, surprising, and honest to Partner B. If Partner B is silent, for any time during their allotted time, Partner A continues to wait until Partner B continues, until their time is up. Partner A then takes a few minutes to read through and rearrange the words and phrases captured to create a poem or rap for Partner B based on the expressed words and responses. The process is then repeated where Partner B asks a question of Partner A and records their responses as described.

This intervention serves as a moment for the couple to hear one another differently, to engage in a listening activity that holds at bay formulation of a preconceived idea of their partner's response, and to cultivate curiosity about their partner's personal experiences of sex and intimacy. Culturally, this intervention prioritizes creative modalities, namely poetry and rap, that are familiar to Black couples, and that often go unused, underutilized, or unrecognized as a skill already possessed by the individuals that can be applied to their current challenge.

It is important to note that whichever partner is speaking must respond from their personal experience and be ready to engage in authentic responses that incorporate "I" statements. It may be helpful for couples to first engage in this activity in a therapy session with a clinician to help the speaker remain focused on their personal experiences and not get caught in the circular recounting of a previous painful history. The questions in this activity should be focused toward helping each partner affirm and articulate what they want rather than what they do not want. Examples of questions that can be asked in this activity are listed at the end of this chapter in Exhibit A. This activity centers Black cultural expression as a valuable tool for playfully cultivating openness and creativity, applied toward a seemingly stuck or rigid challenge.

11.6 Conclusion

Strategies for creating healthy sexually intimate relationships for Black heterosexual couples include balancing power through egalitarian role sharing and decision making; becoming more flexible about traditional gender roles; developing enhanced collaboration by becoming more specific in defining commitments to one another; and engaging in culturally empowered sexual intimacy (Amato, 2011; Senn et al., 2009). Though Black couples face many challenges to develop healthy relational sexual intimacy, through recognition of the systemically based nature of the challenges and working collaboratively from a pro-cultural empowered stance, they can create a new standard of intimacy that provides both emotional and sexual satisfaction.

Discussion Questions

1. How have negative beliefs throughout history about Black men and women impacted relational intimacy for these couples?

2. What are some dangers of contextualizing Black couples through a Euro-American framework?
3. Explain the importance of spirit when conceptualizing intimacy for African American couples.
4. Discuss the connection between communication and intimacy.

Exhibit A

Questions to Open Up Communication and Conversations about Intimacy:

What is your favorite place on the body/thing to taste?
What foods are arousing to you?
What smells turn you on?
In what ways do you like to be touched?
What does arousal look like for you?
How do you feel about public displays of affection?
What is an ideal date for you?
What are some of your turnoffs? How did that come about?
What should I know about your sexual trauma herstory/history?
What areas of sexual intimacy make you nervous?
What areas of sexual intimacy make you uncomfortable?
Would you be open to washing/bathing each other?
Is there anything you dislike about sex?
Are you interested or open to marriage?
How often do you require sex?
What kind of music turns you on?
Do you think getting to know someone is important before engaging in a sexual relationship?
How long do you think a couple should wait before having sex for the first time?
Is it important for you to have an orgasm during every sexual encounter?
Is it important for you to know how many partners I have been with?
What is a sexual intimacy deal-breaker in a relationship?
Is there anything you fear about sex?
What are your favorite body parts to have massaged?
What are some of your erogenous zones?
How can I make you feel safe? What do you need to feel safe sexually?
What sexual fantasies do you have about me? Are you willing to share?
Does being emotionally connected to your partner make you feel more sexually aroused?

What is important for me to know about you sexually?

Are you open to sharing your history of sexually transmitted diseases/ sexually transmitted infections?

What does it mean for you to be sexually satisfied?

Are you interested in sex games?

How does power come into play in your sexual activity?

Are you open to role playing? Have you engaged in role playing before?

Do you like toys? If yes, what's your favorite toy(s)?

Have you had sex with more than one partner at one time?

Are you aroused by watching other people have sex?

Do you find pornography arousing?

What is your favorite genre of pornography?

Where is your favorite place to make love?

What does an orgasm look like for you?

Do you pleasure yourself?

Would you enjoy watching me pleasure myself?

Would you want me to watch you pleasure yourself?

REFERENCES

African Heritage Collection (2016, April 8). *Adinkra corner – sankofa* [Blog post]. Retrieved October 17, 2022, from https://www.africanheritagecollection .com/blogs/main/96430529-adinkra-corner-sankofa

Akbar, N. (1996). *Breaking the chains of psychological slavery*. Mind Productions.

Amato, P. R. (2011). *Marital quality in African American marriages*. National Healthy Marriage Resource Center.

Ani, M. (1994a). *Let the circle be unbroken: The implications of African spirituality in the diaspora*. The Red Sea Press.

 (1994b). *Yurugu: An African-centered critique of European culture and behavior*. Africa World Press.

Baca-Zinn, M., Eitzen, D. S., Wells, B. (2015). *Diversity in families*. Pearson.

Billingsley, A. (1968). *Black families in white America*. Prentice-Hall.

Blee, K. M., & Tickamyer, A. R. (1995). Racial differences in men's attitudes about women's gender roles. *Journal of Marriage and the Family, 57*, 21–30.

Boyd-Franklin, N. (2010). Incorporating spirituality and religion into the treatment of African American clients. *The Counseling Psychologist, 38*(7), 976–1000. https://doi.org/10.1177/0011000010374881

Crook, T., Thomas, C. M., & Cobia, D. C. (2009). Masculinity and sexuality: Impact on intimate relationships of Black men. *The Family Journal, 17*(4), 360–366.

Danieli, Y. (1998). *International handbook of multigenerational legacies of trauma*. Plenum Press.

Drake, D. Y. (2019). *Spiritual creativity among African Americans* (Order No. AAI27666653) [Doctoral dissertation, Fielding Graduate University]. ProQuest Dissertations & Theses Global.

Drake-Burnette, D., Garrett-Akinsanya, B., & Bryant-Davis, T. (2016). Womanism, creativity and resistance: Making a way out of "no way." In T. Bryant-Davis & L. Comas-Diaz (Eds.), *Womanist and mujerista psychologies: Voices of fire, acts of courage* (pp. 173–193). American Psychological Association.

Dunn, A. B., & Dawes, S. J. (1999). Spirituality-focused genograms: Keys to uncovering spiritual resources in African American families. *Journal of Multicultural Counseling and Development, 24*(4), 240–254.

Durodoye, B. A., & Coker, A. D. (2008). Crossing cultures in marriage: Implications for counseling African American/African couples. *International Journal for the Advancement of Counselling, 30*, 25–37.

Frame, M. W., & Williams, C. B. (1996). Counseling African Americans: Integrating spirituality in therapy. *Counseling and Values, 41*(1), 16–28.

Fu-Kiau, K. K. B. (2001). *Self-healing power and therapy: Old teachings from Africa*. African Tree Press.

Gillum, T. L. (2007). "How do I view my sister?" Stereotypic views of Black women and their potential to impact intimate partnerships. *Journal of Human Behavior in the Social Environment, 15*(2–3), 347–366.

Grills, C. (2016, Nov. 8). *Emotional emancipation circles: The community healing network and association of black psychologists*. Presented at the Caribbean Regional Conference of Psychology 2016 Conference, Caribbean Alliance of National Psychological Associations, Promoting Caribbean Health with Multilingualism and Multiculturalism: Challenges and Opportunities, Port au Prince, Haiti.

Hammond, W. P., & Mattis, J. S. (2005). Being a man about it: Manhood meaning among African American Men. *Psychology of Men and Masculinity, 6*(2), 114–126.

Harnois, C. E. (2010). Race, gender, and the black women's standpoint. *Sociological Forum, 25*(1), 68–85.

(2014). Complexity within and similarity across: Interpreting black men's support of gender justice, amidst cultural representations that suggest otherwise. In B. C. Slatton & K. Spates (Eds.), *Hyper sexual, hyper masculine?: Gender, race and sexuality in the identities of contemporary black men* (pp. 85–99). Ashgate.

Hazzard-Gordon, K. (1990). *Jookin: The rise of social dance formations in African-American culture*. Temple University Press.

Hicks, D. S. R. (2017). *Therapeutic interventions: Commissioned thematic briefing paper*. Institute for the Advanced Study of Black Family Life and Culture.

hooks, b. (1993). *Sisters of the yam: Black women and self-recovery*. South End Press.

Hunter, A. G., & Davis, J. E. (1994). Hidden voices of Black men: The meaning, structure, and complexity of manhood. *Journal of Black Studies, 25*(1), 20–40. https://doi-org.ciis.idm.oclc.org/10.1177/002193479402500102

Hunter, A. G., & Sellers, S. L. (1998). Feminist attitudes among African American women and men. *Gender & Society*, *12*(1), 81–99. https://doi.org/10.1177/002193479402500102

Kambon, K. K. K. (2004). The worldviews paradigm as the conceptual framework for African/black psychology. In R. L. Jones (Ed.), *Black psychology* (4th ed., pp. 73–92). Cobb & Henry Publishers.

Kelly, S., Maynigo, P., Wesley, K., & Durham, J. (2013). Black communities and family systems: Relevance and challenges. *Couple and Family Psychology: Research and Practice*, *2*(4), 264–277.

LaTaillade, J. J. (2006). Considerations for treatment of Black couple relationships. *Journal of Cognitive Psychotherapy*, *20*(4), 341–358.

Leary, J. D. (2005). *Post traumatic slave syndrome: America's legacy of enduring injury and healing*. Uptone Press.

Lewis-Coles, M. E. L., & Constantine, M. G. (2006). Racism-related stress, Africultural coping, and religious problem-solving among African Americans. *Cultural Diversity and Ethnic Minority Psychology*, *12*(3), 433–443. https://doi.org/10.1037/1099-9809.12.3.433

Nobles, W. W. (1985). *Africanity and the black family: The development of a theoretical model*. Institute for the Advanced Study of Black Family Life and Culture.

(2013). Fundamental task and challenge of black psychology. *Journal of Black Psychology*, *39*, 292–299.

(2015). From black psychology to *sakhu djaer*: Implications for the further development of a pan African black psychology. *Journal of Black Psychology*, *41*(5), 399–414. https://doi.org/10.1177/0095798415598038

O'Neil, J. M. (2008). Summarizing 25 years of research on men's gender role conflict using the gender role conflict scale: New research paradigms and clinical implications. *The Counseling Psychologist*, *36*(3), 358–45.

Parks, F. M. (2003). The role of African American folk beliefs in the modern therapeutic process. *Clinical Psychology: Science and Practice*, *10*(4), 456–467.

Pinderhughes, E. B. (2002). Black marriage in the 20th century. *Family Process*, *41*(2), 269–282. https://doi.org/10.1111/j.1545-5300.2002.41206.x

Richardson, B. L., & Wade, B. (1999). *What mama couldn't tell us about love*. HarperCollins.

Rouse-Arnett, M., & Dilworth, J. E. L. (2006). Early influences on Black women's sexuality. *Journal of Feminist Family Therapy: An International Forum*, *18*(3), 39–61.

Seal, D. W., Smith, M., Coley, B., Perry, J., & Gamez, M. (2008). Urban heterosexual couples' sexual scripts for three shared sexual experiences. *Sex Roles*, *58*(9–10), 626–638. https://doi.org/10.1007/s11199-007-9369-z

Senn, T. E., Carey, M. P., Vanable, P. A., & Seward, D. X. (2009). Black men's perceptions of power in intimate relationships. *American Journal of Men's Health*, *3*(4), 310–318.

Somé, S. (2000). *The spirit of intimacy: Ancient African teachings in the ways of relationships*. HarperCollins.

Welsh, K. (2017). *Dance in the service of healing: Commissioned thematic briefing paper*. Institute for the Advanced Study of Black Family Life and Culture.

Wilkins, E. J., Whiting, J. B., Watson, M. F., Russon, J. M., & Moncrief, A. M. (2013). Residual effects of slavery: What clinicians need to know. *Contemporary Family Therapy*, *35*(1), 14–28. https://doi.org/10.1007/s10591-012-9219-1

Winek, J. L. (2010). *Systemic family therapy: From theory to practice*. Sage Publications.

Wyatt, G. E., Strayer, R. G., & Lobitz, W. C. (1976). Issues in the treatment of sexually dysfunctioning couples of Afro-American descent. *Psychotherapy: Theory, Research & Practice*, *13*(1), 44–50.

CHAPTER 12

Intimacy, Desire, and Sex in the African American Relationships

Jeshana Avent-Johnson

Where do individuals learn about sex and intimacy? Through what experiences do they form the basis of their perceptions, motivations, and interactions in intimate relationships? The topics of sex, intimacy, and desire are relatively scarce in the literature for marriage and family therapy (Gottman & Schwartz-Gottman, 2012; Schnarch, 1991) and even more limited regarding African American couples (Bryant et al., 2010; Gupta et al., 2015; Helm & Carlson, 2013; Staples, 2006). Yet one of the primary motives for seeking couples therapy is intimacy, sex, and desire. African American couples face unique circumstances when forming and maintaining intimate couple relationships. Black intimacy and sex are dissected and judged based on the norms of a traditional white middle-class framework that implies pathology for African Americans.

To understand the impact of systemic racism on the Black couple and their functioning as sexual beings is to know the context of Black Americans' historical experience around sex and sexuality. The institution of slavery irrevocably altered the sexuality of enslaved Africans for generations (Staples, 1972). The normalized and legal forced breeding, physical breaches of body boundaries, and sexual exploitation of African Americans during enslavement, impacted the ways many African Americans view sex and sexuality. Many myths and stereotypes around African Americans being organically hypersexual and deviant are deeply rooted in American history and culture. Because sexual behavior is highly influenced by sexual stereotypes, historical oversexualized images and beliefs of African Americans in media and the greater society continue to shape the perception of Black sexuality. In fact, Dr. Gail Wyatt (1997), in her book *Stolen Women* discussed how the auction block made room for dangerous views of Black women to either ignore their sexuality altogether or be perpetually sexually available. The internalization of such beliefs and expectations has caused serious disruptions to our identity and plays a significant role in sexual dysfunction when people are unable to live up to the stereotypes

(Wyatt et al., 1976). With little to no sex-positive dialogues in Black institutions such as churches, schools, and families (McGruder, 2009), our mainstream conversations regarding Black sexuality are more about risks and negative sexual outcomes, leaving little room to explore Black pleasure. For many African American men and women, inadequate sexuality education in their homes, schools, and churches also plays a role in how they develop a sexual identity and engage in sexual activity (Rouse-Arnett et al., 2006; Staples, 2006).

12.1   Sex, Intimacy, and Desire

Sex, intimacy, and desire are multicausal and multidimensional with large individual, couple, cultural, and value differences where "one size never fits all" (McCarthy & McCarthy, 2012). Early research on sex and desire focused on sexual behavior rather than sexual experience. It has been assumed that erections and sexual activity reflected sexual desire, intimacy, and pleasure. The increasing clinical attention to problems of pleasure discrepancy (Mintz, 2017) and sexual desire are two of the newest developments in the history of modern sex therapy (Schnarch, 1991). There is a powerful belief about couple sexuality: the closer, more communicative (Kolodny et al., 1988), more intimate the relationship, the better the sex (McCarthy & McCarthy, 2012; Perel, 2006). There is also the belief that the key to resolving sexual dysfunction is stand-alone medical interventions (McCarthy & McCarthy, 2012). The medical model of sex and desire tends to leave out some of the most important aspects of sexual functioning even among clinicians. The lessons individuals learn during their formative years about love, commitment, and relationship maintenance exert influence in their intimate relationships later in life. Although we are born sensual creatures, we are embedded within the larger culture and influenced by it. In this culture we learn early on which parts of sex, intimacy, and desire are acceptable, and as a result we begin to gradually shut those other parts of ourselves down. What does all of this mean for the African American couple? Since we are not only influenced by family but societal norms as well, we must ask the question, what would Black intimacy and sexuality be without white supremacy?

In working with African American couples, therapists must be especially prepared to develop the context of therapy to include the impact of social, political, economic, and environmental conditions (McGoldrick et al., 2005). Social, racial, and historical factors stress the Black relationship beyond what other ethnic groups face and these factors can wreak havoc on the sex lives of these couples. The couple may not be acutely aware of how these factors decrease their desire to want to connect intimately and engage in sex. In fact, couples may not articulate the impact of these factors when seeking treatment (Boyd-Franklin, 2003). Therefore, treatment for African American couples should include an assessment of how these factors impact the couple's presenting problems. We are more aware than ever that the assessment and treatment of intimacy, sex, and desire demand an integrative and holistic approach (Wincze & Weisberg, 2015). Schnarch's (1991) quantum model of sexual function, although not created specifically for African Americans, can be adapted to work with these couples as it integrates physiological (sensations) and psychological aspects (thoughts and feelings) of sexual functioning. It provides an understanding of why bodies function sexually and why sometimes they do not. Ogden's (2018) research also highlighted the importance of feelings and our ability to make meaning of sex and its direct impact on our sexual experience.

12.2 Family Systems Theory: Differentiation

To be human is to be in relationships.

Jenny Brown (2012)

The importance of one's relationships is an understatement. After our basic needs such as food, water, and shelter, the quality of relationships affects the quality of one's life. Who we become is not free from the influence of family, culture, and society. In fact, life within our families of origin is often rehearsal for our adult relationships. Our families influence how we think, feel, and behave according to what is praised, punished, encouraged, and validated early in life. Much of our personalities and patterns around intimacy, sex, and desire can be traced back to one's family emotional unit. These patterns often are inherited from the previous generation and are passed down to the next, and ultimately have an impact on how we love, fight, and engage in intimacy and sex.

One major theoretical approach to understanding how people relate can be looked at through the lens of Bowen Family Systems. Developed by psychiatrist and researcher Dr. Murray Bowen, family systems looks at a broader aspect of becoming an individual. He saw the family as an emotional unit that had a direct impact on becoming who we are. Bowen believed that the basic task of adult life is to differentiate a self in relation to the important relationships in one's life (Titelman, 2008).

Bowen family systems theory discussed eight concepts of this process. These concepts are interconnected, and a thorough understanding of each may be necessary to understand the others. At the core of the Bowenian approach is differentiation of self. Differentiation of self is defined as "the capacity of the individual to function autonomously by making self-directed choices, while remaining emotionally connected to the intensity of a significant relationship system" (Brown, 2012). It is the process of becoming whole as a human being with the ability to separate thinking from emotions and balance the "I" and the "we." When the balance of these two life forces (togetherness and individuality) are healthy, relationships are less likely to be what Bowen calls "emotionally fused."

Fusion, in its most basic form, is the merging of emotional selves due to insufficient interpersonal boundaries between members of the system. Families with low levels of differentiation, whether they are aware or not, typically encourage groupthink and often at the expense of an individual(s) within the system. As a result, the fusion makes it difficult to become an individual because of the emotional pull (Gilbert, 2017). The way one manages the emotional pull may present through relationship patterns such as conflict, over-functioning/under-functioning or triangling. Seen as neither good or bad, the patterns of relating are efforts to solve the anxiety within the relationship (Bowen, 1978; Gilbert, 2017). Those presenting with higher levels of differentiation can stand strong in his or her opinions and principles and respect others' opinions and behaviors without trying to change them. They walk the thin line of becoming extremely close in their unity while holding steadfast onto their separate sense of self.

Families vary in the intensity of the emotional togetherness. Bowen saw the nuclear family as an emotional unit with the ability to pass anxiety and immaturity from one person to the next when living together. The more fused, the easier the transmission of emotions and anxiety. Depending on the intensity of the emotional family unit, each person will either develop a posture or pattern in efforts to manage the anxiety. A posture is developed when an individual experiences the anxiety for a short period of time as opposed to long-term exposure resulting in a pattern.

Sex, intimacy, and desire are separate entities that intersect and influence each other but one may not precipitate the other. However, several studies have indicated differentiation of self as a fundamental prerequisite for intimacy in long-term relationships and marriages (Lerner, 1989; Schnarch, 1997). Other studies have shown differentiation as an important component in couples' overall satisfaction at different stages of marital life (Peleg, 2008). Ferreira et al.'s (2014) research showed differentiation of self as a predictor of desire, intimacy, and couple satisfaction with desire mediating the association between differentiation and couple satisfaction and the association between differentiation and intimacy. Intimacy mediated the association between desire and satisfaction. Their results provide support that differentiation plays an important role in sexual desire, intimacy, and couple satisfaction.

Schnarch (1997) applied Bowen's theory of differentiation to sex therapy. His concept of differentiation includes four points of balance: your ability to maintain a separate self in close proximity to your partner, being nonreactive to their reactivity, emotional self-regulation, and tolerating discomfort for growth. With our relationships serving as a curriculum for what one needs to learn, our connectedness to others provides a mirror for growing the self. Like Bowen, Schnarch stressed the importance of balancing the "I" and the "we" in emotionally committed relationships. They found that couples with higher levels of differentiation are more likely to engage openly despite differences and tolerate high levels of intimacy and closeness without feelings of threat, abandonment, or engulfment anxiety (Bowen, 1978; Schnarch, 1997). Bell and Harsin's (2018) longitudinal research of midlife couples found that strong differentiation was connected to having a healthier and happier relationship. The couples in this study attributed relationship improvements to partners' ability to make room for each other's individuality and show affection.

Kerr and Bowen (1988) argued that those with lower levels of differentiation were likely to engage in highly dependent relationships while wanting to escape each other. A longitudinal study that followed couples for over twenty-five years found that those who were unable to make room for and respect their partner's individuality experienced greater amounts of tension. Lerner's research also shows that when one has not successfully carved out a clear and whole "I" in their nuclear family, couples struggle with the fear of being swallowed up by togetherness. This fear often results in instinctual reactions of distancing or fighting in an attempt not to lose the self (Lerner, 1989) and ultimately impacting intimacy, desire, and sex.

Many calculated factors are in one's level of differentiation. To understand differentiation for African Americans, one must consider developing a self within a context of a gruesome history embedded in a dehumanizing system yet rising above the seemingly impossible obstacles to achieve a sense of self capable of determination and strength. Bowen saw differentiation on a continuum and a natural process not to be pathologized. The Differentiation of Self inventory is used to assess couples' levels of differentiation (Schnarch & Regas, 2012). The information gathered about previous generations may serve as a rich resource for individuals (Brown, 2012).

This concept also aligns with the concept of *Sankofa*. Sankofa is becoming more familiar to the African American community as they develop and learn more about their African identities. Sankofa is derived from King Adinkra of the Akan people of West Africa. Sankofa teaches us to "go back to our roots in order to move forward." It emphasizes the need to reach back and gather the best of what our past has to teach us, so that we can achieve our full potential as we move forward. African American couples are part of interdependent systems that rely on cultural beliefs and community support (Piper-Mandy & Rowe, 2010). Because of the severe realities of discrimination and oppression that African American couples face, strategies to increase levels of differentiation and strengthen intimacy need to be based on a sound understanding of the couple's experience and rooted in their interests, and traditions (Helm & Carlson, 2013). The concept of differentiation should be approached with a multicultural lens and adapted without losing the integrity of the theory or the couple.

12.3   Intimacy

Humans are social beings. We are wired for connection with fellow humans and need love and care to thrive. This makes intimacy vital to the success of human relationships (Bagarozzi, 2014). However, the conversation about intimacy is often hindered simply by defining the phenomenon (Lerner, 1989; Schnarch, 1991). In its modern conceptualization, intimacy is defined as a construct of ideas of self and self in relationship with another. It is neither monolithic nor always consistent. In fact, Perel (2006) states, even in the best relationships, intimacy waxes and wanes. Intimacy entered the field of relationship therapy in the 1960s, as Bowen introduced his concept of "differentiation" as a marker of mental health in the family and the couple system. Looking at intimacy through the lens of differentiation, Lerner (1989) defines it as the "ability to be who you are in a relationship and allow the other person to do the same while staying emotionally connected even in their differences without trying to change or fix the other" (p. 3). Schnarch (1991) defined intimacy as involving our ability to make a self-other distinction, engaging in self-confrontation, self-awareness, and self-disclosure in the context of a partner. It is not always consistent or comfortable, but an understanding of its ebbs and flow in ongoing relationships is essential. Masters and Johnson (1966) saw intimacy as two people sharing a close and trusting relationship, being emotionally vulnerable despite risks.

In Crucible Theory, Schnarch (1997) differentiated between the levels of intimacy: other-validated intimacy and self-validated intimacy. Other-validated intimacy is the most familiar intimacy we come to understand. This level of intimacy is usually experienced in the beginnings of all relationships and rooted in mutuality but often deteriorates as the relationship develops over time. It hinges on sharing vulnerability when it is safe to do so with the expectation that your vulnerability will be validated by your partner through acceptance and understanding. According to Schnarch, this level of intimacy is short term and low level. It is most often seen in couples with lower levels of differentiation as it supports each individual's personal reflected sense of self as a result of fusion.

Fusion begins to replace intimacy when only togetherness is acknowledged and private space is denied (Perel, 2006). When there is a decline in this type of intimacy, couples tend to seek professional help as they chase after what they initially experienced during the "Velcro stage" of the relationship (Lerner, 1989). With validation resting in the hands of the other partner, the partner with the least desire for intimacy controls disclosures and the level of intimacy experienced in the relationship (Perel, 2006; Schnarch, 1997). Perel (2006) argues she is not convinced that unrestrained disclosures foster harmonious and robust intimacy. In fact, she points out that couple's beliefs that they should have unrestricted access to their partner's private thoughts and feelings begin to resemble coercion and force reciprocity. Intimacy becomes more intrusive rather than their desired outcome of closeness (Perel, 2006).

Self-validated intimacy requires greater risks. It means maintaining one's own sense of identity and self-worth when disclosing. There are no expectations of acceptance or forced reciprocity from your partner. It means choosing to show up even if your partner is not open, receptive, or validating. This level of intimacy requires one to have emerged as a full self with the ability to be a self in a relationship rather than what others wish, need, and expect them to be (Lerner, 1989). In fact, Regas (2010) states "maintaining passion in a long-term relationship requires bringing more of your true self into the relationship" (para. 10). For this reason, self-validated intimacy is seen in couples with higher levels of differentiation as they can participate in relationships that do not come at the expense of the self. Self-validated intimacy allows us to fully engage and benefit in the components of intimacy.

For African American couples, there is a unique challenge that can hamper the development of intimacy (Dunham & Ellis, 2010). For one, intimacy requires a level of vulnerability. For many in this community, vulnerability has not only felt unsafe, but the messages of it being unsafe are engrained at an early age in their families. In America, there have been consistent restraints on the intimate relationship of African Americans through racial, sexual, and economic oppression. The development of the African American couple's intimacy has been an adaptation deviated from traditional African principles that valued interdependence, cooperation, unity, and mutual responsibility (Bethea & Allen, 2013). The conditions in which they had to create a new way of relating, under the backdrop of oppression, became significant daily stressors that contribute to the emotional distress of couples and families still today. For African American men, slavery inhibited their ability to actively participate in patriarchal authority, a trait that defined manhood at the time. The inability to challenge a system made room for interpersonal strains within relationships between Black women and men. For African American women, the socialization to be strong and independent may play a key role in their willingness to demonstrate vulnerability and reliance on a partner.

A lifetime of exposure to negative images of one's culture can lead one to hate the qualities they see in themselves and their partner (Helm & Carlson, 2013). Research shows experiences of discrimination are negatively associated with relationship functioning (Lavner et al., 2018). Some of the emotional distress can be witnessed in displaced anger and resentment onto partners in the relationship, accounting for high divorce rates and marital dissatisfaction. But despite the significant challenges, African American men and women still desire to have healthy relationships with one another. This history could be observed on plantations where the enslaved were not allowed the opportunities to exercise agency in bonding with their loved ones, yet male and female relationships endured. The intergenerational transmission processes allowed African Americans to pass down African traditions that valued family and assisted in the development of a collective existence (White & Parham, 1990). Therefore, it is vital that clinicians understand the African worldview as holistic, made up of many interlocking systems. (White, 1984).

12.4 Desire

Desire is one of our most convoluted feelings. It is a mixture of hormones, chemicals, relationships, eroticism, passion, love, and self-awareness. It is often confused with arousal, but desire and arousal are separate. Low desire means you don't want to have sex or at least at a significant decline, while arousal means you're unable to be turned on. For couples, the most common sexual problems that arise in therapy are low desire and desire discrepancy (Leiblum, 2010; McCarthy, 2015). Desire is a core dimension of sex and often a common cause for divorce when couples are unable to work through their desire discrepancies (Schnarch, 2009). However, Schnarch (2009) posits, low desire simply put is a position within the couple system, as it is rare that both partners will have the same appetite for sex at the same time (McCarthy & McCarthy, 2012). In fact, the ebb and flow of desire is natural and to be expected in loving relationships. For some, desire comes spontaneously, while others experience responsive desire: the growing interest in sex that occurs in reaction to sexual stimuli (Penner & Penner, 1993). There is no "normal" or "right" amount of desire for sex. In Nagoski's (2015) study of the dual control model, she explained context is key. Some people want lots of sex, some people have a lower desire for sex, while others want no sex at all. All can be healthy and without issues, but most want to feel as though satisfaction is accessible.

There are numerous internal and external factors to consider when looking at desire that is bothersome to a couple. Those factors can range from shifts that come with age, stress levels, trauma, lack of accurate information, physical health, hormonal changes, and sexual pain. Low desire not only impacts the sense of self, but it can also have significant ramifications on the partner's sense of desirability and the relationship. It is important when working with couples who report desire discrepancies that psychoeducation is provided, and physical exams are encouraged by their primary care physicians to rule out any medical issues or hormonal changes contributing to lack of desire. While it can be widely known that desire is also impacted by relationship satisfaction, including relationship conflict, betrayal, resentment, and neglect, for many, a hefty physiological or medical component will also play a role. The unfortunate thing about our thoughts around desire and improved sex experiences is that we often view it as a switch that is easily turned on or off. Desire is neither static nor monolithic, but a gift that is an ever-changing process requiring work and intentionality. When couples are educated about the possible changes they may encounter, they can better prepare to adapt their sex lives as needed.

In the author's experience working with couples, another significant factor impacting desire includes the level of differentiation and fusion. In the early development of relationships, desire centers on each other's reflected sense of self through other-validated intimacy. Perel (2006) argues that the collapse of intimacy into fusion creates too much closeness, and a lack of desire is the result. This common desire killer of "abandonment of our own identity" is a result of us being so focused on our partner's needs that we lose our own sense of self and deny our own wants. Owning our wants is the backbone of true desire.

12.5   Sex and Sexuality

Tell me how you were loved, and I'll tell you how you make love.
Esther Perel (2006)

Our sexuality holds valuable information about who we are and how to act to get our needs met. It contains our fantasies, our fears, trauma, body esteem, techniques, and communication between sexual partners. As African Americans enter intimate relationships, they bring a historical context that includes not only intergenerational processes but also long-standing and overlapping racial and gender stereotypes that have been internalized and often displaced onto their significant other. Sex is perhaps the area of human experience in which we can feel the most vulnerable. In sex, we are visibly naked before another human being, both literally and symbolically. And there is no doubt, our society has socialized us through movies, songs, and poetry about sex and sexuality. These socializations rarely include the complexity of sexuality, which has led us to believe sex is natural, easy, uninhibited, and always spontaneous (McCarthy & McCarthy, 2012). So, when an individual or couple experiences sexual difficulty, it is often experienced with shame. Yet, all couples will experience some sort of sexual difficulties at one time or another during their relationship experience.

Sexuality is complex. It is shaped by one's family (Gupta et al., 2015) religion, laws, politics, and culture. It encompasses nearly every aspect of our being, from attitudes and values to feelings and experiences (Dailey, 1981; McCarthy & McCarthy, 2012; Ogden, 2018; Schnarch, 1991). Yet when people think about sex, it is narrowly focused on intercourse and orgasms, overshadowing pleasure, touching, and sensual feelings (McCarthy & McCarthy, 2012). In an age of accessibility, we presume people are sexually knowledgeable, comfortable, and having the best sex in history. The truth is sexual awareness and satisfaction have not grown much after the sexual revolution (McCarthy & McCarthy, 2012). Prior to 1960, we lacked scientific information about sexual functioning and dysfunction.

With poor quality of educational materials, many people developed a misunderstanding around sex and sexual functioning (McCarthy & McCarthy, 2012) in the West. Masters and Johnson's research made significant contributions to our understanding of sex and sexual dysfunction (Gottman & Schwartz-Gottman, 2012). Their work resulted in what is widely known as the model of human sexual response. The four phases of physiological arousal include excitement, plateau, orgasm, and resolution (Masters & Johnson, 1966). Their work has been invaluable in understanding orgasms through masturbation and penetration.

Many other researchers such as Helen Singer Kaplan, Bernie Zilbergeld, and Rosemary Basson followed Masters and Johnson's work. Kaplan (1974) added the concept of sexual desire to the model and condensed it to three phases: desire, arousal, and orgasm. Her revision was a result of taking a closer look at the treatment failures of her own clients and realizing they lacked interest in sex (Nagoski, 2015). Kaplan's model dominated the field for decades and was the standard in the American Psychiatric Association's Diagnostic and Statistical Manual. Basson's (2002) model was nonlinear and incorporated the importance of emotional intimacy, sexual stimuli, and relationship satisfaction.

Studies show that sexual activity, including our thoughts and emotions, involve the entire brain (Ogden, 2018). Because the brain stores our memories and cultural values, the influence of the brain greatly impacts our sexual arousal. (Crooks & Baur, 2008). In fact, the quantum model, developed by Dr. David Schnarch demonstrates how our brains may be one of our most important organs in human sexual arousal. His model is an alternative model to Masters and Johnson's linear model of sexual functioning. His model has two thresholds that address the complex aspects of human sexuality and sexual functioning across genders. The first threshold is the arousal threshold, followed by the orgasmic threshold. At its most basic, the model addresses how one functions sexually. A combination of physical stimuli (sensations) and psychological stimuli (feelings and thoughts) create the total sexual experience (Schnarch, 1997). When an individual is sufficiently aroused, their genitals will respond, meeting the first threshold of arousal. For men, this means an erect penis and for women, vaginal lubrication and breast sensitivity. As one becomes more aroused the body has the potential to reach the second threshold of orgasm.

Where things differ for humans from any other animal on the planet is the addition of the neocortex. The neocortex allows us to make meaning of our experiences. The meaning we ascribe to our experience can be the cause of us either experiencing great sex or diminishing our satisfaction. Our meanings are a combination of how we feel about what we are experiencing and with whom we are experiencing it with. Simply put, our feelings have a greater impact on genital functioning than our physical sensations (Schnarch, 1997). Recent focus on the relationship between differentiation and a couple's sex life has found those with greater levels of differentiation had an ability to openly talk about sex more effectively, which is connected to heightened satisfaction in sex and marriage (Ferreira et al., 2015). This indicates the significance of how we feel about our personal sexuality and our partners, which can determine how we engage in and enjoy sex.

The concepts of sex and race are inextricably interwoven (Butts, 1977), yet, for African Americans, much of their sexual experiences and concerns are left out of the research (Rouse-Arnett et al., 2006). For various reasons they may be excluded from studies, whether African Americans are not participating in studies because of possible distrust of historically oppressive systems (Townes et al., 2020) or researchers not being interested in Black intimacy, one must ask the question, are we effectively treating Black couples? The research shows exposure to high levels of racial stress and discrimination detrimentally impacts mental and physical health (Pavalko et al., 2003). Anything that impacts our mental and physical health will also have an impact on our sexual health. This is tremendously important when working with Black couples who experience ongoing stress given that stress can be an inhibitor or "brake" in our sex life.

Additionally, it is important to note a large portion of the African American community identify as having a religious belief or spiritual practice. While in most cases this can be a protective factor in the community, it is wise to consider the ideas that also come from our religious influence. There are strong messages, not only in church but in society as a whole, that the only "normal" or "natural" expression of erotic feelings is sex between a man and a woman (Ogden, 2018). This may leave the lesbian, gay, bisexual, transgender, queer (LGBTQ) community to wonder where they fit. Until recent years, homosexuality was a psychiatric disorder and no attention was given to treating same-sex sexually dysfunctional partners – either male or female. The marginalization of LGBTQ African Americans perpetuates a clear message of "otherness." This constant battle of otherness can have a direct impact on their self-worth, sense of self, levels of differentiation, and sexual identity.

As clinicians, we must be mindful and vigilant of the destructive portrayals and stereotypes that present Black women as promiscuous, lustful, wild, and exotic and Black men as violent, dangerous, and pred-atory (Collins, 2000) and the LGBTQ community as deviant. It may be helpful to assist individuals and couples deconstruct the negative messages around sex and sexuality while developing a more fitting sexual identity around truth and understanding.

12.6 Using the PLISSIT Model for Treatment Planning

Clinicians using the Permission, Limited Information, Specific Suggestions, and Intensive Therapy (PLISSIT) model, an evidence-based practice for identifying causes of sexual dysfunction, find it helpful for effective treatment planning and determining what the couple may need. It is often stated that the happiest people are those in good relationships while the next happiest are those not in romantic relationships, but the least happy are the ones in bad relationships. The backbone of Black families is rooted in the emotional health of committed partnerships. As clinicians assessing Black couples, it is critical to use assessments with a systemic lens and describe the systemic impact of how cultural narratives affect one's view of romantic relationships. Therefore, an assessment that looks at the impact of sociocontextual and ethnocultural factors that include gender and gender roles, economic and financial status, racial and ethnic considerations, religious and spiritual practices as well as interactional styles are essential.

In a society where sex is considered a private matter, a sex-positive approach that encourages and makes space for couples to explore dysfunc-tion and their capacity for better sex starts with PLISSIT.

P – Permission; clinicians are encouraged to ask for the couple's permission to engage in a discussion regarding their sexual feelings and relationship. The clinician is nonjudgmental, while normalizing and validating the couple's concerns. It is also important to keep in mind that the permission phase of this model should be used throughout the rest of the phases as well.

LI – Limited Information; clinicians provide limited and specific information on the topic, offering resources, organizations, support, and books needed to function sexually or on the effect their condition has on their sexuality. Clinicians may also need to dispel any myths.

SS – Specific Suggestions; clinicians offer specific suggestions, interventions, and or assignments to enable clients to engage in sexual activity according to their desired level.

IT – Intensive Therapy; clinicians either provide or refer to another health care professional if necessary to address the complex issues related to their sexual concerns.

Using the PLISSIT model following initial intake is helpful to get an understanding of the politics surrounding the couple's intimacy, desire, and sexual functioning. It is recommended to utilize an elicitation window approach of their most recent sexual encounter. It allows for the clinician to examine each partner's sexual script (sexual behaviors, context, and repertoire that has been negotiated and played out in the relationship). The elicitation approach evokes the multidimensional aspects of the couple's concerns and unresolved emotional development by exploring each partner's sexual style and attitude (Schnarch, 1991). The individual meanings attached to their sexual style and attitudes are used to highlight each partner's emotional needs and family inheritance.

12.7   Clinical Implications for Working with African American Couples

Since all sexual issues are multicausal, the therapist will gain insight into the multiple causes of the couple's sexual issues when thoroughly assessing and exploring their family dynamics and gathering meanings of their experience that pose barriers to intimacy, desire, and sexual fulfillment. The assessment should also include a clear understanding of the current baseline, the couple's optimal sexual functioning (their ideal sex life at the end of treatment), sexual desire, sexual satisfaction, level of distress they are experiencing due to the sexual problem and the problem's impact on the intimate relationship.

Lance and La Nia are both thirty-nine years old. They have been married for fourteen years. La Nia works as a medical professional and Lance is a respiratory therapist. They met through mutual friends. When La Nia became pregnant, they made the decision to marry. The couple had very little support from their families. They described their first year of marriage as "two kids raising kids without resources." The couple began having problems in their marriage after Lance lost his first job due to racism. La Nia described being frustrated with Lance's lack of motivation to get back in the field of respiratory therapy. He had worked "different odd jobs" to help make ends meet." His underemployment status is the subject of many of the couple's disagreements. Given the historical oppression of African American males, the fact that his wife is currently the "breadwinner," and he does not fit the gender role modeled by society or his family of origin, Lance's insecurities as a man are frequently triggered. As a result, Lance displays signs of depression and drinks regularly. La Nia is frustrated with his drinking. She has resorted to kicking him out of the house on several occasions. La Nia disclosed feeling dismissed and emotionally unsafe with Lance as she did with her father. La Nia reported her parents married young and were heavily affiliated with the church. She described her father as intense, controlling the bills, money, and household. Her mother is quiet and submissive. La Nia and her father often clashed when she was a teen. She harbors some resentment toward her mother for not speaking up on her behalf when her father was harsh in his parenting. Lance's parents remain married to date and moved to California. from Mississippi, leaving Lance behind when he was young. Lance spent a lot of his time with his grandmother and cousins since his parents worked to make a better life for him and the family. Lance reports his family is more "laid back" in comparison to La Nia's family. He describes his family as close without a lot of conflict.

In addition to financial strains, the couple reports a lack of intimacy. La Nia has been disappointed in their sex life. Lance reports "she seems uninterested," and he often feels rejected. Lance and La Nia report their parents never talked to them about sex except to scare them into celibacy. They described their intimate encounters as emotionally disconnected. During the elicitation window of the couple's most recent intimate encounter, La Nia discussed Lance's rush to penetrative sex before she was ready and finished before she had time to warm up. He was embarrassed he finished "quicker" than he wanted to. The couple spends little to no time engaging in intimacy and foreplay. She explains most of their sexual encounters are similar. Until now, she had not told Lance about her frequent frustrations around sexual pleasure or lack thereof. La Nia is aware of his insecurities as a man, therefore she acquiesces to keep his ego intact, but feels resentful that she does not feel "taken care of."

Providing Limited information (LI) to the couple may include helping La Nia increase her total stimulation. It is important to educate the couple on how their bodies work sexually and the benefits of foreplay and outercourse. Provide information on how desire and arousal are impacted by her thoughts, feelings, and emotions, as well as encourage her to hold on to herself (differentiation). Her ability to hold on to herself will make room for her to disclose her desires in her sexual encounters, without feeling the need to soothe Lance at the expense of her pleasure. Wyatt (1997) found that Black women found sexual communication critical to sexual satisfaction. La Nia will need to be able to convey her sexual needs verbally and non-verbally.

Specific Suggestions (SS) include referring Lance to his primary care physician to rule out any medical concerns (premature ejaculation). Health problems are a big factor in Black male sexual dysfunction. Black men have considerably higher rates of hypertension, heart disease, diabetes, and prostate cancer in comparison to their white counterparts. Other suggestions may include helping Lance to direct his focus away from his erection by focusing on deep breathing to address anxiety around his performance and tune into his own experience with La Nia. Assisting the couple to explore new elements of their sexual connection by encouraging them to expand their sexual repertoire and push the limits beyond their typical boundaries can help them to increase their sexual potential and ability to express their wants and desires.

Intense Therapy (IT) will include increasing the couple's levels of differentiation. Intimacy deepens as they increase their ability to manage emotional reactions when differences cause tension. Helping La Nia and Lance in committing to relating to each other in ways that are true to their deeply held values and beliefs are fundamental to their harmony. Processing La Nia's anger and resentment will be essential since anger is often a message that our needs or wants are not being adequately met. Assisting La Nia in seeing how her learned coping strategies of "doing things herself," only makes room for her to push through things, and not ask for help or believing she is worthy of getting help. She has learned to survive by dimming her needs to keep the peace, but it comes at the expense of her. In session, La Nia has realized her perpetual need for validation from Lance, and at times the therapist, when she is unable to do it for herself (reflected sense of self).

When the couple both experience emotional intensity, he copes through drinking, leaving her feeling uncared for and unprotected, and she reacts through unproductive efforts to change him, making him feel inadequate. Her habituated pattern of kicking him out of the house can mimic a parent–child dynamic that creates distance and colludes with his own narrative that he is easily disposable and unwanted, a narrative he has held since his parents moved to California without him. Addressing Lance's insecurities and the impact it has on his sex life is essential. Lance appears to have sex in a way that colludes with his inadequacies. His rush to penetrative sex is often associated with his fears of "being enough" to please La Nia. Her narrative of not being emotionally cared for, makes her pull back instead of leaning into his touch and letting herself be felt by him, ultimately inhibiting the emotional connection she desires during sex.

In working with this couple, a genogram may also be useful. It can be used to explore the couple's familial history It can assist in seeing patterns of bonding in the previous generations that impact attachment, differentiation, and intimacy, as well as family illness (physical and mental), medical and genetic concerns that may impact sexual functioning. This tool looks for multigenerational patterns that also include exploring the impact of religion, political affiliations, critical incidents, and lived trauma.

Clinicians exercise significant influence on treatment outcomes. Our behaviors with clients are shaped by our thinking and personal beliefs and not always in the best interest of our clients. Our ability to understand our clients and implement interventions will depend heavily on our own self work. As with any client or couple, rapport is vital to the work you will do. However, what may be more fundamental to the progress of this couple or any client is the clinician's own perceived notions about intimacy, desire, and sex, as well as a clear understanding of one's own level of differentiation. We cannot assist clients to a level of differentiation we have yet to achieve.

Discussion Questions

1. How might religiosity in the Black community impact a couple's expressions of intimacy and sexual desire?
2. How might experiences of racism and oppression impact intimacy, desire, and sex for Black couples?
3. What are some pros and cons with using the PLISSIT model for treatment planning with Black couples?
4. How would you describe your level of differentiation and your ability to effectively work with Black couples?

REFERENCES

Bagarozzi, D. (2014). *Enhancing intimacy in marriage: A clinician's guide*. Routledge.
Basson, R. (2002). A model of women's sexual arousal. *Journal of Sex and Marital Therapy, 28*, 1–10.
Bell, L., & Harsin, A. (2018). A prospective longitudinal study of marriage from midlife to later life. *Couple and Family Psychology: Research and Practice, 7*, 12–21.
Bethea, S., & Allen, T. (2013). Past and present societal influences on African American couples that impact love and intimacy. In K. M. Helm & J. Carlson (Eds.), *Love, intimacy and the African American couple* (pp. 20–59). Routledge.
Bowen, M. (1978). *Family therapy in clinical practice*. Jason Aronson.
Boyd-Franklin, N. (2003). Race, class, and poverty. In F. Walsh (Ed.), *Normal family processes: Growing diversity and complexity* (pp. 260–279). Guilford Press.
Brown, J. (2012). *Growing yourself up: How to bring your best self to all life's relationships*. Exisle Publishing.
Bryant, C. M., Wickrama, A. S., Bolland, J., Bryant, B. M., Cutrona, C. E., & Stanik, C. E. (2010). Race matters, even in marriage: Identifying factors linked to marital outcomes for African Americans. *Journal of Family Theory and Review, 2*(3), 157–174.

Butts, J. D. (1977). Inextricable aspects of sex and race. *Contributions in Black Studies: A Journal of African and Afro-American Studies, 1*, Article 5. https://scholarworks.umass.edu/cibs/vol1/iss1/5

Collins, P. H. (2000). *Black feminist thought: Knowledge, consciousness, and the politics of empowerment*. Routledge.

Crooks, R. L., & Baur, K. (2008). *Our sexualities* (10th ed.). Wadsworth.

Dailey, D. M. (1981). Sexual expression and aging. In F. J. Berghorn & D. E. Schafer (Eds.), *The dynamics of aging: Original essays on the processes and experiences of growing old* (pp. 311–330). Westview Press.

Dunham, S., & Ellis, C. M. (2010). Restoring intimacy with African American couples. In J. Carlson & L. Sperry (Eds.), *Recovering intimacy in love relationships: A clinician's guide* (pp. 295–316). Routledge.

Ferreira, L. C., Fraenkel, P., Narciso, I., & Novo, R. (2015). Is committed desire intentional? A qualitative exploration of sexual desire and differentiation of self in couples. *Family Process, 54*, 308–326.

Ferreira, L. C., Narciso, I., Novo, R. F., & Pereira, C. R. (2014). Predicting couple satisfaction: the role of differentiation of self, sexual desire and intimacy in heterosexual individuals. *Sexual and Relationship Therapy, 29*(4), 390–404.

Gilbert, R. M. (2017). *Extraordinary relationships. A new way of thinking about human interactions* (2nd ed). Leading Systems Press.

Gottman, J., & Schwartz-Gottman, J. (2012). *The art and science of lovemaking: Research-based skills for a great sex life*. Gottman Institute.

Gupta, R., Pillai, V., Punetha, D., & Monah, A. (2015). Love experiences of older African Americans: A qualitative study. *Journal of International Women's Studies, 16*(3), 277–293.

Helm, K. M., & Carlson, J. (2013). *Love, intimacy and the African American couple*. Routledge.

Kaplan, H. (1974). *The new sex therapy*. Brunner-Mazel.

Kerr, M. E., & Bowen, M. (1988). *Family evaluation: An approach based on Bowen theory*. W. W. Norton.

Kolodny, R., Johnson, V. E., & Masters, W. H. (1988). *Masters and Johnson on sex and human loving*. Little, Brown.

Lavner, J. A., Barton, A. W., Bryant, C. M., & Beach, S. R. H. (2018). Racial discrimination and relationship functioning among African American couples. *Journal of Family Psychology, 32*(5), 686–691. https://doi.org/10.1037/fam0000415

Leiblum, S. (2010). *Treating sexual desire disorders*. Guilford Press.

Lerner, H. (1989). *The dance of intimacy: A woman's guide to courageous acts of change in key relationships*. Harper & Row.

Masters, W. H., & Johnson, V. E. (1966). *Human sexual response*. Little, Brown.

McCarthy, B. (2015). *Sex made simple. Clinical strategies for sexual issues in therapy*. PESI.

McCarthy, B., & McCarthy, E. (2012). *Sexual awareness* (5th ed.). Routledge.

McGoldrick, M., Giordano, J., & Garcia-Preto, N. (2005). *Ethnicity & family therapy*. Guilford Press.

McGruder, K. (2009). Pathologizing Black sexuality: The U.S. experience. In J. Battle & S. Barnes (Ed.), *Black sexualities: Probing powers, passions, practices, and policies* (pp. 101–118). Rutgers University Press.

Mintz, L. B. (2017). *Becoming cliterate: Why orgasm equality matters-and how to get it*. HarperOne.

Nagoski, E. (2015). *Come as you are. The surprising new science that will transform your sex life*. Simon & Schuster.

Ogden, G. (2018). *Expanding the practice of sex therapy: The neuro update edition* (2nd ed.) Routledge.

Pavalko, E. K., Mossakowski, K. N., & Hamilton, V. J. (2003). Does perceived discrimination affect health? Longitudinal relationships between work discrimination and women's physical and emotional health. *Journal of Health and Social Behavior, 44*(1), 18–33.

Peleg, O. (2008). The relation between differentiation of self and marital satisfaction: What can be learned from married people over the course of life? *American Journal of Family Therapy, 36*(5), 388–401.

Penner, C. L., & Penner, J. J. (1993). *Restoring the pleasure. Complete step-by-step programs to help couples overcome the most common sexual barriers*. W. Publishing.

Perel, E. (2006). *Mating in captivity: Unlocking erotic intelligence*. Harper Collins.

Piper-Mandy, E., & Rowe, T. D. (2010). Educating African-centered psychologists: Towards a comprehensive paradigm. *Journal of Pan African Studies, 3* (8), 5–23.

Regas, S. (2010). *Beyond the erotic*. http://www.susanregas.com/floral-design

Rouse-Amett, M., Dilworth, J. E. L., & Stephens, D. P. (2006). The influence of social institutions on African American women's sexual values and attitudes. *Journal of Feminist Family Therapy, 17*(2), 1–15.

Schnarch, D. (1991). *Constructing the sexual crucible: An integration of sex and marital therapy*. Norton.

(1997). *Passionate marriage: Love, sex, and intimacy in emotionally committed relationship*. Norton.

(2009). *Intimacy & desire: Awaken the passion in your relationship*. Beaufort Books.

Schnarch, D., & Regas, S. (2012). The crucible differentiation scale: Assessing differentiation in human relationships. *Journal of Marital and Family Therapy, 38*(4), 639–652.

Staples, R. (1972). Research on Black sexuality: Its implication for family life, sex education, and public policy. *The Family Coordinator, 21*(2), 183–188.

(2006). *Exploring Black sexuality*. Rowman and Littlefield.

Titelman, P. (2008). *Triangles: Bowen family systems theory perspectives*. Haworth Press, Taylor & Francis.

Townes, A., Guerra-Reyes, L., Murray. M., Rosenberg, M., Wright, B., Long, L., & Herbenick, D. (2020). "Somebody that looks like me" matters:

A qualitative study of black women's preferences for receiving sexual health services in the USA. *Culture, Health & Sexuality*, *30*, 1–15. https://doi.org/10.1080/13691058.2020.1818286

White, J. L. (1984). *The psychology of Blacks*. Prentice-Hall.

White, J. L., & Parham, T. A. (1990). *The psychology of Blacks* (2nd ed). Prentice-Hall.

Wincze, J. P., & Weisberg, R. B. (Eds.). (2015). *Sexual dysfunction: A guide for assessment and treatment* (3rd ed.). Guilford Press.

Wyatt, G. E. (1997). *Stolen women: Reclaiming our sexuality, taking back our lives.* Wiley.

Wyatt, G. E., Strayer, R. G., & Lobitz, C. W. (1976). Issues in the treatment of sexually dysfunctioning couples of Afro-American descent. *Psychotherapy. Theory, Research and Practice*, *13*(1), 44–50.

CHAPTER 13

Wearing a Mask in Love: Implications for Covering and Infidelity in Black Relationships

Laura Dupiton & Cynthia Chestnut

The mainstream narrative of relationships in the Black community has been largely pathologized (Eyre et al., 2012; Utley, 2011). The fragility and instability of Black committed relationships in America bends under the weight of internalized negative messaging and the reality of social injustice, stubbornly rooted in the effects of racism. Statistically, Black women are least likely to get married and have higher rates of marital instability (Raley et al., 2015). According to Caucutt et al. (2019), "in 2016 only 29% of African Americans were married compared to 48% of all Americans, half or 50% of African Americans have never been married compared to 33% of all Americans" (p. 1). In addition, Black women are also "three times as likely as white women never even to live with an intimate partner" (Banks, 2011, p. 2). Scholars have correlated the decline of Black marriages with "structural factors, for example, declining employment prospects and rising incarceration rates for unskilled black men" (Raley et al., 2015, p. 89). Research has shown that the mass incarceration of Black men is directly correlated to the decline in marriages and is represented in the imbalanced sex ratio, in which there are more Black women than Black men (Banks, 2011; Caucutt et al., 2019; Raley et al., 2015).

African American couples face many systemic and socioeconomic obstacles in the United States; however, the common phenomenon of infidelity also poses a threat to the safety and stability of Black relationships. Penn et al. (1997) explained that the "forces" that are working against African American committed relationships "include the legacy of slavery, the impact of racism and discrimination, economic hardships, and imbalanced sex ratios" (p. 173). Despite the dearth of research regarding infidelity in Black committed relationships, scholars have drawn correlations between infidelity, poverty, the disproportionate sex ratio of Black men and women (eighty-five Black men for every one hundred Black women), and the incarceration of Black men (Eyre et al., 2012; Utley, 2011). However, it is important to recognize that due to the institution of slavery "marital and familial units were not allowed to develop and exist in their traditional manner. For example, mothers, fathers, and children could be sold away from each other, disrupting any semblance of family security or stability" (Penn et al., 1997, p. 173). Despite the unique experience of the Black community, Utley (2011) highlighted that mainstream researchers continue to "normalize infidelity as a black community pathology," calling into question the cultural norms of Black relationships (p. 66).

The discussion of infidelity and Black relationships typically "focus[es] on why men cheat, public apologies from who have strayed, and salacious details from mistresses" (Utley, 2011, p. 67). However, it seems the narrative has largely been driven by "dehumanizing mythological constructions and stereotypes of black male masculinity as well as Black womanhood and sexuality" (Slatton & Spates, 2014, p. 4). These stereotypes and narratives have an inherent impact on how Black men and women view themselves and one another in relationship. Racialized and gendered stereotypes often point to the Black male as insatiably seeking sex from multiple partners and Black women as the hypersexual Sapphire. In a study completed with low-income Black males from New York City, Slatton and Spates (2014) found that several Black male respondents shared that "'faithful' men are sometimes ridiculed socially as 'fools' or 'suckers,' or 'cuffed,' but when asked for their own opinions virtually all endorsed faithful monogamy as a legitimate choice to be respected" (p. 179). Though the study is limited due to the number of participants, the responses refute the ideology that monogamy is outside the realm of possibility for Black couples.

Slatton and Slates (2014) explained that it is often necessary for marginalized identities to utilize "counter-narratives as a critical tool of social science research that amplifies the voices of marginalized groups" (p. 170). In 2019, renowned radio personality Lenard McKelvey also known as "Charlamagne tha God" began trending in social media due to his attempt of creating a counternarrative by stating "Black men don't cheat." Williams (2019) described McKelvey's creation of the hashtag and song "Black Men Don't Cheat" as a strategic method to author a new narrative for black men that sheds positive light on their role as committed partners. According to Williams (2019), the song sparked tense debates between those that questioned the veracity of the statement "Black men don't cheat" and Black men and women who utilized the hashtag to intentionally highlight positive long-lasting Black relationships. The quote "Black men don't cheat" emphasizes the internalized messaging that is a part of the majoritarian narrative regarding Black relationships and the inherent duplexity in the discussion of infidelity in the Black community.

Slatton and Spates' (2014) study as well as the trending statement "Black men don't cheat" showcase a significant duality in the thought processes of Black men and women's perspective of infidelity. The narrative regarding infidelity has been one that is proverbially stuck between wanting and respecting the safety and security of monogamy and the societal expectation/stereotype of the hypermasculine and hypersexual Black male. Though scholars are able to highlight the systemic injustice and circumstances that remain as barriers in Black marriage and relationships, it is also important to highlight emotional and racial trauma, attachment injuries, internalized stereotypic messages, and the inherent distrust that occurs within Black relationships.

13.1   Definition of Covering

Black relationships carry the invisible baggage of transgenerational, historical, and relational trauma. Historically, Black people have been forced to suppress and repress their needs, wants, and vulnerabilities for survival purposes. With the primary goal of moving through their world safely, Black people have had to mute their stigmatized identities to remain palatable for the status quo and to conform to white normativity. This act is known as "covering." Covering is a sociological phenomenon coined by Erving Goffman in 1963. It is the act of "keeping the stigma of their identity from looming large" (Yoshino & Smith, 2013, p. 4). Covering is the intentional act of hiding one's authentic self/emotions, due to having a stigmatized identity (e.g., person of color, lesbian, gay, bisexual, transgendered, queer or questioning, physically handicapped etc.). Individuals who stray from white normativity tend to distance themselves from any behavior, feeling, or thought that highlights their "otherness." Therefore, one who "covers" changes or modifies their appearance, language, emotional needs, and response to effectively assimilate to societal expectations.

Literature has specifically focused on covering and the distress of not being able to be one's authentic self in the workplace. Weaver (2015), a Black female clinical psychologist, described her visceral experience with covering in the workplace. Weaver (2015) explained that she covered by minimally being transparent with her white co-workers and described relenting to her identity as a "stigmatized minority" (para. 2). The fear of being discredited and stereotyped silenced Weaver and minimized her ability to be transparent with her white colleagues. According to Yoshimo and Smith (2013), in a study exploring the impact of covering among 3,129 respondents, 79 percent of Black people, 67 percent of women of color, and 81 percent of individuals identifying as lesbian, gay, bisexual, transgendered, queer or questioning, or asexual reported experiencing the deleterious effects of covering (p. 4). Black respondents described various manners by which they covered, including not speaking up when hearing racist comments in the workplace, not wearing natural hairstyles, repressing feelings of anger etc. (Yoshino & Smith, 2013). Goffman (1963) emphasized that covering is used "to reduce tension, that is, to make it easier for himself and the others to withdraw covert attention from the stigma" (p. 102). Therefore, Black people are often in a state of double consciousness to protect themselves from the inevitability of racial trauma. Hardy (2013) explained that "racial oppression is a traumatic form of interpersonal violence which can lacerate the spirit, scar the soul, and puncture the psyche" (p. 25). This level of trauma inherently impacts the identity of Black people. It is asserted that due to the complex historical trauma of slavery and the continued experience of racism in America, Black men, women, and children have hidden internal wounds that continue to impact their well-being. Hardy (2013) explained that racial oppression has led Black people to have "internalized devaluation, [an] assaulted sense of self and internalized voicelessness" (p. 25). The internalization of these wounds is precipitated by the constant mistreatment and detrimental messages that Black children and adults receive daily. It is no surprise that the response to such an onslaught of trauma and abuse is to resort to behaviors and attitudes that allow Black people to survive and protect themselves from the dangers of racism. Therefore, covering as a sociological concept sheds light on the reality that Black individuals often exist within a double consciousness, suppressing one's true thoughts, feelings, and beliefs while attempting to take on a persona that is deemed as culturally acceptable.

13.2   Impact of Covering on Black Couple Relationships

The daily act of covering and the detrimental psychological and emotional impact on Black men and women may transcend the arena of the workplace and infiltrate the relational dynamics of Black couples. Covering or wearing a mask in relationship may precipitate the maladaptive behavior of infidelity. With stereotypes of the Strong Black Woman and the hypermasculine and hypersexual Black man, it is necessary to question whether Black men and women can be their true and authentic selves with one another and whether covering is not allowing for trust and honesty to occur in Black relationships. Ultimately, it is a question of how Black couples are able to delineate when it is possible to lay down their burden of covering versus when and with whom is it safe to be vulnerable/intimate when their daily experience requires them to wear a mask for their own protection and survival. Black men and women are accustomed to muting their emotional needs and vulnerability. Therefore, they hide from one another to protect themselves from seemingly inevitable loss. This is evidenced by the statistical data about infidelity and Black relationships. Parker and Campbell (2017) explained that Black men are reported to have the highest instances of infidelity. Though this is often explained by the imbalanced sex ratio and other pressing contextual factors that are rooted in racism, one cannot ignore the intracultural mistrust that becomes inherent in relationships between Black men and women. Macauda et al. (2011) explained that,

> since everyone is always "on the move" to survive emotionally and physi-cally and can be involved with several different people on different emo-tional levels, they expect that even in a committed relationship their partner likely has someone on the side. Thus, to prevent emotional injury, the cultural norm is having someone on the side or waiting in "the wings' even though they recognize this is a violation of trust that can undermine the development of the very relationships they yearn for. (p. 362)

Parker and Campbell (2017) articulated the effectual residue of emotional and physical survival that Black men and women face in their relation-ships. The constant state of protecting oneself from emotional hurts highlights that covering is occurring in Black relationships that cannot seem to find secure attachment because they are built on a foundation that is often ruptured by racial trauma.

Black men and women safeguard their vulnerability with the expecta-tion of inevitable infidelity (Parker & Campbell, 2017). The tangible distress of not being able to trust in the monogamy and commitment of relationships creates disconnection and raises the intensity of fear in many Black relationships. This is problematic, as research has indicated that "attachment anxiety and avoidance predict greater likelihood of infidelity" (Parker & Campbell, 2017, p. 173). Attachment avoidance often causes "emotional repression and suppressive coping during stressful situations. Individuals with high avoidance are "characterized by a lack of emotional investment, a value for self-reliance, and over-all avoidance of emotional intimacy. Infidelity may be used in an effort to [create] distance from a committed partner" (Parker & Campbell, 2017, p. 174). Attachment avoidance is symbiotic with the act of covering. It is a defense from increased risk of emotional pain. Black men and women face the threat of trauma and subjugation frequently, therefore, increasing their level of self-reliance and the need to operate from a stance of survival. Sun et al. (2019) further stressed that studies analyzing Black relationships found that "external stressors, including economic strain and racial discrimination, were linked to poorer couple relationship quality" (p. 83). The racial experience of Black couples in America plays an inherent and imperative role in their relational dynamic. This is reminiscent in the way racialized gendered stereotypes of Black men and women continue to impact the self-perception and narratives of Black people. Hardy (2013) explained that the phenomenon of "internalized devaluation" begins in the experience of Black children. Internalized devaluation is "a direct by-product of racism, inextricably linked to the deification of whiteness and the demonization of non-white hues" (Hardy, 2013, p. 25). The internal messages that are sent to Black children who suffer at the hands of a broken system tend to create a message of "I am bad" or "unworthy" of better treatment. Black men and women are often subject to having their identity assaulted by racist assumptions and ideologies that date back to slavery.

Dickens (2014) further emphasized the distinctive gendered experience of Black women by stating that "young Black women have a unique racialized gender identity in that some are raised to have both feminine and masculine characteristics as a navigation skill through various life experiences" (p. 15). Black women have not had the privilege of maintaining the mainstream ideology of fragility that is often associated with being feminine. This factor is significant when considering gender assignments in Black relationships and the ways in which the racial experience of both Black men and women impact their interpersonal and intimate relationships. Ultimately, the survival tactics that Black men and women have developed in response to racism have the potential to become inherent and visible in their relationships.

13.3   Wearing a Mask in Black Relationships and the Many Ways Covering Relates to Infidelity

The exploration of the sociological concept of covering and the traumatic experience of infidelity in Black relationships is inextricably bound to how Black men and women perceive themselves and one another in relationship, as well as their ability to trust each other interpersonally. Nunnally (2012) posited that "trust indicators include the following (1) behavior, (2) context, (3) perceived outcomes, and (4) perceived risks" (p. 25). In relationships, trust is a significant factor of a successful relationship; therefore, in deciding whether one can trust another individual in relationship, often individuals are observing behavior and anticipating a successful outcome depending upon the risks and how the individual presents himself or herself. However, Nunnally (2012) stressed that when determining someone's trustworthiness, "people either consider others' reputation or make a prediction about their prospective behavior on the basis of the information available to them. If information is scarce, then stereotypes convey data about others" (p. 25). Therefore, when considering Black relationships, one must keep in mind the stereotypes that have been internalized and projected upon the Black community.

Black women often feel that they must safeguard/protect their vulnerability due to the consistency of seeing failed relationships within the Black community. Black women are often impacted by implicit messages that were passed down trans-generationally. Richardson and Wade (1999) emphasized that "Black people were not completely immune to messages of black inferiority and white superiority, for we also were bombarded by the media, as the whole culture was with ideas about how we should look, and we have internalized some of them" (p. 25). The experience of denigrating images of Black people has impacted their beliefs and assumptions about love. Richardson and Wade (1999) detailed instances of Black women attempting to convince themselves that they "like being single" or that they are "destined to be alone" due to the idea that "there are no good ones" when considering Black men (p. 26). Black women tend to engage in rationalization and a series of other defense mechanisms in order to support their unconscious beliefs that are rooted in traumatic experiences of historical trauma. Richardson and Wade (1999) asserted that Black women have received an "emotional inheritance of anti-intimacy beliefs" (p. 19). Some of these beliefs included "There will never be enough of anything I need, especially love," "I'm not good enough to be loved," "I'll lose anyone who gets close to me," "It's not safe for me to face my anger," and "I have to control everyone and everything around me to protect myself from being hurt again" (pp. 20–21). Richardson and Wade's (1999) list of inherited beliefs are rooted in the tragic losses Black women faced during slavery. These internalized messages continue to reverberate throughout generations, directly impacting Black committed relationships.

Therefore, it is imperative to shed light upon stereotypes that continue to create distance in Black relationships. The gendered racialized

stereotypes that have been projected upon the Black woman have functioned to create a rigid sense of self that is dehumanizing in nature. The
stereotypes imposed upon Black women range from the hypersexual
Sapphire "who cannot control her sexual impulses" to the "morally mas-
ochistic Mammy" (Kelly & Green, 2010, p. 426). However, specific
stereotypes such as the Strong Black Woman (SBW) can be internalized
and transformed into schemas and ways of thinking and being for Black
women. The strong Black woman has been deemed as a source of pride in
the Black community (Beauboeuf-Lafontant, 2009). However, the schema
tends to maintain the Black woman's fear of expressing anger, fear,
vulnerability, and her overall need for support. The SBW ideology maintains that the Black woman can experience tragedy, trauma, and hardship
without relying on external resources, and holds self-sacrifice as a significant value (Beauboeuf-Lafontant, 2009; Donovan & West, 2014; Watson
& Hunter, 2016).

Furthermore, Black men also experience the deleterious effects of being
stereotyped and prejudged. Brooms and Perry (2016) explained that "the
perceptions of Black men are in a constant battle where Black men have to
struggle and fight for opportunities to define themselves" (p. 172). The
societal construction of the Black man's identity is typically seen through
the muddied lens of stereotypes. Black men are frequently seen as angry,
threatening, criminalized, hypermasculine, and hypersexual (Hester &
Gray, 2018). Theorists assert that "racism is a conditional variable that
adversely affects Black male-female relationships [specifically,] when couples internalize the negative images of themselves portrayed by society for
the purpose of establishing and maintaining White dominance" (Kelly &
Floyd, 2001, p. 110). These stereotypes can create a deep schism within
Black relationships. As previously mentioned, trust within all relationships
is a significant factor; however, Black relationships have the added stressors
of cultural mistrust that inherently impacts their view of one another
(Kelly & Floyd, 2001). The dichotomous and conflictual messages that
Black men and women receive about their identity versus their personal
perception of self, causes extreme distress, frustration and anger, that is
likely to create behaviors that are in alignment with the concept of
covering. Kelly and Floyd (2001) further highlighted that for Black individuals in relationships "the feeling of inferiority has engendered a rage
that is unsafe to vent toward white society, and thus that rage is displaced
toward each other, leading to mutual mistrust and disrespect" (p. 111).
This dysfunctional projection of anger and mistrust in Black relationships
can cause disconnection and sever opportunities of secure attachment.

Unfortunately, racism has served as the backdrop of conflict in Black relationships and must be viewed within the context of the many external factors that Black couples face. Kelly and Floyd (2001) explained that "society's treatment of Blacks has caused a higher percentage of Blacks to face poverty, health problems, crime, and drug abuse as compared with Whites" (p. 11) The insidious effects of racism continues to encourage the mutual lack of trust in the Black community. With the inability to escape feelings of powerlessness and frustration, Black men and women may be protecting their vulnerability due to their exposure to infidelity, pecking order status, feelings of inferiority, and protection from further attachment injury. Therefore, it is important to consider that both the Black man and woman have been socialized in convoluted messaging, further diminishing their trust in one another.

Black couples covering in relationships can manifest in several maladaptive ways and can provide couple's therapists with a roadmap in addressing the subtlety of covering when treating Black men and women. It is important to explore fears around self-expression, being vulnerable with others and one's self, communicating needs, and responding in emotionally open ways that indicate healthy coping skills. Signs of covering in Black relationships that may lead to infidelity include silence, avoidance of vulnerability, avoidance in seeking help, hiding pain, self-abdication, and survival mechanism.

13.3.1 Silence

Covering is an act of willful self-abdication (Dupiton, 2019). Therefore, one can decide to remain silent when one's needs are not met and feelings are not considered. Silence can act as a strategic form of avoidance in relationship. The fear of rejection and/or abandonment may cause individuals to shrink into silence as a form of protection. The need to protect against any threat or harm to one's vulnerability may cause individuals to grow detrimentally silent toward one another. It is important to consider the fact that Black men and women operate in a form of double consciousness causing them to continuously assess whether it is safe to share their authentic feelings. For example, when Black women and men are angry in white spaces, he/she must determine the safest way to emote as he/she does not want to be seen as a potential threat. Silence can also include holding/keeping secrets, which continues to erode the trust in the relationship. It is essential to consider the significance of internalized stereotypes with this emotional response of silence. The SBW schema tends to "promote a rigid sense of self whereby Black women are bound by the concept of uncompromising strength, which limits their ability to be congruent" (Dupiton, 2019, p. 40). The internalization of this stereotype may cause Black women to feel that sharing vulnerability can be deemed as a weakness.

13.3.2   Avoidance of Vulnerability

Brené Brown (2013) described vulnerability "as the catalyst for courage, compassion, and connection" (p. 11). Though understanding the emotional risk of vulnerability Brown cautioned us that by "spend[ing] our lives waiting until we're perfect or bulletproof before we walk into the arena, we ultimately sacrifice relationships and opportunities that may not be recoverable, we squander our precious time, and we turn our backs on our gifts" (p. 11). Black men and women who avoid vulnerability due to distrust do not seek to be perfect or bulletproof. Rather, it is a necessity to be as close to perfect as possible in order to adapt to the status quo and to remain safe in white spaces. Therefore, vulnerability for Black men and women can be deemed as a double emotional risk that is being taken because being one's authentic and true self is often not permitted in all spaces. It is also imperative to consider that there are Black men and women who have internalized stereotypes and project them upon one another. For example, a Black woman emoting in her relationship can still cause her paramour to assign her the role of being an "angry Black woman." Therefore, avoiding vulnerability as an act of covering is not limited to white spaces but can also be employed within Black relationships. Covering is enacted when an individual refuses to say that they love someone first, avoids sharing that he/she/they feels lonely, admitting that their sexual needs are not being met, pretending to be happy in a relationship that is falling apart etc. These individuals wear a mask not for egotistical gain, but in fear of being overly exposed to potential hurts. Therefore, in these instances of avoiding vulnerability, rather than sharing one's feelings openly with their mate, one may resort to engaging in cheating.

13.3.3   Avoidance in Seeking Help

There may be circumstances where individuals do not seek assistance or support in their relationship, specifically married and/or cohabitating Black couples. Typically, couples tend to maintain privacy regarding relational difficulties. Wischkaemper et al. (2020) stressed that many couples are accustomed to turning toward other sources of support, such as "close friends, or relatives, primary care providers, or clergy, instead of trained relationship professionals" (p. 2). Historically, Black people have underutilized mental health services. According to Liao et al. (2020), "African American women are more likely than European American women to report depression symptoms. Loneliness, defined as feeling isolated and disconnected from others, is positively associated with depressive and anxious symptoms among African American women" (p. 86). The paucity of psychological research and literature regarding Black couples must be emphasized. Research has largely focused on the experience of the Black single parent or challenges around parenting (Wischkaemper et al., 2020). Therefore, the reasoning behind Black men and women not seeking assistance with their relational challenges is tied to multiple contextual layers that range from the impact of racialized and gendered stereotypes of Black men and women not being allowed to show signs of "weakness," as well as a lack of trust for the mental health field due to many psychological precepts being rooted in white normativity.

However, refusing to seek assistance can manifest in many ways in Black relationships. One may decide not to admit to their partner that they are feeling symptoms of depression or hopelessness, not acknowledging or disclosing that you need assistance with parenting, having difficulty achieving a work/life balance, or reaching out to a couple's therapist to address relational stress. Liao et al. (2020) explained "that in a quantitative study completed by Watson and Hunter (2015), the Strong Black Woman schema positively predicted depressive symptoms" (p. 86). Therefore, with the awareness that Black women are susceptible to depression and the lack of trust and resources that are accessible to Black men and women, this form of covering can be detrimental to the healthy functioning of a Black couple.

13.3.4   Hiding Pain

Infidelity tends to begin with acts of secrecy. However, the process of infidelity is preceded by covering. This occurs via avoidance of emotional pain and the experience of disconnection with one's partner. This lack of communication is extremely detrimental as there are many concerns around having multiple sex partners. Utley (2011) explained that "not only are black men more likely to have multiple sex partners, but black women are less likely to control condom use in their relationship" (p. 68).

According to Bowleg et al. (2004), cultural scripts and messaging around gender norms in the Black community is significant in understanding how Black men and women conceptualize their relationships. Bowleg et al. (2004) interviewed fourteen Black women to assess their interpersonal relationship scripts and found that infidelity was considered normative among a majority of the participants. One of the participants in the study stated that she "was willing to tolerate [her partner of 8 years] cheating "as long as he just don't flaunt it in my face [and] don't give me no sexual diseases or anything" (p. 76). The reality of infidelity and contracting sexual diseases is an unfortunate reality. Bowleg et al. (2004) reported that "the HIV/AIDS epidemic, continues to rage disproportionately among African American women. [In 2001,] Black women accounted for 58% of reported AIDS cases among women" (p. 70). These statistics tell a damning story of covering that occurs in the Black community. Infidelity being deemed as "normative" provides insight into the hidden emotional, mental, and potentially physical pain that Black men and women endure in silence.

13.3.5   Self-Abdication

Self-abdication is the act of disowning one's self. The tragedy of racial oppression and the many internal messages that Black men and women have received as a result, can manifest into self-abdication or the suppression of one's true emotions and needs. Parker and Campbell's (2017) study found that "fearful attachment indicated a positive association with extradyadic interaction (EDI) [or infidelity] for African American/ Black participants, indicating that the higher a participant scored on fearful attachment, the more infidelity reported" (p. 177). There was also a positive correlation with dismissive attachment among African American couples in this study. African American couples who presented with high anxiety and high avoidance were linked to experiencing infidelity (Parker & Campbell, 2017). An individual with fearful attachment exists within an internal paradox of both being afraid of getting too close and being too distant from their loved one. The anxiety of losing oneself and experiencing loss is extremely significant in Black relationships, specifically when acknowledging the historical trauma of Black people which is filled with narratives of loss and devastation. The negative messaging around Black relationships also impacts the trust that is foundational to commitment. The lack of trust in the attachment leads to suppression of one's authentic self and can result in seeking out others to fill a void. Therefore, the willful and intentional self-abdication of Black men and women can be seen as a form of self-protection from the risk of attachment injuries.

13.3.6 Covering as a Survival Mechanism

Though covering can be detrimental to one's psyche, creating willful distance between one's true self and another in a relationship that is lacking in emotional maturity, safety, and experiencing infidelity may paradoxically be a healthy response to avoid further attachment injury and emotional trauma. Black men and women tend to cover with the intent of protecting themselves and to soften the blow of racial stigmatization. However, in relationship, covering can be a way to create healthy boundaries in relationship, to hold self and others accountable in the way one would like to be treated, and to allow one to understand and pay attention to the narrative of their life's story. Covering may be appropriate during the beginning stages of building an intimate relationship to fully assess whether a partner can be reliable long term. People often cover to manage their vulnerability in a relationship. They show up masking the intensity of their attraction in romantic exchanges. In this sense covering is seen as a protective factor managing parts of self-avoiding exposure. Shame, fear, guilt, insecurity, lack of confidence, and poor self-esteem are sometimes managed with covering, in order to wait for the opportunity to feel safe in relationship. Therefore, in order to safekeep one's vulnerability, an individual may seek out quick fixes such as extra sexual encounters with many or more than one partner because the individual lacks the courage to do the work that demands action toward healing using infidelity as a symptom when the major problem or issue is not being addressed.

13.4 Case Study and Further Conceptualization of Covering

Covering shows up in many interactions couples have in their relationships. This vignette demonstrates the covert and overt constructions of covering in the dynamics Danielle and Dorian internalized and projected in their coupling. The multigenerational effects of the transmission of trauma have impacted this couple's feelings of inferiority which depleted their self-esteem and confidence in each other.

Narrative Therapy (Guise, 2018) will be used to highlight what is true to each member and assess whether it matches their historical truth, which focuses on the effects of the problem, examining how the problem impacts them as individuals and a couple, while not emphasizing the problem as a cause. The constructs of Narrative Therapy that are addressed in this vignette include addressing the personal experiences that show up as ambiguous while attending to the language used to describe their experience and examine how it is shaping their reality. This example is used to demonstrate how the story organizes their experience and shapes behavior. This will also show how change comes by finding an alternative solution by helping members to open themselves up to other possibilities to expand their sense of self and each other. Although not all the details to demonstrate the process of their therapy experience will be described, the overall story will reflect some of the changes that occurred in their relationship.

13.4.1   Dorian and Danielle's Vignette

Danielle, thirty-five years old, and Dorian, thirty-eight years old, are an African American married couple. The couple has faced several hurdles in their seven years of marriage. Both are alumni of Delaware State University where Danielle graduated with her degree in business and Dorian graduated with a bachelor's in psychology. Danielle within the past year has attained her MBA and has been promoted at her workplace, which has increased her pay to making six figures. Dorian has been working as a tech in a residential treatment facility and working overnight as security for over three years and makes about half of Danielle's salary.

Early in their marriage, Dorian was caught texting an ex-girlfriend. Dorian admitted to Danielle that he was immature, and he was "just messing around with her" not meaning for it to go anywhere yet the attention was entertaining. Danielle reminded him that being flirtatious has gotten him into trouble before they got married and that he promised he would not act it out with others. Danielle was unable to shake her feelings of discomfort due to the text message exchanges being with an ex-girlfriend. Danielle became consumed with anxiety and frustration because she felt she could not trust that Dorian would set the appropriate limits. Dorian emphatically apologized and explained that he realized he took a risk and promised to remain committed to Danielle.

Danielle agreed to forgive Dorian, although lingering mistrust tends to resurface, specifically during heated arguments. Recently, Danielle noticed that ever since announcing her pay increase, Dorian has been behaving differently. Danielle has been confiding in Ray, a Black male friend at work, in order to process her feelings about Dorian's flirtatious behaviors. Dorian has become short tempered, frustrated, and angry specifically with

Danielle. Whenever Danielle and Dorian disagree and begin debating about a topic, Dorian tends to assert himself and make statements such as "stop interrupting me," "you're always trying to challenge somebody, I'm the man in this house." Dorian also makes snide remarks such as "that's why y'all Black women stay single, ya'll don't know how to act." Furthermore, Dorian also complains about his job. He believes that he deserves a pay raise and feels like management is undercutting him due to being a Black man. Dorian becomes angry whenever individuals in his family suggest that he goes back to school to further his career as a potential therapist. Dorian insists that people, including Danielle, are trying to "run his life." Danielle recently asked Dorian if he needed help with paying the bills in the home, as she is now making more money, which caused Dorian to not speak to Danielle for three days. Within this time of Danielle receiving the silent treatment, she became suspicious about how Dorian is spending his time and decided to look through his phone while he was asleep. Danielle found text messages between Dorian and a female co-worker. Their discussion was flirtatious and filled with sexual innuendos. These text messages seem to have been going back and forth for two months. Danielle has now decided that marital counseling is necessary to rebuild their trust and to determine whether they are able to stay married.

13.4.2   *The Narrative of Dorian and Danielle's Therapy Experience*

When implementing Narrative Therapy theory in Dorian and Danielle's case, it is necessary to consider that Dorian and Danielle's narrative is reflective of their personal story based on how they expressed their experience. Probing this couple brought out feelings of betrayal, disloyalty, deceitfulness, disrespect, insecurity, fear, and worry for Danielle. Dorian expressed feelings of neglect, emasculation, belittling, disrespect, sneakiness, not feeling like a leader, and racial disparity. The language they both used to describe the function of exiles within demonstrated the couple's need for protection, healing, and resolution.

Both were asked to discuss how they understood the language used by the other and to put what they heard in context of how they understand the other. Danielle described Dorian as a fun-loving person who has a great sense of humor, charm, and swag. She said she could see as a Black man how he would feel disrespected by his job, as they continue to ignore his talents and hard work, thereby making him feel demeaned and emasculated. She further stated she tries hard to make him feel like the man of the house and not like a "boy" by following his rules to allow him to pay the bills and keep up the house, so that he won't feel like she is neglecting her responsibilities to help out. Danielle said she did not understand how he used "sneaky" because she does not see herself as ever being sneaky in their life together.

Dorian stated he understood how Danielle felt betrayed and viewed him as disloyal because of his affair early in their relationship. He said he was not the stereotypical Black man who would cheat and have girlfriends on the side like the behaviors she witnessed from her father. Dorian acknowledged he was immature and shared that he realizes he cannot have old friends in his life. In the past, he was not taking his relationship with Danielle seriously and ended up in a sexual experience with his ex. He lied to Danielle about it; however, Danielle found old emails between Dorian and his ex. Dorian explained that he understands that his past actions most likely fuels why Danielle is worried that he would do it again since she caught him texting his female co-worker. Dorian continues to emphasize that he is not engaging in sexual relations with this female co-worker. Dorian also explained that he feels violated because Danielle is now going through his things in search of more evidence.

Both took a defensive response discussing the other in context of themselves. Further probes enabled them to validate each other's point of view and decrease their defensiveness. The couple was asked what story they would use to contextualize the other's experience in how these feelings became real? The couple was then asked to externalize each feeling they described about themselves and personify that feeling to tell how that lives in their life.

For example, Dorian spoke of feeling emasculated. He stated that he was acquainted with emasculation for quite some time. He recalled being introduced to this feeling as a teenager. His parents often told him that he was going to be a "Black bum" because he was lazy and not ambitious like his sisters. He was criticized when he did not do things well and when he was unable to remember something that his parents and sisters felt was pertinent, they called him stupid and slow. Dorian explained that emasculation eventually became his friend when he decided he was going to become numb to the affects he experienced. It did not get in the way of him getting attention from girls and his sense of humor would act as a catalyst to distract emasculation from taking up much room in his thoughts. Dorian reported, when he and Danielle were married, his father made remarks about Danielle seeming "smarter" than he. After Danielle received her master's degree, Dorian's father called to congratulate

Danielle and made a big deal out of her accomplishments that Dorian never experienced. She shared with him that she was interviewing for an executive position, which was eventually offered to her and accepted. After their conversation, Dorian's father warned him that Danielle was going to "outdo him" and that if Dorian "wasn't so lazy, he could try to make some real money too."

This story gave Danielle some insight into Dorian's development that she did not previously consider. She knew his family was hard on him, but she expressed this story gave her a deeper awareness of his pain and grief on not measuring up to the standards of the people in his life. Danielle understood that Dorian often felt he had to aim to please and did not fully understand the extent Dorian would go to hide or cover his pain and disappointment.

Danielle was beginning to see an alternative story about Dorian and in turn Dorian was in awe that Danielle responded to him with such openness to hear and connect to his experience. Danielle was asked to externalize her feelings as well and she described betrayal as the greatest fear she has and how she swore to herself that she would never allow it to overcome her. Danielle said that her father betrayed his family by leaving her mother for another woman while she was a teenager. She saw her mother grieve the loss of her dad and was often exposed to her father flirting with other women. Danielle shared that betrayal was a badge of honor for her because she knew she would never betray the man in her life and would never give him reason to consider that she was that kind of woman. She said she would work hard in her relationship to show she could be trusted. Danielle explained that she believed that Black men would sleep with other women on the side because "many Black women don't mind being a side chick." She shared that she vowed that she would do whatever she had to do and become whoever she needed to be to make sure her man would not have a need to step outside of their relationship. Danielle declared that betrayal is something she would not surrender to if it happened in her relationship and would fight to keep her marriage.

Danielle internalized betrayal as something she needed to manage not only with herself but with her partner. Although she would hold her partner responsible for his actions, she believed she needed to manage anything that seemed to lead to his betrayal and protect him as well as herself from experiencing it. Danielle was also willing to shift and adapt to Dorian's needs with the hope that changing who she is and compromising would protect her from the betrayal that she so desperately was attempting to avoid.

After hearing Danielle's story, Dorian explained that he knew Danielle's father left her mother for another woman and started a new family and that it was an extremely difficult time for Danielle and her mother. He shared that he noticed that Danielle's mother still grieves the loss of her relationship with Danielle's father and continues after all these years to express feelings of bitterness. However, Dorian shared that he did not realize Danielle felt that she had to be responsible for maintaining the fidelity in their marriage by trying to manage other people, in particular other women in his life. Dorian expressed that he always saw her as trying to control and treat him like a child. Dorian shared that he could see Danielle trying to repair her relationship with her father in and through him and that is not her job. Dorian further stated that his playfulness and flirtatious innuendos might cause her to believe he is not mature and maybe using the word "sneaky" to describe Danielle has more to do with his behavior than hers.

Another narrative that this couple needed to deconstruct was money and career. Danielle expressed to Dorian the changes she noticed in his behavior toward her when she got a pay increase and his angry response when family members suggested he needed to go back to school to be a therapist, as if his current employment was not sustaining their lifestyle. Dorian said he was insulted that she would think her money increase made him feel inferior because he supported her to get her MBA and knew it would help their family. Dorian explained that this assumption is another sting that seemed to suggest that he had a deflated ego as a Black man because of his wife's success. Dorian elaborated on Danielle's success as something he cherished and is proud of her accomplishment. Dorian expressed feelings of disdain and disappointment because he felt like his wife was seeing him like the white leaders at his job who refuse to give him the opportunity he feels he deserves. Dorian was able to connect that this makes him feel emasculated by her and less than.

Danielle shared that she is aware that Dorian is proud of her which is why she felt that if she discussed this issue with another Black man (Ray, her co-worker) that it would help her to not internalize the projections she had toward Dorian. Danielle felt that she would get objective feedback to help her to not see her husband in a disparaging way because she realized that feeling of emasculation may be what is driving Dorian to feel the need to get attention from other women. Danielle also referenced Dorian taking a cheap shot that continues to resonate with her in his statement about "Black women staying single" as if he were saying she could end up like her mother. That highlighted her fears of how that could eventually become a reality.

It is important to acknowledge the effects that Dorian's and Danielle's narratives were having on themselves and each other. Due to unpacking their previous narratives, an alternative story was created as Dorian began to realize that Danielle is trying to heal her injuries with her dad through Dorian, therefore, struggling to trust Dorian to do his own work. Although Danielle needs to heal from her attachment injuries with her dad, she also needs to trust her ability while in her vulnerability to be resilient when those injuries are bruised by Dorian. Danielle will need to set boundaries around her vulnerability while she learns whether Dorian is able to grow into a husband who can honor the trust, she yields to him. Dorian needs to learn to honor her trust by learning to trust himself to uphold his integrity and dignity to maintain the fidelity in his marital contract. Working through these challenges will help them determine the status of their commitment to each other.

Dorian's alternative story is that his flirtatious behavior is used to shield him (or cover him) from feeling less than. Getting attention from other women was being used to inform him of his self-worth and also served to prove to himself, his parents, his boss at his job, Danielle, and society as a whole, that he is more than what everyone believes him to be. Dorian believes he doesn't doubt his competence and worthiness, but everyone significant in his life does. He recognizes that it is his work to change that image and reveal the confidence he has in himself. He expressed his desire to align himself to operate authentically and not be fearful while tapping into his own vulnerability. Dorian also recognizes the negative stereotypical labels he internalizes and projects in being a Black man and acknowledges that he does not want to project these feelings on to his wife.

Danielle's alternative story was to do her own work and pay attention to how she assigns her feelings about her dad to Dorian. Although Danielle has a right to be concerned about Dorian's flirtatious behaviors, she will need to refocus her energy on setting boundaries by sharing what she needs rather than remaining verbally silent and passive aggressive in her anxiety. Danielle must be aware that Dorian cannot be responsible to make up for what she did not receive from her father and cannot rectify what she believes her mother should have received from her father as well. Danielle must recognize that her mother's story does not have to be her own; therefore, she needs to attend to her projections while learning and recognizing negative stereotypical assignments projected to Dorian. Dorian and Danielle must own and live in their own truth. They must reauthor the narrative they desire about who they are individually and as a couple while defining their commitment.

Dorian and Danielle were able to express an alternative truth about themselves that enabled them to see how their feelings invade and preoccupy their relationship. Both Danielle and Dorian continued to discuss how they participated in maintaining the problems in their narrative by constructing the stories around the feelings they externalized and personified to learn the power and their engagement to these truths. They also discussed how to put their feelings in context historically and reflect on the stories they internalized for themselves. Much of the dialogue continued in unpacking these stories, assessing, and acknowledging negative stereotypical labels, injuries, and projections, while making new meaning of their experiences.

13.5   Conclusion

In closing, Dorian and Danielle's narrative demonstrates many of the signs of covering that were previously defined in this chapter. Their narrative depicts the many struggles that Black men and women face in their committed relationships when working through historical traumas. The act of covering also enables people to avoid the emotional risk of being vulnerable and subsequently feeling the aches of betrayal and hurt within their committed relationships.

When treating Black love, it is important to acknowledge the ways in which slavery, internalized racial and gendered stereotypes, and oppression impact and show up in Black relationships. Historical oppression has led many Black people to develop feelings of powerlessness and has amplified avoidance as a survival mechanism in order to suppress their raw feelings of retribution, which sometimes show up in their intimate relationships. Covering one's authentic self, though viewed as detrimental to the psyche, acts as a subtle, yet powerful protective force that allows Black men and women to shield themselves from the cognitive and emotional injuries of oppression. Helping them externalize the problems, personify them to acquaint themselves with their etiology, and raise dilemmas about the meaning while constructing new meaning can enable a journey of discovering other parts of themselves that can lead them to internalizing their liberty (Chestnut, 2009).

Discussion Questions

1. How do stereotypes impact how Black men and women view themselves and one another in relationships?

2. How might the invisible baggage of transgenerational, historical, and relational trauma impact Black couple relationships?
3. Describe the connection between the sociological concept of covering and the traumatic experience of infidelity in Black relationships.
4. What is the benefit of a Narrative Therapy approach to work with Black couples experiencing infidelity?

REFERENCES

Banks, R. R. (2011). *Is marriage for white people? How the African American marriage decline affects everyone.* Dutton.

Beauboeuf-Lafontant, T. (2009). *Behind the mask of the strong black woman: Voice and the embodiment of a costly performance.* Temple University Press.

Bowleg, L., Lucas, K. J., & Tschann, J. M. (2004). "The ball was always in his court": An exploratory analysis of relationship scripts, sexual scripts, and condom use among African American women. *Psychology of Women Quarterly, 28,* 70–82.

Brooms, D. R., & Perry, A. R. (2016). "It's simply because we're Black men." *Journal of Men's Studies, 24*(2), 166–184. https://doi.org/10.1177/1060826516641105

Brown, B. (2013). *Daring greatly: How the courage to be vulnerable transforms the way we live, love, parent and lead.* Gotham Books.

Caucutt, E., Guner, N., & Rauh, C. (2019, April 6). *Incarceration, unemployment, and the black-white marriage gap in the U.S.* VoxEU. https://voxeu.org/article/incarceration-unemployment-and-black-white-marriage-gap-us

Chestnut, C. (2009). *The study of internalized stereotypes among African American couples* [Unpublished doctoral dissertation]. Drexel University.

Donovan, R. A., & West, L. M. (2014). Stress and mental health: Moderating role of the strong Black woman stereotype. *Journal of Black Psychology, 41*(4), 384–396. https://doi.org/10.1177/0095798414543014

Dickens, D. D. (2014). *Double consciousness: The negotiation of the intersectionality of identities among academically successful black women* (Order No. 3635597) [Doctoral dissertation, Colorado State University]. ProQuest Dissertations & Theses Global: The Humanities and Social Sciences Collection. https://www.proquest.com/docview/1615129358

Dupiton, L. M. (2019). *Wearing a mask to supervision: A phenomenological exploration of Black female therapists and covering in cross-racial supervision* (Order No. 13859390) [Doctoral dissertation, Eastern University]. ProQuest Dissertations & Theses Global. https://www.proquest.com/openview/2e767f253812d9373ddee62090b9c497/1?pq-origsite=gscholar&cbl=18750&diss=y

Eyre, S. L, Flythe, M., Hoffman, V., & Fraser, A. E. (2012). Concepts of infidelity among African American emerging adults: Implications for HIV/STI prevention. *Journal of Adolescent Research, 27*(2), 231–255. https://doi.org/10.1177/0743558411147865

Goffman, E. (1963). *Stigma: Notes on the management of spoiled identity*. Simon & Schuster.

Guise, R. W. (2018). *Study guide for the marriage & family therapy national licensing examination*. Family Solutions.

Hardy, K. (2013). Healing the hidden wounds of racial trauma. *Reclaiming Children and Youth, 22*(1), 25–28.

Hester, N., & Gray, K. (2018). For Black men, being tall increases threat stereotyping and police stops. *Proceedings of the National Academy of Sciences of the United States of America, 115*(11), 2711–2715.

Kelly, S., & Floyd, F. (2001). The effects of negative racial stereotypes and Afrocentricity on Black couple relationships. *Journal of Family Psychology, 15*(1), 110–123.

Kelly, J. F., & Green, B. (2010). Diversity within African American, female therapists: variability in clients' expectations and assumptions about the therapist. *Psychotherapy Theory, Research, Practice, Training, 47*(2), 186–197. https://doi.org/10.1037/a0019759

Liao, K. Y., Wei, M., & Yin, M. (2020). The misunderstood schema of the strong Black woman: Exploring its mental health consequences and coping responses among African American women. *Psychology of Women Quarterly, 44*(1), 84–104.

Macauda, M. M., Erickson, P. I., Singer, M. C., & Santelices, C. C. (2011). A cultural model of infidelity among African American and Puerto Rican young adults. *Anthropology & Medicine, 18*(3), 351–364. https://doi.org/10.1080/13648470.2011.615908

Nunnally, S. C. (2012). *Trust in Black America: Race, discrimination, and politics*. New York University Press.

Parker, M. L., & Campbell, K. (2017). Infidelity and attachment: The moderating role of race/ethnicity. *Contemporary Family Therapy, 39*, 172–183. https://doi.org/10.1007/s10591-017-9415-0

Penn, C. D., Hernandez, S. L., & Bermudez, M. (1997). Using a cross-cultural perspective to understand infidelity in couple's therapy. *American Journal of Family Therapy, 25*(2), 169–185. http://dx.doi.org/10.1080/01926189708251064

Raley, R. K., Sweeney, M. M, Wondra, D. (2015). The growing racial and ethnic divide in U.S marriage patterns. *Future Child, 25*(2), 89–109.

Richardson, B. L., & Wade, B. (1999). *What mama couldn't tell us about love: Healing the emotional legacy of racism by celebrating our light*. HarperCollins.

Slatton, B. C., & Spates, K. (Ed.). (2014). *Hyper sexual, hyper masculine?: Gender, race and sexuality in the identities of contemporary Black men*. Routledge

Sun, X., McHale, S. M., & Crouter, A. C. (2019). Perceived underemployment and couple relationships among African American parents: A dyadic approach. *Cultural Diversity and Ethnic Minority Psychology, 26*(1), 82–91. https://doi.org/10.1037/cdp0000285

Utley, E. (2011). When better becomes worse: Black wives describe their experiences with infidelity. *Black Women, Gender Families, 5*(1), 66–89.

Watson, N. N., & Hunter, C. D. (2015). Anxiety and depression among African American women: The costs of strength and negative attitudes toward psychological help-seeking. *Cultural Diversity & Ethnic Minority Psychology*, *21*(4), 604–612. https://doi.org/10.1037/cdp0000015

(2016). I had to be strong: Tensions in the strong black woman schema. *Journal of Black Psychology*, *42*(5), 424–452. https://doi.org/10.1177/0095798415597093

Weaver, V. J. (2015, May 16). *Uncovering your authentic self.* Diversity & Inclusion Television. https://ditv-media.com/uncovering-your-authentic-self/

Williams, J. (2019, June 12). Why is "black men don't cheat" trending on Twitter? Lil Duval and Charlamagne tha God spark new trend. *Newsweek.* https://www.newsweek.com/black-men-dont-cheat-day-charlamagne-tha-god-1443628

Wischkaemper, K. C., Fleming, C. J. E., Lenger, K. A., Roberson, P. N. E., Gray, T. D., Cordova, J. V., & Gordon, K. C. (2020). Attitudes toward relationship treatment among underserved couples. *Couple and Family Psychology: Research and Practice*, *9*(3), 156–166. https://doi.org/10.1037/cfp0000142

Yoshino, K., & Smith, C. (2013). *Uncovering talent: A new model of inclusion.* Deloitte. https://www2.deloitte.com/content/dam/Deloitte/us/Documents/about-deloitte/us-about-deloitte-uncovering-talent-a-new-model-of-inclusion.pdf

PART V

Special Topics

CHAPTER 14

Weathering the Storm: Fertility and the Black Lesbian Experience

Tenika L. Jackson

> Their children are not their children. They are the sons and daugh-
> ters of life's longing for itself. They come through them but not from
> them, and though they are with them, yet they belong not to them.
> Khalil Gibran (2019, p. 19)

Sadly, not every woman who longs to be a parent receives the gift of motherhood. To those women, Khalil Gibran's words are not poetic or powerful: They evoke pain and sorrow. Experiencing infertility can cause psychological, emotional, and physical distress. Feelings such as being defective, unworthy and/or of being punished are not uncommon and may lead to diagnosable disorders such as depression and anxiety (Yager et al., 2010). Additional feeling of guilt and shame may arise causing the woman to suffer in silence, even if partnered. Although infertility can impact any woman, disproportionality does exist.

Infertility impacts about 12 percent of women, up to age forty-four, but that number is twice as high for Black women. Black women are more likely to have tubal disease, fibroids, and preexisting medical challenges like obesity, heart disease, or hypertension, which can increase challenges with conception and impact fertility (Lister et al., 2019). Additionally, Black women are less likely to seek assistance from fertility specialists for various reasons such as socioeconomic status, fear of medical professionals, and stigma. For Black women, the fertility journey is further compounded by staggering rates of infant mortality and higher rates of death after childbirth. Nationally, the Black infant mortality rate is twice as high as white or Asian infants (MacDorman et al., 2013). Additionally, Black women are four times more likely to die after childbirth than their white or Asian counterparts (Lister et al., 2019).

Black women who identify as lesbian face even greater challenges. Although a lesbian woman could be fully capable of conceiving and carrying a child to term, her egg has to be fertilized by sperm in order to produce an embryo that grows into a baby (Johnson, 2017). Hence, regardless of her health status, she is labeled as infertile and must undergo medical procedures to become a parent. Although this is true for any lesbian woman, Black lesbian women face all of the aforementioned barriers during the process. For these women, the fertility process is often simultaneously challenging, scary, painful, and rewarding. For her dream of motherhood to be realized, she must attempt to weather the storm and cling to hope.

14.1   Case Study: The Impact of Gender Expression

Andrea and Erica are an African American lesbian couple entering therapy to discuss their challenges during the "fertility process." Andrea discusses the heaviness of the term "infertility." She stated that their file at the obstetrics and gynecology office was stamped with that label before any tests were conducted and it made her feel "less of a woman." She stated that she began to feel as if something was wrong with her or that she would not be able to fulfill her dream of having children. Erica was able to remind her that the doctor needed to examine her first and that they should not jump to conclusions.

Andrea and Erica explained that they had to make some decisions about who would actually carry their child and move past the labels associated with that decision. Erica is a feminine identified lesbian woman. Physically, her appearance checks the typical boxes of femininity in American society. She is quite curvy, wears her hair long, wears traditionally feminine clothing and makeup. She often carries a purse and accessorizes. When looking at her, most people would label her as a woman and even assume that she is heterosexual. She chooses to express her gender identity in this way. Andrea tends to be closer to the other end of the spectrum. She has broad shoulders and lacks a curvaceous body. She wears her hair short and typically feels most comfortable in a suit purchased from the male section of the department store. It is rare for the world to see her in makeup and when she does wear it, it is because her wife has asked her to do so for red carpet appearances. She generally carries a wallet or a "man bag," not a purse. From behind many people have mistakenly called her a man. As such, she does not neatly fit into the box of "woman" or "Mama" according to Western standards (Moore, 2006). Andrea has consciously chosen her outward presentation. She considers herself a gender nonconforming lesbian woman.

Discussion Questions

1. How might gender expression impact Black lesbian women who seek to conceive children?
2. What are some important clinical and cultural considerations when working with this couple therapeutically?
3. What transference/countertransference issues would you encounter?

14.2   Conception in a Black Lesbian Relationship

There are multiple medical procedures to assist a couple in conception. Each procedure varies in level of preparation, invasiveness, and cost. Although this chapter is not intended to be a medical guide, the author feels that it is important to review common medical procedures often endured by lesbian couples as they attempt to conceive. Knowledge of these procedures can assist the clinician in understanding the psychological, emotional, physical, and financial stressors that the couple might experience during this journey to pregnancy and ultimately motherhood.

To begin, in order to conceive a child within the context of a Black lesbian relationship or any lesbian relationship, the couple must go through the process of artificial insemination or invitro fertilization. Artificial insemination or intrauterine insemination (IUI) is a process where the doctor uses a syringe to insert sperm into a woman's uterus to facilitate fertilization (Johnson, 2017). The goal is to increase the number of sperm that reach the egg and subsequently increase the likelihood of fertilization. Although the procedure gives the sperm a head start, the sperm must travel to and penetrate the egg on its own. It simulates what would happen if a woman and a man engaged in sexual intercourse. The major difference is that the doctor prepares the woman's body to receive the sperm before inserting it, which would typically not happen if impregnation occurred as a result of intercourse with a man. Before undergoing the IUI procedure, several medical tests must be conducted including blood tests, vaginal ultrasounds, and a hysterosalpingogram (HSG) test. The tests are designed to ensure that her eggs are viable, she does not have any cysts or fibroids, and her fallopian tubes are open to allow for the releasing of an egg. The process is completed on a specific timetable to optimize the likelihood of pregnancy. If her ovarian reserves are low as determined by the blood test, it might be difficult to conceive. If she has cysts or fibroids as determined by the vaginal ultrasound, that could impact

3

the embryos ability to implant into her uterus. In some cases, women have had to have surgery to remove the cysts or fibroids first. If she has the HSG test and her fallopian tubes are blocked, the entire process of IUI is no longer possible. Blocked fallopian tubes inhibit the sperm from reaching the egg needed for fertilization. If she does not have any blockages, the doctor will provide instructions on how to give herself a series of injections designed to prepare her eggs for fertilization. She must take the right dosage for her body type because if she becomes overstimulated, she has to stop the cycle and start all over. That could be costly and time consuming.

If she is not able to conceive a child using IUI, one of the next options would be in vitro fertilization (IVF). The process of IVF involves another series of blood tests and vaginal ultrasounds. Again, they are testing for ovarian reserve levels and the presence of cysts and/or fibroids. After the tests, she is then instructed to take a series of shots over a carefully planned time period. The purpose of these injections is to enlarge her eggs and prepare them to be surgically removed from her body. Once her eggs are ready, she must go into the hospital or clinic and while she is under general anesthesia the doctor performs an egg retrieval. After the retrieval, the eggs are evaluated and fertilized with the sperm she provides. Some women choose to freeze their eggs at that point to stop their biological clock because they have not identified a donor. Other women do not begin the IVF process until they are ready to conceive. Once the doctor fertilizes her eggs, they allow them to grow to a certain stage. The eggs are graded and labeled. They even give her a picture showing their level of growth. She then has the option to do a live transfer or a frozen transfer. With a live transfer, the doctor calls her back into the clinic to have the embryos transferred into the uterus soon after the egg retrieval. At that point, the hope is that an embryo implants into her uterus and grows into a healthy baby. In numerous cases, the embryo does not implant or stops growing for a variety of reasons resulting in the lack of a viable pregnancy. Another option, which also has financial implications, is to freeze the embryos for implanting at a later date. Once she is ready, the embryos are thawed, and the procedure moves forward in the same manner as the live transfer (Futeral et al., 2014).

The woman can experience many challenges at various points along the way. For example, a woman could have an egg retrieval and not get any viable eggs. She could get a few eggs but have them reject the sperm she provides, and they do not fertilize. In some cases, the eggs do fertilize, and she chooses a frozen cycle and the eggs dissipate once they are thawed. Finally, she could go through the entire process and not get pregnant. The cost is the same regardless of the outcome. Some women have taken out loans and others have had to stop the process because they did not have any more money to continue. The process is an emotionally, financially, and physically taxing ordeal. It often places a strain on the couple, causing increased conflict and couple discord.

The third option available is adoption. Adoption is not a new concept. Families have served as foster parents and adopted children for many years. Adoption is the action or fact of legally taking another person's child and raising her/him as your own (Roszia & Maxon, 2019). There are several steps in the process. The couple must prepare themselves mentally, emotionally, and financially. They must decide the age, gender, and ethnicity of the child they want to adopt. They then must choose an agency. There are private and public agencies available. Some women chose to serve as a foster parent first through the department of children and family services. They can then adopt the child they have been fostering for a period of time, if the parental rights have been severed by the court. That process tends to be less expensive than private adoption. The next step in public adoption is a home study where a licensed professional, usually a social worker, evaluates the home and their fitness to adopt. Once they are deemed eligible, they wait until a birth mother is found, gives birth and signs her rights over to them. They then get to take the child home. That process is typical for most women. The challenge in the Black lesbian community is the presence of discrimination. On June 26, 2017, the Supreme Court reversed an Arkansas Supreme Court ruling and ordered all fifty states to treat same-sex couples equal to opposite-sex couples in the issuance of birth certificates. Those same court rulings have made adoption by same-sex couples legal in all fifty states. (Roszia & Maxon, 2019). That was only a little over five years ago. Prior to those rulings, adoption laws varied by state. Some states banned same-sex adoption and only allowed the partner in a same-sex relationship to adopt the biological child of the other partner. There are also numerous stories of how applications were initially accepted based on what was written on paper but then rejected after the home study even though there was nothing wrong with the home. The social workers allowed their bias against Black lesbian couples to deem their homes inappropriate for children (Devault & Miller, 2019).

Discussion Questions

1. How might the label of infertility impact Black lesbian couples?
2. What are some challenges Black lesbian couples face in conceiving children? Adopting?

3. How can clinicians assist Black lesbian couples as they attempt to maneuver through this emotionally difficult and financially taxing process?

14.3   Medical Professionals' Insensitivity to the Needs of Black Lesbian Woman

> We now know, where we could only surmise before, that we have contributed to their ailments and shortened their lives.
>
> Oliver Clarence Wenger, MD, U.S. Public Health Service, 1950
> (Washington, 2006)

There is a long history of medical inefficiency and insensitivity toward Black women in Western society. By the mid-nineteenth century, Black people had already correlated Western medicine with punishment and brutal violence by physicians who refused to acknowledge their pain (Washington, 2006). Whether women are attempting to relay their level of pain, describe a symptom, or survive childbirth, the needs of women in the Black community have been overlooked, misunderstood, and flat out ignored in some cases. The tennis star Serena Williams endured biased treatment with the birth of her daughter in 2018. She has a history of blood clots and was experiencing similar symptoms. She told the doctors and nurses what she was experiencing, but they did not believe her and chose to run tests on other parts of her body. After finally giving her the CT scan that she repeatedly requested, it was determined that she did have a series of blood clots in her lungs. She was experiencing a pulmonary embolism, which is a sudden blockage of an artery in the lung by a blood clot (Salam, 2018). According to the Centers for Disease Control and Prevention (CDC), about 700 women die each year in the United States as a result of pregnancy or delivery complications. Complications impact more than 50,000 women annually. For African American women, the rate is three to four times higher than that for white women (Salam, 2018). There were 17.8 deaths per 100,000 live births in African American communities in 2009 and 2011, according to the CDC; add the additional aspect of sexual orientation to the long history of challenges in receiving good-quality medical care and they have quite the conundrum (Romanelli & Hudson, 2017).

14.4   Case Study: Insensitive Medical Professionals

Jessica and her wife Rhonda were having challenges with the fertility process. The couple reported that they had doctors and nurses ask about their husbands or wanted to know which name they wanted on their paperwork. Jessica reported frustration because she had to explain that they are a married lesbian couple and that they do not have a husband. Both of their names should be listed on the documents because they would both be the parents of the child(ren). This explanation came after the couple had given their entire medical history to the doctor. It was as if the medical professionals had not listened to anything that they had stated previously. Rhonda reported that after one of Jessica's IUI procedures, she had a nurse to tell her to go home and have sexual intercourse with her husband to increase the chances of Jessica getting pregnant. The couple reported feeling unseen and vulnerable.

Discussion Questions

1. What challenges did the clients face in the vignette?
2. What cultural components were present?
3. How would you work with the clients in the therapy room? What issues would you address first?

14.5 Case Study: Imbalance in the Lesbian Couple Relationship

Mary is a forty-two-year-old cisgender, African American, queer, lesbian woman. She has been married to her wife Krystal for 12 years. Mary and Krystal have been attempting to manage their fertility journey for eight years by the time they walk into your office. This is their first time in therapy. They currently have two children conceived through IVF using donor sperm. The process to conceive their first child took five years. Krystal began the journey of getting pregnant but after three years of trying, she was not successful. It was discovered that her fallopian tubes were blocked and her ovarian reserve was low. The couple decided to have Mary attempt to carry their children. After two years of trying and two miscarriages, Mary gave birth to their first child. The couple was extremely happy. The baby was healthy and happy. Mary gave birth to their second child almost two years later without incident. Again, the birth was joyful and free of any health challenges.

The couple presents with marital issues. They are fighting over money, parenting styles, and issues of intimacy. Mary believes that the children are a blessing and that the relationship must change to focus on their needs. Krystal believes that Mary does not have enough time for her anymore. She also feels left out because she did not conceive the children. She watches Mary breastfeed and feels detached. She reports that the children seem to be more connected to Mary. She wants to be supportive and an active parent but she finds herself pulling away. Mary does the majority of the parenting while Krystal appears to be a passive observer. Mary recognizes Krystal's sadness but feels powerless to assist. She also becomes frustrated with Krystal because of her lack of involvement. She states repeatedly that she did not think she was going to be a single mom while in a relationship. In the meantime, she throws herself into her new role of "Mama." She even asks Krystal if she could have one more child. Krystal responds by saying "no" which Mary interprets as "not right now."

Discussion Questions

1. What challenges do the clients face in the vignette?
2. What cultural components were present?
3. How would you work with the clients in the therapy room? What issues would you address first?
4. Would you offer any referrals to the clients?
5. What transference/countertransference issues might be present?

14.6   Summary

In working with Black lesbian women who are going through the fertility process, clinicians must be aware of the biological, psychological, social, and emotional factors impacting the couple. They must address the stress that the couple may be experiencing and effectively work with the couple to sustain the relationship despite the challenges. It is extremely important that the clinician understand the basics of the fertility process and what procedures the couple may discuss in the therapy room. It is critical that the clinician understand the nuisances of how the process impacts Black lesbian women differently than their white or Asian counterparts. They must keep in mind that there may be a heightened level of anxiety or discomfort in Black woman in reference to this process due to the higher rates of Black infant mortality and increased rates of deaths of Black women after childbirth.

Despite the numerous challenges, there are many women who are able to conceive children or adopt in the Black lesbian community. However, in addition to seeking clinical treatment, it is extremely important that both individuals in the relationship have a strong support system. Clinicians may refer them to support groups in their communities. They may recommend that they read certain literature to gain more insight into the process. They may also recommend various self-care regimens to reduce stress. It can also be helpful to have lesbian friends who are raising children to be a part of their support system. It shows them that they are not alone and that there is a light at the end of the tunnel. It is helpful to have healthy outlets such as exercise, reading, listening to music, journaling, artwork, etc. Clinicians can assist their clients in utilizing the coping skills that work best for them. On the other hand, therapists must be ready to work with clients who go through the fertility process and are not able to conceive. That also can have a negative impact on the Black lesbian relationship and can lead to possible breakups. Being an informed, nonjudgmental clinician while working with Black lesbian clients maneuvering the fertility process can help them weather the storm.

14.7 Implications for Clinical Practice

1. Recognize that every lesbian couple will have a different fertility journey that is unique to them. A counselor or therapist who is able to listen with a nonjudgmental ear and engage in a variety of therapeutic styles would be able to assist diverse populations.
2. Become knowledgeable about various fertility options and their potential impact on their clients.
3. Become aware of your own bias and beliefs about fertility.
4. Recognize the toll the fertility journey can have on Black lesbian relationships and potential therapeutic techniques that can assist the couple in working through those challenges together.

REFERENCES

DeVault, A., & Miller, M. K. (2019). Justification-suppression and normative window of prejudice as determinants of bias toward lesbians, gays, and bisexual adoption applicants. *Journal of Homosexuality*, *66*(4), 465–486. https://doi.org/10.1080/00918369.2017.1414497
Futeral, A., Dugay, L., Stafford Bell, M., Greindl, J., Kadoch, I.-J., Ajayi, A., Patel, S., Baccino, G., Nunez, R., & Tan, S. L. (2014). In vitro fertilization (IVF) patients' online behaviors: how do they browse the web about infertility issues and what are they looking for online? *Fertility & Sterility*, *102*(3, Suppl.), e57. https://doi.org/10.1016/j.fertnstert.2014.07.196
Gibran, K. (2019). *The prophet*. Penguin Books.
Johnson, M. (2017). *Human biology: Concepts and current issues* (8th ed.) Pearson Education Limited.

Lister, R. L., Drake, W., Scoot, B. H., & Graves, C. (2019). Black maternal mortality – The elephant in the room. *World Journal of Gynecology & Women's Health*, 3(1). https://doi.org/10.33552/wjgwh.2019.03.000555

MacDorman, M. F., Hoyert, D. L., & Mathews, T. J. (2013). *Recent declines in infant mortality in the Unites States, 2005–2011* (NCHS data brief, no 120). National Center for Health Statistics.

Moore, M. R. (2006). Lipstick or timberlands? Meanings of gender presentation in Black lesbian communities. *Signs: Journal of Women in Culture & Society*, 32(1), 113–139. https://doi-org.proxy1.ncu.edu/10.1086/505269

Romanelli, M., & Hudson, K. D. (2017). Individual and systemic barriers to health care: Perspectives of lesbian, gay, bisexual, and transgender adults. *American Journal of Orthopsychiatry*, 87(6), 714–728. https://doi.org/10.1037/ort0000306

Roszia, S., & Maxon, A. (2019). *Seven core issues in adoption and permanency: A comprehensive guide to promoting understanding and healing in adoption, foster care, kinship families and third-party reproduction*. Jessica Kingsley Publishers.

Salam, M. (2018, January 11). For Serena Williams, childbirth was a harrowing ordeal. She's not alone. *The New York Times*. https://www.nytimes.com/2018/01/11/sports/tennis/serena-williams-baby-vogue.html

Washington, H. A. (2006). *Medical apartheid: A dark history of medical experimentation on Black Americans from colonial times to the present*. Anchor Books.

Yager, C., Brennan, D., Steele, L., Epstein, R., Ross, L. R., (2010). Challenges and mental health experiences of lesbian and bisexual women who are trying to conceive. *Health & Social Work*, 35(3), 191–200. https://doi.org/10.1093/hsw/35.3.191

CHAPTER 15

African American Men and Infertility: Biopsychosocial Considerations

Brian R. Humphrey

15.1 Operational Definitions for Discussing Male Factor Infertility

The biopsychosocial model is a paradigm for conceptualizing how illness is impacted by a myriad of factors ranging from societal to molecular (Borrell-Carrió et al., 2004). The model also purports that the subjective experience of the individual is a salient component of health outcomes (Borrell-Carrió et al., 2004). It is from this framework that this chapter explores dimensions of male factor infertility as experienced by African American men. It is also of this framework that terms such as "male," "men," and "African American" are used to operationalize discussion of topics presented in this chapter. These terms are not exhaustive as there are certainly alternatives that may be more optimal. For the purposes of discussion, the term "male" or "man" is used to describe cisgendered men (independent of sexual orientation or preferences) and the term "African American" refers to persons of color in the United States who are a part of the African Diaspora.

Infertility is defined as failure to conceive after at least six to twelve months of unprotected sexual intercourse (Barratt et al., 2017; Kumar & Singh, 2015). Male infertility and male factor infertility are often used interchangeably and is defined as the inability for a male to produce pregnancy in a fertile female. Research shows that infertility may affect approximately 15 percent of couples of which nearly 50 percent of these cases are due to male infertility (Agarwal et al., 2015; Naz & Kamal, 2017). Male factor infertility may have either known or unknown causes.

Fertility with an unknown cause and otherwise unremarkable health history is called idiopathic infertility. Idiopathic infertility accounts for approximately 30 to 40 percent of cases of male factor infertility (Friedman & Dull, 2012). In many cases of idiopathic infertility, a completed semen analysis reveals the presence of spermatozoa (sperm) albeit with issues such as abnormal forms of sperm, decreased number of available sperm, and reduction in the motility of sperm (Friedman & Dull, 2012). Potential causes of idiopathic infertility may include environmental factors (i.e., pollution), genetic abnormalities, and reactive oxygen species (an unstable molecule containing oxygen which reacts with ease to other cellular molecules; Friedman & Dull, 2012). There is a lack of consensus on efficacious treatment of cases of idiopathic infertility, but proposed options include pharmacological treatments such as clomiphene citrate, anastrozole, and human chorionic gonadotropin (Friedman & Dull, 2012).

Assistive reproductive technology (ART) is a fertility treatment where eggs and embryos are managed in a laboratory with the purposes of achieving pregnancy (Kissin et al., 2016). ART treatments may include intrauterine insemination, in vitro fertilization (IVF), and intracytoplasmic sperm injection (ICSI; Kissin et al., 2016). Surgical ART treatment for men include percutaneous epididymal sperm aspiration), microsurgical epididymal sperm aspiration, testicular sperm aspiration, testicular sperm extraction (TESE), and microsurgical-testicular sperm extraction (micro-TESE; Esteves et al., 2011). The aim of these procedures is to retrieve an adequate number of sperm for cryopreservation and immediate use, acquire the best sperm available, and minimize injury to the reproductive system to prevent jeopardizing future testicular function or sperm retrieval attempts (Esteves et al., 2011).

15.2 Medical Variables of Male Factor Infertility

Male factor infertility may be diagnosed using methodologies such as hormone tests, physical examinations, testicular biopsies, and semen analyses (Naz & Kamal, 2017). In cases of sterility, reversing infertility may not always be feasible. There are however instances where infertility may be reversed and restored through pharmacological interventions, assistive reproductive technologies, and surgical procedures (Barak & Baker, 2016; Naz & Kamal, 2017).

Male infertility that is caused by an absence of sperm within seminal fluid is defined as azoospermia. Categories of azoospermia include pretesticular, testicular, and posttesticular. Pretesticular deficiency, also referred to as hypogonadotropic hypogonadism (HH), results when there are insufficient amounts of gonadotrophin-releasing hormone (GnRH) and/or follicle-stimulating hormone (FSH) as well as luteinizing hormone resulting in deficient spermatogenesis and androgen secretion (Friedman & Dull, 2012). Causes of HH include systemic disorders (chronic illnesses), congenital GnRH deficiency, genetic disorders (i.e., Klinefelter's syndrome, XX and XYY male karyotypes), hemochromatosis (iron overload from food digested), tumors of the hypothalamus and pituitary (two areas of the brain responsible for coordinating the endocrine system), hormonal abnormalities, and select medications (to be discussed later) (Friedman & Dull, 2012).

As Friedman and Dull (2012) discuss, there are several treatment options for pretesticular deficiency. Given that the endocrine disorder hyperprolactinemia is a known cause of HH, treatment often focuses on normalizing concentrations of prolactin with the use of dopamine agonists (i.e., bromocriptine or cabergoline). For cases of HH not caused by hyperprolactinemia but that are the result of hypothalamic or pituitary factors, gonadotropins may be a treatment option. For treatment of HH caused by hypothalamic disease, Pulsatile GnRH therapy may be used as an off-label hormonal treatment. Additional treatment choices for pretesticular deficiency include human menopausal gonadotropin and recombinant human FSH (r-hFSH).

Another category of azoospermia is testicular deficiency also known as nonobstructive azoospermia. Nonobstructive azoospermia is defined as failure of spermatogenesis resulting from a cause other than hypothalamic–pituitary–gonadal (HPG) axis dysfunction and/or obstruction. There are three types of nonobstructive azoospermia. The first is congenital failure, which results from testicular dysgenesis (a congenital derangement of the functioning and structure of seminiferous tubules), genetic abnormalities, cryptorchid, and anorchia (disorder where the male is born without testes; Friedman & Dull, 2012).

The second type of nonobstructive azoospermia is acquired testicular failure, which is caused by exogenous factors (i.e., enlarged veins inside of the scrotum called varicocele), trauma, surgeries, orchitis (inflammation of the testicles), and testicular torsion (Friedman & Dull, 2012). Of note, approximately 40 percent of men with male factor infertility and nearly 15 percent of men in the general population have varicoceles (Friedman & Dull, 2012). One treatment possibility is a varicocelectomy if there are palpability of the varicocele, presence of one to several sperm or semen parameters, female fertility, and a clinical diagnosis of infertility. The third type of nonobstructive azoospermia entails idiopathic variables (akin to the aforementioned discussion on idiopathic infertility) (Friedman & Dull, 2012). Current research indicates that for many instances of testicular deficiency, IVF-ICSI may be essential to achieve successful fertilization.

The third category of azoospermia is called obstructive azoospermia. Obstructive azoospermia is caused by an obstruction of sperm delivery and ejaculatory dysfunction. Approximately 40 percent of men with azoospermia have obstructive type. Obstructions may be present in the vas deferens, epididymis, and ejaculatory duct (Friedman & Dull, 2012). The obstruction may also be either congenital or acquired.

Treatment options for obstructive azoospermia are limited to surgical procedures and medication. Surgical procedures include microsurgical procedures (i.e., vasectomy reversal) or IVF-ICSI (Friedman & Dull, 2012). For cases of emission failure associated with ejaculatory dysfunction, an alpha-adrenergic agonist may be utilized by converting emission failure to a scenario of retrograde ejaculation for sperm retrieval to be used with insemination (Friedman & Dull, 2012).

15.3   The Impact of Substance Use on Fertility

Substance use is defined as the consumption of any substance that alters ones physiological and/ or psychological functioning. Ordinarily, the substance is used in moderation and is less likely to result in significant deleterious life impairments. Examples include appropriate use of medication prescribed by providers and caffeine contained in soda products. In contrast, substance abuse is an excessive use of a prescribed or illicit substances that results in negative effects such as physical and/or psychological dependence, legal issues, relational challenges, and negative health consequences (Alozai & Sharma, 2020; Griffin, 1990). Recreational substances that are commonly abused include narcotics, cocaine, methamphetamines, cannabis, and anabolic androgenic steroids.

Recreational substance abuse has been found to adversely impact male fertility. These substances are risk factors that may affect sperm functioning, HPG axis, and the testicular architecture of men (Durairajanayagam, 2018; Sansone et al., 2018). Current research appears to disagree on the impact that the aforementioned substances may have with casual/nonabusive use (Durairajanayagam, 2018; Sansone et al., 2018).

Although available research directly correlating tobacco and alcohol use to infertility is conflicting, most agree that both are certainly risk factors to consider. For example, tobacco use has been shown to affect spermatogenesis, sperm maturation, and subsequent sperm functionality due to variables such as DNA damage, sperm mutations, and aneuploidies (Durairajanayagam, 2018). Alcohol has been shown to have determinantal effects on sperm morphology and semen volume (Durairajanayagam,

2018). Most research suggests that increased use of alcohol and tobacco individually or in tandem increases the risk factor of infertility in men.

15.4 Additional Risk Factors

Another risk factor of male factor infertility is psychological stress. Because the stress response system involves the hypothalamus-pituitary-adrenal (HPA) axis, Durairajanayagam (2018) indicates that both the HPA axis and gonadotropin inhibitory hormone inhibits HPG and testicular Leydig cells. This results in lowered testosterone levels and subsequent suppression of spermatogenesis resulting from alterations in Sertoli cells and the blood–testis barrier (Durairajanayagam, 2018). Research also reveals that psychological stress may be associated with abnormal sperm morphology, decreased progressive sperm motility, and lower sperm concentration (Durairajanayagam, 2018).

Lifestyle risk factors such as obesity, diet, and nutritional factors may also affect male factor infertility. Fainberg and Kashanian (2019) demonstrated that obesity causes hormonal changes that are secondary to excess amounts of adipose tissue. Durairajanayagam (2018) observed that certain diets may negatively or positively correlate with sperm quality. For example, diets consisting of coffee, beverages with high sugar content, full fat dairy products, and processed meats are associated with low fecundity rates and poor semen quality. In contrast, diets that include vegetables and fruits, both fish and poultry, and low-fat dairy products are positively correlated with sperm quality (Durairajanayagam, 2018).

Research also shows that another risk factor is advanced paternal age. As men age, the testes experience age-related morphological changes (i.e., decreased germ, Leydig, and Sertoli cells) and structural changes (i.e., narrowing of seminiferous tubules). There is also a decrease in both free and total testosterone levels. Lowered testosterone levels are greatly involved in primary hypogonadism which also impacts male fertility. Alterations of the HPG axis, accumulation of reactive oxygen species, and apoptosis are all impacted by age and contribute to the deterioration of sperm quantity and quality. There are a number of additional lifestyle variables that contribute to male factor infertility such as genital heat stress, sleep issues, and the use electronic devices such as cell phones.

Genital heat stress is caused by excessive sitting, exposure to radiant heat, cryptorchidism, and varicocele (Durairajanayagam, 2018). Elevated scrotal temperature associated with genital heat stress may result in a number of negative fertility outcomes including germ cell apoptosis, sperm DNA damage, oxidative stress, and spermatogenic arrest (Durairajanayagam, 2018). Sleep may play a role in male factor infertility. In one study, semen volume was discovered to be lower in participants who experienced challenges initiating sleep (Durairajanayagam, 2018). Electronic devices have been found to adversely contribute to male infertility. In one study, cell phones were found to emit radiofrequency electromagnetic wave radiation resulting in reduced sperm viability and motility (Durairajanayagam, 2018).

15.5 Men and Health

Men's health is an ongoing public health concern. Research indicates that in the United States, men have a higher death rate than women in fourteen of the fifteen leading causes of death (Ornelas et al., 2009). African American men have even greater health disparities; the average lifespan of an African American man is seven years less than that of a white male (Ornelas et al., 2009). African American men are less likely than other ethnicities to receive preventative care, seek medical care only when ill and/or in poor health, and are more likely to delay medical attention (Ornelas et al., 2009). Many of these statistics are caused by a number of social determinants.

Social determinants are defined as risk factors at community and societal levels that impact and influence health variables through proximal determinants such as socioeconomic status (SES), gender, racism and discrimination, environment, and geography (Ornelas et al., 2009). For example, societal inequalities create an imbalance of opportunities and resources in the physical, social, and economic environments of the African American community (Ornelas et al., 2009). Studies reveal that African American men's attitudes about social determinants of health, specifically, dynamics of socioeconomic status, racism, and male gender socialization, adversely impact their health behaviors (Ornelas et al., 2009).

Ornelas et al. (2009) performed an analysis of race and racism. Findings from this study exposed the adverse impacts of race and racism on health behaviors including the stark reality that the social and physical environments in which African American men reside often lack the resources and conditions for optimal health; the daily stressor of interpersonal racism and its impact on health; the marketing of unhealthy foods and substance use marketed to African American men by commercial industries; and the physical environment's constant reminder of institutional racism due to mainstream society's abandonment and neglect of community institutions that serve African Americans (Ornelas et al., 2009). Ornelas et al. (2009) also showed that aspects of male gender identity impacted health behaviors. For example, African American men had a tendency to deprioritize health due to expectations that they are healthy and strong. They also contend with the demands of life, which may create challenges with healthy eating, exercise, and routine health care.

Research shows that males across most demographic groups possess limited knowledge about factors contributing to male infertility (Daumler et al., 2016). In a study by Daumler et al. (2016), men could identify roughly only 51 percent of risk factors for male infertility and 45 percent of the 51 percent were able to identify health issues linked to male factor infertility. A lack of knowledge about factors of infertility is problematic because males may miss opportunities to engage in preventive and interventive strategies that may alter the trajectory of infertility. Coupling the health and racial disparities that African American men experience with the general lack of knowledge, one could argue that African American men are more at risk to go without medical or psychological treatment in the presence of an infertility diagnosis.

15.6 Constructs of Masculinity

There exist cultural, biological, anthropological, and societal norms that collectively impact how men view themselves with respect to both concepts of masculinity and infertility. Courtenay (2011) purports that men actively reject ideals and perceptions of femininity in lieu of cultural and societal ideals of masculinity. As Griffith et al. (2015) state, "Hegemonic masculinity is the idealized cultural standard of masculinity that exists in a specific time, place and culture; it sets the ideal of how to be a man and sets the standard by which all men are judged" (p. 2).

Many men create ideological beliefs of gender and masculinity based on Western constructs that create, shape, and perpetuate said beliefs. These ideals are the product of both intrapersonal and interpersonal variables. Specific examples of westernized stereotypes of masculinity include emotional control, stoicism, tough exterior, preoccupation with sex, and minimization of the need to request assistance from others (Courtenay, 2011; Fisher & Hammarberg, 2012). As a result, a dissonance between male factor infertility and stereotypical Western perceptions of masculinity develops. This dissonance may make it difficult for men to be vulnerable and experience vulnerable emotions thus resulting in deleterious consequences that adversely affect men's health.

Masculine norms are class and racially bound and include values such as economic success, acquisition and utility of consumer products, and both physical and sexual virility (Griffith et al., 2015). As a result, African American men are not always able to subscribe to hegemonic masculine norms. African American men experience marginalization, racism, segregation, class differentials, and discrimination that prevent them from the social, economic, and political benefits ordinarily awarded to being male (Griffith et al., 2015). Similar to the previously discussed social determinants of health, there also appear to be social determinants of masculinity and manhood (Griffith et al., 2015). Additionally, there are many barriers to African American men receiving health care and their health-seeking behaviors such as SES, racism, societally defined masculine norms, peer influences, and environmental variables. All these factors must be considered when exploring dimensions of infertility and African American men.

15.7   Infertility and African American Men

Compared to women, available literature is scarce regarding the subjective and objective realities and experiences of men dealing with infertility (Barratt et al., 2017). Further, there is a disproportionate degree of available data pertaining to African American men and infertility. Known risk factors for issues of infertility with African American men include the aforementioned lifestyle variables, dynamics of social determents of health (i.e., availability and access to reproductive technologies and resources), and disproportionate health disparities between African American men and other ethnicities (Bruce et al., 2015; Dieke et al., 2017; Gilbert et al., 2016).

African American men may be at greater risk for developing male factor infertility than other ethnicities based on incidences of previously discussed risk-factors. With regard to health issues, one study demonstrated that up to 40 percent of African American men aged forty and older are considered obese, a known risk-factor for male infertility (Griffith et al., 2011). Considering substance abuse as a risk-factor for infertility, Pacek et al. (2012) found that marijuana use alone and comorbid marijuana and alcohol abuse occurred at a higher rate with African Americans than whites and Latinx. As already discussed, issues of discrimination and racism significantly impact stress levels of African American men. This stress adversely affects the stress response system and associated HPA axis thus contributing to infertility. African American men are also more likely to receive poor sex education, less preventative care, and less protection against the transmission of sexually transmitted disease, which adversely impact the reproductive health of men.

15.8 Coping with Male Factor Infertility

Independent of gender, the psychological response to infertility may include experiences of distress, anxiety, depression, and grief for both males and females. Research does, however, indicate that males may react differently than females in response to being infertile (Patel, Sharma, & Kumar, 2018). Psychological variables impacting a male's response to infertility include personality factors, social support (actual or perceived), cognitive appraisals of the circumstances, and health perceptions (Patel, Sharma, Kumar, & Binu, 2018). Another study compared two groups of men in relationships: one with fertility challenges and the other without. Findings indicated that the men who had male factor infertility had more negative relational, social, personal, sexual experiences than men without infertility challenges (Smith at al., 2009).

The manner in which a male copes with infertility impacts their psychological distress with being infertile. Psychologically speaking, coping describes the manner by which a person invests in efforts and behaviors to resolve both interpersonal and personal issues allowing them to manage and tolerate conflict and stress (Gopinath, 2019). The efficacy of coping is influenced by a variety of factors including the person and their respective circumstances, personality attributes, environment, and the type and degree of stress (Gopinath, 2019).

Psychological coping typically consists of positive coping strategies and maladaptive coping. Positive coping strategies alleviate psychological stress and promots positive psychological outcomes. Examples of positive coping resources include positive cognitive restructuring (changing one's perception of a stressful situation as to view the situation more positively); self-compassion (showing the same kindness and compassion to others who are suffering to one's self); social support (comfort, advice, and support from one's social and faith communities); and passive adaptive coping resources (i.e., listening to music, watching television, etc.; Allen & Leary, 2010). In contrast, maladaptive coping strategies exacerbate psychological stress while promoting negative or adverse psychological outcomes. Examples of maladaptive coping resources include negative displays of negative emotions (i.e., physically or verbally harming someone), denial, self-blame; substance abuse, and behavioral disengagement (Allen & Leary, 2010; Moore et al., 2011; Smith et al., 2016). This chapter provides a variety of coping recommendations for African American men, their partners, and collective community to consider regarding managing experiences of infertility.

15.9   Grief and the Grief Response

Loss describes the experience of having something taken away or losing something of importance and meaning. Historically, it is thought of as the death of a loved one. Loss, however, is not limited to a person; it may also be considered a response to the termination of a circumstance or experience. Many men who learn that they are unable to conceive experience this reality as a loss and may undergo a psychological and emotional response to the loss. This experience may be categorized into three constructs: grief, mourning, and bereavement.

The constructs of grief, bereavement, and mourning are all rooted in loss and impacted by one's culture, faith, and ideological belief (Casarett et al., 2001). Grief describes emotional and psychological processes (intrapsychic and internal) that one experiences in response to loss. Mourning describes the process of adapting to loss. "Bereavement" is a broad term that describes the period of time following a loss when both grief and mourning occur. Commonly, both grief and mourning overlap and exacerbate the other. Of the three terms, grief will be utilized in the operational conceptualization of loss that men experience with male factor infertility.

As there is variance and fluidity with regard to an individual's experience of grief, there are many models that exist to explain its mechanisms and processes. Although models such as Bowlby and Parkes' Four Phases of Grief Model, Worden's Four Basic Tasks in Adapting to Loss Model, and Kübler-Ross' Five Stages of Grief Model offer sound perspectives on dealing with grief, no singular model exists that takes all of the factors associated with loss into account. Kübler-Ross' Five Stages of Grief model is used in this chapter due to its credibility and applicability to other types of losses such as male factor infertility. Kübler-Ross' model consists of five stages often referred to by the acronym DABDA (denial, anger, bargaining, depression, and acceptance). It is important to note that the stages of Kübler-Ross' model do not always occur in sequential order and in fact, some stages may not occur altogether. Each stage of Kübler-Ross' model is impacted by sociodemographic variables and beliefs.

The first stage of the Kübler-Ross model is denial. Denial describes one's refusal to accept the reality of their loss (Tyrrell et al., 2020). The infertile male in this stage may believe that the diagnosis is incorrect or in error. The second stage is anger, which describes the state where an individual is unable to deny the loss and responds to self and others in frustration and/or anger (Tyrrell et al., 2020). Behaviors exhibited by infertile men in this phase may include statements and actions rooted in anger toward others or self. The third stage is bargaining, which describes personal attempts to negotiate, often with a higher power, in hopes of circumventing the reality of the loss (Tyrrell et al., 2020). An example of a behavioral response in this phase is an infertile man asking "God" for a change in their fertility diagnosis in exchange for a change in lifestyle.

The fourth stage is depression, which describes the despair and sadness associated with the inevitability of the loss (Tyrrell et al., 2020). Men in this stage display depressive symptoms including sadness, tearfulness, avoidance, and negative self-perception. The final stage is acceptance, where the person accepts the reality of their circumstances and as a result becomes overall more psychologically and emotionally stable and at peace (Tyrrell et al., 2020). Infertile men in this stage may begin to explore other options for family expansion including procreation via technologically assisted methods, adoption, and/or foster care.

To illustrate the applicability of the Stages of Grief model, take as an example the depression stage. Feelings of depression may not be related to the circumstances directly but rather the interpretations of what the circumstance means. If the infertile male defines the construct of his masculinity on the ability to biologically procreate, his identity may come under assault given the inability to conceive. Additionally, many men may not be able to readily identify feelings associated with any of the aforesaid stages let alone express them. For example, the infertile male may not say that he is sad or depressed but may cry, isolate, or lose interest in once enjoyable things in life.

15.10   Managing Relationships with Infertility Challenges

Couples dealing with infertility may experience challenges that impact the relationship. Building on the previous discussion of grief, the relationship as a whole may encounter the stages of grief within DABDA. In the denial stage, the couple may both be in denial, unable to accept their reality, and in some instances blame the other for the circumstances. During the anger stage, the couple may have communicated in anger to one another. In the bargaining stage, the couples may agree to negotiating hopeful outcomes with their spiritual beliefs and also with treating doctors in an effort to change the trajectory of their reality. During the depression stage the couple may jointly experience sadness and depressive symptoms. In the fifth and final stage, acceptance, the couple may begin to explore alternative options for allowing family expansion.

For some couples, the unit may experience an identity crisis in terms of competence, ability, and adequacy (Alamin et al., 2020). For many, procreating is a deeply rooted expectation and hope of the relationship unit. Not being able to conceive naturally may impact the prospect of parenting in the traditional sense and thus impact the building and meaning of the unit. Couples may also contend with cultural and societal expectations, stigmas, and stereotypes that impact the lens of how the couple may view themselves (Alamin et al., 2020). Unfortunately for many, an inability to conceive life with their partner may be interpreted as a failure in other domains including the relationship itself. As a result, the creation of an alternative identity may be quite challenging for some couples (Alamin et al., 2020).

The couple may also face challenges with the dynamics of sexual intimacy. Sexual intimacy within the relationship affects the couple's general sense of well-being and quality of life. Many studies show incidents of sexual dysfunction by men. This sexual dysfunction has been found to be the product of perceived loss of masculine identity, mechanical demands of sexual performance for the purpose of conception (i.e., scheduled postcoital tests), and psychological and emotional factors (Tao et al., 2011). As such, sexual intercourse within a given relationship may cause separation as opposed to connectedness and may contribute to negative self-esteem and confidence for the unit as a whole (Tao et al., 2011).

ART treatments also impact dynamics of the couple relationship. In a study by Moura-Ramos et al. (2016), findings revealed that both the number of ART cycles and duration of infertility affected men and women differently during their adjustment to infertility and the prospect of childlessness. Men receiving multiple ART treatments when confronted with the prospect of not being able to conceive resulted in reduced distress and increased acceptance (Moura-Ramos et al., 2016). Moura-Ramos et al. (2016) demonstrated that the opposite was true with females where each ART cycle was perceived as an experience of hope that decreased with each unsuccessful result.

Other considerations such as the cost, duration, cultural, spiritual, and personal beliefs about ART treatment may impact the well-being of the relationship. For example, lengthy ART treatment incurs greater financial costs and prolonged psychological distress. Crawford et al. (2016) indicated that in 2016, the approximate cost for a fresh ART cycle was $15,715 and the cost of a frozen cycle was $3,812.

Despite the challenges that exist for the infertile couple to conceive a child, there are alternative options to experiencing parenthood other than the aforementioned medical procedures. One option is gamete donation. This option allows one parent to have a genetic connection to the child given the circumstances of the infertility. For male factor infertility, the donor would provide sperm and in the case of the infertile woman, the donor would provide an egg. Further, an embryo donation is an option that involves adoption of a fertilized egg.

A second option for parenthood is surrogacy. With this option, an embryo is created from donor gametes and transferred into the uterus of a surrogate who will carry the child to term through traditional or gestational surrogacy. With traditional surrogacy, the egg is provided by the surrogate themselves and the surrogate is the biological mother. With gestational surrogacy, the egg is provided by the couple and thus preserves a biological connection with the person/couple who donates the egg.

A third option for parenthood is adoption. Adoption is the process by which the infertile individual/couple chooses a child to raise. There are two primary types of adoption: private domestic and fostering. Private domestic adoption is the process where the biological mother gives their child up for adoption and transfers legal authority of the child to the adoptive family. The child may/may not have relational ties to their biological family. The second is a foster care adoption, which entails inviting a child into the infertile couple's family from the foster care system. It is important to note that unlike private adoption, legal guardianship does not belong to the foster parents but to the government.

15.11 Recommendations for Support

It has been demonstrated that male factor infertility causes difficulties for both the individual and the couple as a whole. Despite gendered notions of masculinity that may serve as a barrier to treatment, men nonetheless desire an outlet for discussing challenges associated with their infertility (Miner et al., 2019). Unfortunately, many men perceive that there is less psychosocial support available to them including support from their partner (Agostini et al., 2011). Despite there being limited research about infertility and men, especially African American men, there are a number of recommendations available to both men and their relationship unit. One major source of support for males dealing with infertility is the medical support they receive.

Research shows that African American men both appreciate and value their significant others accompanying them to medical appointments (Mitchell et al., 2019). Having a companion present may reduce feelings of alienation and loneliness while simultaneously offering an opportunity to have another set of eyes and ears for information provided. Men who prefer to enter the medical appointment alone may appreciate and benefit from having their companion accompany them to and from the encounter but not participate in the session with the physician.

The essential best practices for rendering mental health treatment to men are comparable to those of any physical health medical care. Practices such as developing trust through a collaborative clinical partnership, mobilizing kinship and social networks (including, if applicable, input from trusted persons in their faith community), exploring and discussing available treatment options within a holistic framework, and increasing cognizance and awareness of gender and racial biases help to foster a more meaningful exchange between the male and the provider (Hankerson et al., 2015).

Education and open dialogue are two key steps to destigmatizing and demystifying male factor infertility, especially within the African American community. Encouraging open discussion can help to normalize the situation and provide opportunities to educate the male, his partner, family, and community. By doing so, the male is able to better integrate a healthy identity within the context of societal and cultural norms.

Support from a mental health professional is another resource that may offer benefit to men. Masoumi et al. (2019) demonstrated that Cognitive Behavioral Therapy (CBT) and mindfulness (i.e., yoga, mindfulness training) are efficacious support options for men and their partners who may be coping with male factor infertility. CBT may help men and couples examine and modify problematic perceptions and beliefs of infertility dynamics and the interplay of said perceptions and beliefs on the emotions and subsequent behaviors of the male. Incorporating mindfulness into the treatment plan allows the male and his partner to decrease emotional and psychosocial distress and arousal by focusing their attention on the reality and experiences of infertility in the present moment sans judgement. Additional psychotherapeutic support options including counseling (i.e., grief counseling), traditional psychotherapy, emotion-focused therapy, problem-focused therapy, and marital therapy (Masoumi et al., 2019; Patel, Sharma, & Kumar, 2018).

Spiritual support is another resource that men may consider when dealing with individual and collective impacts of infertility. Given the significance that one's faith and spirituality may have in their lives, a faith community for the African American male may provide opportunities for experiencing a degree of peace and acceptance with being infertile via interpersonal support from other parishioners and guidance from spiritual leaders.

Intentional communication strategies should be used to support African American men struggling with male factor infertility. Components of healthy communication must include empathy, alliance, active listening, respect, self-awareness, and patience. In contrast, negative communication that minimizes expressed thoughts and feelings, offers clichés and platitudes (i.e., "What is meant to be will be"), judgment, crude comments and jokes, and unrequested solutions (i.e., "just adopt or use science") should be avoided. Also, adapting one's language to fit the cultural and societal norms surrounding the male and their unique personality and preferences is also key in increasing the receptivity of communication and support from African American men (Courtenay, 2011). Arguably, these components are essential factors of most healthy communication strategies.

Findings from a study conducted by Schmidt et al. (2005) indicated that men preferred active-confronting coping to receive and deliver communication about their infertility. Active-confronting coping entails a number of methodologies including accepting sympathy and compassion from others, opportunities to express feelings, discussing with others emotional reactions to their being infertile, and seeking advice from others (Schmidt et al., 2005). It stands to reason that these coping approaches may also be used toward the male himself, for example, the male showing compassion and sympathy to himself and allowing himself the space and opportunity to release feelings about their being infertile. These strategies also serve as a medium for coping with the aforementioned stressors that African American men experience.

In conclusion, African American men suffer silently while experiencing male factor infertility. There are not many available resources to support infertile men. Male factor infertility and its effects on African American men remains silent and often not spoken of in the African American community. Feelings of inadequacy, shame, and hopelessness (among others) may often produce depression, anxiety, and angst as they compare themselves to community and societal norms (especially with regard to expectations of virility). This in turn impacts the operational definition of manhood as well as relational dynamics with their partner.

The discussed dynamics of the sexual health of African American men requires dialogue and attention. This chapter may serve as an opportunity for this to occur by bringing awareness to the often misunderstood or unspoken aspect of infertility that is male factor. It is hoped that this needed dialogue will serve as an impetus to change in terms of self-perspective within the relationship dynamic, within the larger African American community, societally, and within the medical landscape.

Discussion Questions

1. How do the intersections of gender and race impact perceptions of African American men and infertility?
2. What factors contribute to African American male infertility?
3. How might beliefs about masculinity impact the psychological and emotional well-being of African American men who experience infertility?
4. Discuss the importance of various support systems when working with this population.

REFERENCES

Agarwal, A., Mulgund, A., Hamada, A., & Chyatte, M. R. (2015). A unique view on male infertility around the globe. *Reproductive Biology and Endocrinology*, *13*, 37.

Agostini, F., Monti, F., De Pascalis, L., Paterlini, M., La Sala, G. B., & Blickstein, I. (2011). Psychosocial support for infertile couples during assisted reproductive technology treatment. *Fertility and Sterility*, *95*(2), 707–710.

Alamin, S., Allahyari, T., Ghorbani, B., Sadeghitabar, A., & Karami, M. T. (2020). Failure in identity building as the main challenge of infertility: A qualitative study. *Journal of Reproduction & Infertility*, *21*(1), 49–58.

Allen, A. B., & Leary, M. R. (2010). Self-compassion, stress, and coping. *Social and Personality Psychology Compass*, *4*(2), 107–118.

Alozai, U. u., & Sharma, S. (2020). Drug and alcohol use. [Updated 2022, June 21]. In *StatPearls* [Internet]. StatPearls Publishing. Retrieved October 24, 2022, from https://www.ncbi.nlm.nih.gov/books/NBK513263/

Barak, S., & Baker, H. W. G. (2000). Clinical management of male infertility. [Updated 2016, February 5]. In K. R. Feingold, B. Anawalt, A. Boyce, G. Chrousos, W. W. de Herder, K. Dhatariya, K. Dungan, J. M. Hershman, J. Hofland, S. Kalra, G. Kaltsas, C. Koch, P. Kopp, M. Korbonits, C. S. Kovacs, W. Kuohung, B. Laferrère, M. Levy, E. A. McGee, ... D. P. Wilson (Eds.), *Endotext* [Internet]. MDText.com, Inc.

Barratt, C., Björndahl, L., De Jonge, C. J., Lamb, D. J., Osorio Martini, F., McLachlan, R., Oates, R. D., van der Poel, S., St John, B., Sigman, M., Sokol, R., & Tournaye, H. (2017). The diagnosis of male infertility: an analysis of the evidence to support the development of global WHO guidance-challenges and future research opportunities. *Human Reproduction Update*, *23*(6), 660–680.

Borrell-Carrió, F., Suchman, A. L., & Epstein, R. M. (2004). The biopsychosocial model 25 years later: principles, practice, and scientific inquiry. *Annals of Family Medicine*, *2*(6), 576–582.

Bruce, M. A., Griffith, D. M., & Thorpe, R. J., Jr. (2015). Social determinants of men's health disparities. *Family & Community Health*, *38*(4), 281–283.

Casarett, D., Kutner, J. S., Abrahm, J., & End-of-Life Care Consensus Panel. (2001). Life after death: A practical approach to grief and bereavement. *Annals of Internal Medicine*, *134*(3), 208–215.

Courtenay, W. (2011). *Dying to be men: Psychosocial, environmental, and biobehavioral directions in promoting the health of men and boys*. Routledge.

Crawford, S., Boulet, S. L., Mneimneh, A. S., Perkins, K. M., Jamieson, D. J., Zhang, Y., & Kissin, D. M. (2016). Costs of achieving live birth from assisted reproductive technology: A comparison of sequential single and double embryo transfer approaches. *Fertility and Sterility*, *105*(2), 444–450.

Daumler, D., Chan, P., Lo, K. C., Takefman, J., & Zelkowitz, P. (2016). Men's knowledge of their own fertility: A population-based survey examining the awareness of factors that are associated with male infertility. *Human Reproduction*, *31*(12), 2781–2790. https://doi.org/10.1093/humrep/dew265

Dieke, A. C., Zhang, Y., Kissin, D. M., Barfield, W. D., & Boulet, S. L. (2017). Disparities in assisted reproductive technology utilization by race and ethnicity, United States, 2014: A commentary. *Journal of Women's Health*, *26*(6), 605–608.

Durairajanayagam, D. (2018). Lifestyle causes of male infertility. *Arab Journal of Urology*, *16*(1), 10–20.

Esteves, S. C., Miyaoka, R., & Agarwal, A. (2011). Surgical treatment of male infertility in the era of intracytoplasmic sperm injection – new insights. *Clinics (Sao Paulo, Brazil)*, *66*(8), 1463–1478.

Fainberg, J., & Kashanian, J. A. (2019). Recent advances in understanding and managing male infertility. *F1000Research*, *8*, F1000 Faculty Rev-670.

Fisher, J. R., & Hammarberg, K. (2012). Psychological and social aspects of infertility in men: An overview of the evidence and implications for psychologically informed clinical care and future research. *Asian Journal of Andrology*, *14*(1), 121–129.

Friedman, S. K., & Dull, R. B. (2012). Male infertility: An overview of the causes and treatments. *US Pharmacist*, *37*(6), 39–42.

Gilbert, K. L., Ray, R., Siddiqi, A., Shetty, S., Baker, E. A., Elder, K., & Griffith, D. M. (2016). Visible and invisible trends in Black men's health: Pitfalls and promises for addressing racial, ethnic, and gender inequities in health. *Annual Review of Public Health*, *37*, 295–311.

Gopinath, A. V. (2019). Perceived control, coping and subjective wellbeing among infertile men and women. *Liberal Studies: A Bi-Annual Journal of School of Liberal Studies, Pandit Deendayal Petroleum University*, *4*(1), 45–60.

Griffin J. B., Jr. (1990). Substance abuse. In H. K. Walker, W. D. Hall, & J. W. Hurst (Eds.), *Clinical methods: The history, physical, and laboratory examinations* (3rd ed., Chapter 206). Butterworths. https://www.ncbi.nlm.nih.gov/books/NBK319/

Griffith, D. M., Brinkley-Rubinstein, L., Bruce, M. A., Thorpe, R. J., Jr., & Metzl, J. M. (2015). The interdependence of African American men's definitions of manhood and health. *Family & Community Health, 38*(4), 284–296.

Griffith, D. M., Gunter, K., & Allen, J. O. (2011). Male gender role strain as a barrier to African American men's physical activity. *Health Education & Behavior, 38*(5), 482–491.

Hankerson, S. H., Suite, D., & Bailey, R. K. (2015). Treatment disparities among African American men with depression: implications for clinical practice. *Journal of Health Care for the Poor and Underserved, 26*(1), 21–34.

Kissin, D. M., Boulet, S. L., Jamieson, D. J., & Assisted Reproductive Technology Surveillance and Research Team. (2016). Fertility treatments in the United States: Improving access and outcomes. *Obstetrics and Gynecology, 128*(2), 387–390.

Kumar, N., & Singh, A. K. (2015). Trends of male factor infertility, an important cause of infertility: A review of literature. *Journal of Human Reproductive Sciences, 8*(4), 191–196.

Masoumi, S. Z., Parsa, P., Kalhori, F., Mohagheghi, H., & Mohammadi, Y. (2019). What psychiatric interventions are used for anxiety disorders in infertile couples? A systematic review study. *Iranian Journal of Psychiatry, 14*(2), 160–170.

Miner, S. A., Daumler, D., Chan, P., Gupta, A., Lo, K., & Zelkowitz, P. (2019). Masculinity, mental health, and desire for social support among male cancer and infertility patients. *American Journal of Men's Health, 13*(1). https://doi.org/10.1177/1557988318820396

Mitchell, J., Williams, E. G., Perry, R., & Lobo, K. (2019). "You have to be part of the process": A qualitative analysis of older African American men's primary care communication and participation. *American Journal of Men's Health, 13*(4), 1557988319861569.

Moore, B. C., Biegel, D. E., & McMahon, T. J. (2011). Maladaptive coping as a mediator of family stress. *Journal of Social Work Practice in the Addictions, 11*(1), 17–39.

Moura-Ramos, M., Gameiro, S., Canavarro, M. C., Soares, I., & Almeida-Santos, T. (2016). Does infertility history affect the emotional adjustment of couples undergoing assisted reproduction? The mediating role of the importance of parenthood. *British Journal of Health Psychology, 21*(2), 302–317.

Naz, M., & Kamal, M. (2017). Classification, causes, diagnosis and treatment of male infertility: a review. *Oriental Pharmacy and Experimental Medicine, 17*, 89–109.

Ornelas, I. J., Amell, J., Tran, A. N., Royster, M., Armstrong-Brown, J., & Eng, E. (2009). Understanding African American men's perceptions of racism, male gender socialization, and social capital through photovoice. *Qualitative Health Research, 19*(4), 552–565.

Pacek, L. R., Malcolm, R. J., & Martins, S. S. (2012). Race/ethnicity differences between alcohol, marijuana, and co-occurring alcohol and marijuana use disorders and their association with public health and social problems using a national sample. *American Journal on Addictions, 21*(5), 435–444.

Patel, A., Sharma, P., & Kumar, P. (2018). Role of mental health practitioner in infertility clinics: A review on past, present and future directions. *Journal of Human Reproductive Sciences, 11*(3), 219–228.

Patel, A., Sharma, P., Kumar, P., & Binu, V. S. (2018). Illness cognitions, anxiety, and depression in men and women undergoing fertility treatments: A dyadic approach. *Journal of Human Reproductive Sciences, 11*(2), 180–189.

Sansone, A., Di Dato, C., de Angelis, C., Menafra, D., Pozza, C., Pivonello, R., Isidori, A., & Gianfrilli, D. (2018). Smoke, alcohol and drug addiction and male fertility. *Reproductive Biology and Endocrinology, 16*(1), 3.

Schmidt, L., Holstein, B. E., Christensen, U., & Boivin, J. (2005). Communication and coping as predictors of fertility problem stress: Cohort study of 816 participants who did not achieve a delivery after 12 months of fertility treatment, *Human Reproduction, 20*(11), 3248–3256.

Smith, J. F., Walsh, T. J., Shindel, A. W., Turek, P. J., Wing, H., Pasch, L., Katz, P. P., & Infertility Outcomes Program Project Group. (2009). Sexual, marital, and social impact of a man's perceived infertility diagnosis. *Journal of Sexual Medicine, 6*(9), 2505–2515.

Smith, M. M., Saklofske, D. H., Keefer, K. V., & Tremblay, P. F. (2016). Coping strategies and psychological outcomes: The moderating effects of personal resiliency. *Journal of Psychology, 150*(3), 318–332.

Tao, P., Coates, R., & Maycock, B. (2011). The impact of infertility on sexuality: A literature review. *Australasian Medical Journal, 4*(11), 620–627.

Tyrrell, P., Harberger, S., Schoo, C., & Siddiqui, W. (2020). Kubler-Ross stages of dying and subsequent models of grief. [Updated 2022, July 20]. In *StatPearls* [Internet]. StatPearls Publishing. Retrieved October 24, 2022, from https://www.ncbi.nlm.nih.gov/books/NBK507885/

CHAPTER 16

Couples Therapy with Black American Couples Facing Medical Illness: Considerations for Treatment

Lekeisha A. Sumner

Enduring romantic partner relationships, particularly marital relationships, face many shifts and stressors throughout the course of the relationship. Yet, few challenges are as demanding and potentially turbulent to a couple's relationship as when a partner experiences a substantial change in health status or medical illness. Medical illness is a shared experience that affects both patients and partners individually and collectively. Moreover, substantial changes in health status unfold in dynamic, contextual systems, underscoring the need for a consideration of a broader treatment approach (Berg & Upchurch, 2007). Amid recognition of the increasing role of familial caregivers in patient care and public health discussions, considering the couple's needs in the provision of health care, especially mental health care, is necessary to optimize treatment outcomes and quality of life of patients.

Expanding health care beyond the individual to the couple dyad is particularly relevant for Black American couples who, despite having considerable heterogeneity and cultural strengths, are differentially influenced by unique historic and current sociocultural, economic and environmental health determinants that contribute to mental, relational, behavioral and physical health functioning, the provision and access of high-quality health care, and health outcomes.

To date, the majority of clinical focus on medical populations have centered on conceptualizing and treating patients individually but a compelling body of literature has emerged that demonstrate the profound impact of relationship quality and functioning of couples on health and illness (Farrell & Simpson, 2017; Kiecolt-Glaser & Newton, 2001; Robles et al., 2014). Despite these findings, the majority of research examining the influence of couples functioning, relationship quality, and associated consequences for health, coping, and adjustment when dealing with medical illness have not centered on Black American couples nor applied theoretical frameworks relevant to Black Americans. Yet, the application of existing data is likely to have utility for the treatment of Black American couples dealing with medical illness *if* applied within culturally relevant conceptual frameworks along with the basic principles of couples therapy. In other words, treatment interventions for Black American couples must consider the sociocultural landscape in which they function.

The intergenerational effects of sustained anti-Black discriminatory government policies – at local, state, and federal levels – that have engendered violence, exploitation, marginalization, and exclusion across numerous domains (e.g., social, economic, medical, psychological) of Black Americans spans the history of the United States. Such race-based policies have cemented ongoing structural social and economic barriers that persist. Today systematic inequities that target Black Americans (e.g., redlining, employment discrimination and exposure to unemployment, predatory banking, racism in health care, residential segregation, mass incarceration, unequal resources in education, disproportionate exposure to environmental pollutants, and restrictive covenants) exert social-psychological effects that cripple opportunities across the lifespan and contribute to familial dynamics and emotional and physical health functioning (American Psychological Association, 2017; Williams & Collins, 2001; Williams et al., 2019). Mental health professionals providing treatment interventions for Black American couples facing medical illness are uniquely suited to aid their patients in adjustment, alleviate emotional suffering, and bolster relational functioning, particularly when utilizing conceptual frameworks and tailored treatment interventions that consider the strong reciprocal associations among macro-level and micro-level determinants of health and functioning within historic and current social structures.

The primary objectives of the current chapter are to (a) familiarize clinicians with the sociohistorical experiences and current social positioning of Black Americans in the United States that shape experiences and health, (b) provide a brief overview of research findings on couples and health, (c) describe theoretical and empirical findings on Black American couples, and (d) offer clinical strategies and considerations to guide psychotherapists working with Black American couples facing chronic illness. Notably, this chapter is not intended to be an exhaustive study but a primer for mental health professionals treating Black American heterosexual couples facing medical illness. Black American immigrants, same-gender loving couples and members of the lesbian, gay, bisexual, trans, queer, intersex community also possess unique yet shared experiences in terms of their unique strengths, social positioning, and health experiences in the United States and warrant specialized consideration in the approach and provision of couples therapy. Given that other chapters in this book center these populations, the current chapter focuses on Black American heterosexual couples facing a health concern or medical illnesses.

16.1   Sociohistorical Context and Health

Social and economic conditions contribute to health risks that render Black Americans vulnerable to a range of medical illnesses and poorer health outcomes relative to their counterparts from other racial backgrounds and receive inequitable treatments in health care (Centers for Disease Control and Prevention, 2021). For example, relative to white women, Black women are two to three times more likely to die from pregnancy related complications, even among Black women with high levels of education (Petersen et al., 2019). In the health care system, Black Americans are often provided with substantially less pain relief – and in a fair number of cases no pain medications at all – due to stereotypes about the likelihood of illicit prescription misuse and abuse and providers are more likely to offer lifesaving procedures to their white counterparts (Meghani et al., 2012; Singhal et al., 2016). When considering common beliefs about Black American health and treatment of Black Americans by the medical establishment in the nineteenth century, one finds striking parallels between the past and present that further underscore the need to consider historic contexts in formulating case conceptualization and treatments.

Racial residential segregation – a primary cause of racial disparities in health and a determinant in access to educational and employment opportunities associated with adverse social and environmental conditions – remains high for most Black Americans, demonstrating one type of pervasive and enduring institutional racism (Williams & Collins, 2001). It should be of little surprise then, that African American households hold only ten cents in wealth for each one dollar held by white households resulting in white families of low and middle income having four times as much wealth as their African American counterparts (Kochhar & Cilluffo, 2017). In sum, residential segregation and vast disparities in wealth render African Americans at heightened risks for chronic strain and health risks that extend to familial strain.

For populations such as African Americans who experience an usually high level of chronic stressors across multiple domains throughout the lifespan along with racism at institutional and interpersonal levels, the need to harness the strengths of one's partner may be especially important in coping with and adjusting to the illness. As previously discussed, social context is imperative in considering the health and treatment of African Americans as these factors contribute not only to access to resources but the significantly high levels of chronic strain including family stress and subsequent impact on health behaviors, immune system responses, and cellular aging (American Psychological Association, 2012; Chae et al., 2020). For example, the higher prevalence of hypertension among African Americans is not attributable to genetics but rather societal and environmental conditions (Cooper et al., 2005). As it relates to mental health, African Americans are more likely to be misdiagnosed at higher rates with more severe psychiatric diagnosis, such as schizophrenia, than whites, and less likely to be successful in accessing specialty mental health care (Schwartz & Feisthamel, 2009).

16.2 Couples and Health

Couples' relationships influence health in both positive and negative ways for both partners (Shrout, 2021). There is now ample evidence that close intimate relationships influence health through both direct and indirect pathways such as lifestyle behaviors, mental health, and physiological mechanisms and that these relationships influence both health process and outcomes (Kiecolt-Glaser & Newton, 2001). Positive relationship functioning (e.g., intimacy, responsiveness, support) confers a protective effect on the stress process and overall health, whereas negative functioning (e.g., frequent hostility, conflict, attachment insecurity) elicits a more profound stress response and is associated with worsened health over time (Farrell & Simpson, 2017). The chronic strain of distressed relationships elevates risk for medical and psychiatric conditions (Kiecolt-Glaser & Wilson, 2017). Moreover, several relational factors such as marital cohesion, marital functioning, and couples characteristics not only affect health, coping, and adjustment of patients with medical illness but also contributes to well-being and distress of the partner (Martire et al., 2010). Available data show promise for the utility of couple-based interventions among medical populations and suggest better outcomes on multiple domains than patient-only interventions (Berry et al., 2017).

Psychological treatment with African American couples requires an approach that is culturally sensitive, system oriented and strength based (Kelly & Boyd-Franklin, 2009). Understanding the dynamic and contextual factors that contribute to risks, onset, maintenance, and outcomes is also useful. Tailoring couples intervention for medical illness can be guided by conceptual and theoretical frameworks that address these multifaceted cultural, psychosocial, and biological problems. As Pinderhughes (2002) argues, differences in African American couples are magnified by contextual dynamics, which must be considered but if too much focus is given, could reinforce maladaptive ways of coping. In the next paragraphs, two appealing models are reviewed for use as a conceptual tool in guiding practice and organizing approach that offers a map for appreciating unique dynamics without reinforcing potentially harmful schemas and ways of coping.

The biopsychosocial model as credited to cardiologist George Engel (1977) is a useful approach in conceptualizing both disease and illness with appreciation of the complex interactions of biological, psychological, and social factors. In this model, psychological factors, such as stress and affective distress, may impact when a patient reports symptoms, adherence to treatment, and response to treatment. Notably, many scholars have advanced this model to consider the role of both *illness*, which refers to more subjective experiences of the patient's presentation and functioning such as how they, their family, and immediate social networks adjust, respond to symptoms of disability, and *disease*, which focuses heavily on the objective biological events that interfered with specific bodily systems and structures (Gatchel et al., 2007). This biopsychosocial framework, rooted in systems theory, allows for consideration of the role of multiple dimensions of a person's life to be considered in coping and adjustment, including cultural factors in the construction of individual and family subjective understanding and response to medical illness. As it is rooted in systemic theory, similar to the practice of family and couples therapy, it recognizes the reciprocal interactions and associations of individual, interpersonal, and micro systemic factors over a period of time.

Clark and colleagues (1999) advanced the biopsychosocial model to consider the psychological, social, and physiological effects of racism among African Americans. The underlying principle in their model is that environmental stimuli perceived as racist result in pronounced psychological and physiological stress responses that are shaped by sociodemographic, psychological, and behavioral factors; coping responses; and other constitutional factors (Clark et al., 1999). The authors assert that several factors, such as social class and skin tone, contribute to an individual's perceptions of an event as racist and that coping strategies used in the face of racist events have the potential to compound the distress (Clark et al., 1999). This may occur through several pathways. For example, poor eating habits or tobacco consumption to soothe distress may not only perpetuate negative societal stigma but have a negative physiological response. Moreover, race-related stress is associated with psychological distress, cardiovascular activity, immune and neuroendocrine responses, and other physiologic indices of stress response over time (Chae et al., 2020; Geronimus et al., 2006; Williams et al., 2019).

But how does all of this talk about racism relate to developing psychological interventions for African American couples facing medical illness? The impact of anti-Black racism and racism-related stressors extends to couples functioning as it negatively impacts communication (Kelly & Floyd, 2006), drives conflict in the dyad and perceptions about one's partner, and drains ability to effectively cope with existing stressors (Awosan, 2014; Hardy & Awosan, 2019). Thus, therapists should recognize that racism is experienced by most Black Americans either directly or indirectly and this unique chronic and traumatic stressor steeped in sociocultural trauma is often present, even if unspoken and not the primary objective of treatment. Accordingly, in a context in which partners may have already endured chronic strain, the presence of a medical condition may present both as a compounding stressor for the couple and a threat to emotional bonds. Yet, with the aid of psychological intervention, the medical illness may also present an opportunity for deep relational healing and restoration for the couple and promote adaptive coping with illness, improved medical management, and relationship functioning.

The Ecological Systems Theory developed by developmental psychologist Urie Bronfenbrenner (1977) is another framework that offers utility in tailoring couples interventions with Black American couples facing medical illness. Originated with the goal of offering a theoretical perspective to foster understanding of human development in one's environment, the theory has undergone significant revisions since initial development and is now applied in many fields, including health and psychology. In brief, this multidimensional, comprehensive ecological perspective considers the role of environmental and developmental factors and meaning of contexts on individuals both simultaneously and over time within four systemic levels of risk: (a) the ontogenetic system that includes personal factors such as histories of trauma and psychological distress; (b) the microsystem, which emphasizes interrelations and relational contexts, such as relationship dynamics and those between an individual and their immediate environment such as work and home (Bronfenbrenner, 1977; El-Bassel et al., 2009); (c) the exosystem, which centers interrelations between major environmental settings that impact individual settings and high-risk health

354 LEKEISHA A. SUMNER

behaviors, such as poverty, neighborhood, and access to preventive health care; and (d) macrosystems, which includes laws, cultural values, and beliefs systems that influence all other systems. As the theory was revised and advanced to better understand developmental outcomes, the interactions of biological, psychological, and environmental factors were considered (Bronfenbrenner & Ceci, 1994). Accordingly, it has been used with African American populations, including couples, at heightened risk for medical illness (El-Bassel et al., 2009).

African American couples dealing with medical conditions may not be consciously aware of or concerned with the influence of systems or sociohistorical factors in treatment as their most immediate and pressing threat is medical illness, management of care, adjusting to functional impairments, and role changes. Nonetheless, consideration of these factors will assist the therapist in understanding the processes that maintain and exacerbate symptoms of distress in the relationship along with difficulties with adjustment and coping with the demands of the relationship and management of their medical condition.

16.3   Couple-Based Psychological Treatment Interventions and Medical Conditions

As scholars note, couple-based interventions for medical conditions differs from traditional couple therapy and despite a growth in research on the integral role of intimate relationships and health, studies on the effectiveness of interventions for couples facing medical illnesses continue to grow (Baucom et al., 2012). As Baucom et al. (2012), point out, the focus and primary objectives in couple-based interventions for medical problems are not to alleviate relationship distress and enhance relational functioning but rather assist the patient facing the health or medical condition while also recognizing the importance of being attuned to the well-being of the other partner along with the dyad relationship, as the presence of the medical or health concern affects the partner's well-being. Further, the therapist recognizes that the partner's well-being and relationship functioning foster the patient's adjustment to the medical condition, changes in behavioral health, and the patient's view of their bodies and beliefs about their ability to manage and effectively cope. Incorporating a partner appears to bolster a patient's ability to reduce health risk behavior through many pathways, including communication.

Couple-based therapy still requires use of the common principles and processes as nonmedically focused couples therapy. It is important that therapists attempting to work with African American couples with medical illnesses should possess fundamental competencies for couples, along with knowledge of the medical illness. For example, essential in treatment is an in-depth assessment of the couple's relationship in general, communication, and mutual partner support that is usually gathered across sessions for couples facing illness. We now briefly review a couples-based intervention therapy that may be tailored to working with African American couples facing medical illness.

Emotionally focused couples therapy (EFT), developed by Greenberg and Johnson (1988), is a time-limited intervention based on attachment theory. EFT asserts that relationship distress stems from partners maladaptive responses to emotional threats that trigger reactivity in the other partner (Johnson & Greenberg, 1985). An empirically validated approach, in EFT relational patterns are both dynamic and reciprocal and posits that triggered couples are both limited in emotional flexibility and become engaged in negative reactive patterns that reinforce continuing misunderstanding and disconnection (Johnson & Greenman, 2006). As such, the EFT therapist works with the couple to help them understand their problems as difficulties in processing emotional experiences and the individual emotions and motivations that contribute to interactions. Accordingly, they also foster the couple's appreciation for attachments, interdependence, and their ability to reframe their problems as emotional needs. Attention is given to negative interactions and the reprocessing of such experiences in developing more positive interactions in the relational cycle through honest and authentic communication, which strengthens each partner's feelings of a secure base in the relationship.

In EFT, attachment injuries can impede the creation of new and positive interactions between couples as they erode trust. Because what constitutes an attachment injury may vary from couple to couple and their interpretation; treatment seeks to address such injuries. For couples facing medical illness, especially terminal illness, the presence of illness may be a threat to the attachment bonds (McLean & Nissim, 2007). While a review of attachment theory and adults is beyond the scope of this chapter, interested readers are encouraged to read the work of Shaver and Hazan (1987) who discuss attachment theory in romantic relationships. Of note, EFT is composed of nine steps in three stages (Johnson et al., 2005). Stage I (cycle deescalation), focuses on the therapist establishing alliance with the couple through empathic attunement and observing patterns of responses and expressions and identifying negative cycles. In Stage 2 (structuring new interactions) the therapist expands upon unmet attachment needs and seeks to increase accessibility and responsiveness in the couple dyad. Stage 3 (consolidation) encourages the couple to integrate newly developed ways of engaging and problem solving. EFT works best for couples in which there is an emotionally safe base to work from. For couples who lack such a secure base for both individuals to feel vulnerable and safe, this intervention would not be appropriate.

Integrative approaches are likely the most commonly used by therapists working with couples with medical illness. In this approach, therapists may utilize more than one psychotherapeutic technique, such as those found in behavioral and systems couples therapy.

16.4   Practical Clinical Considerations

The intervention the therapist chooses to use with Black American couples facing medical conditions may vary, based on the nature of the illness, duration, caregiving demands, and couple's needs. Yet despite the intervention used, therapists are encouraged to include a component of psychoeducation in treatment, take a collaborative role with the couple, and be willing to consult with other health care providers (Shields et al., 2012). Psychoeducation has the benefit of facilitating adjustment, emotional processing of the couple, and preparation for anticipated changes in lifestyle and relational dynamics and empowering them in medical decision making (Baucom et al., 2012). The psychoeducation component should focus on the medical condition, illness trajectory, symptoms, treatment, and prognosis and offer the couple the opportunity to externalize the threats brought forth by the condition instead of blaming one another or internalizing responsibility for illness onset. Therapists who are willing to consult with health care providers are likely to be better positioned to answer questions, facilitate the couple's understanding of individual health prognosis, and promote health-related communication skills with their providers.

Given the magnitude of uncertainty couples often face when dealing with medical conditions, anticipating changes in roles, responsibilities, and expectations may help alleviate anxiety. The therapist is tasked with assisting couples in understanding the medical problem and its psychological and physical consequences and the fears it evokes. For instance, patients affected by many medical conditions often report disabling fatigue, diminished sexual functioning, sleep disruptions, and changes in bodily appearances all of which creates fear and anxiety about engaging in activities that impact the couple dyad. An understanding of the medical condition and how it may necessitate changes in role and relational dynamics helps the couple navigate these changes and facilitate adaptation.

While the couple may have started treatment for a health or medical concern and much of treatment does center on illness, the psychotherapist is tasked with striking a delicate balance of addressing and attending to the role of illness while simultaneously helping the couple maintain at least a modicum of normalcy in their relationship that does not center on illness. According to Rolland (1994), onset, disease course, outcome, and level of functional impairments impact the degree to which illness affects the couple. Whether the course of illness tends to fluctuate or relapse, chronic or terminal illness dictates the flexibility needed for partners to adapt to changes in role demands, stress on the caregiving system, and uncertainty experienced. As such, the therapist continually considers how couples communicate their concerns and fears, their responsiveness to each other's needs, and how to help them best adjust to the condition while understanding how the condition affects the relationship.

Specific to treating Black American couples in any capacity, there are also fundamental questions for the therapist to consider: What images and assumptions does one hold when considering Black love, bodily agency of Black Americans, and attributions of their illness and presentation? Psychotherapists must interrogate what they believe they know about Black Americans and the lens through which they view them before the provision of any psychological assessment and intervention to Black couples facing chronic illness. The psychotherapist also recognizes that despite unique challenges, African American couples possess numerous strengths that have positive associations on health and can be harnessed in couples therapy to bolster relationship quality. Noting that the mental health field has historically viewed African Americans through a deficit model, Boyd-Franklin (2003), has highlighted the flaws and harms perpetuated by antiquated frameworks and identified five major strengths inherent among Black American families that can be integrated in couples interventions: (a) the bond of extended family, (b) adaptability of familial roles, (c) religious orientation, (d) strong beliefs and values on work ethic and education, and (e) the ability to develop and utilize effective coping when dealing with economic hardships. Another strength centers on familial support, which extends beyond the nuclear family to extended family members and close relational ties formed in communities (Boyd-Franklin, 2003). African Americans often value egalitarian role sharing, which may reduce couples' conflicts about challenges posed by decreases in physical functioning. As such, therapists are encouraged to welcome Black American couples with a respectful curiosity, explore strengths and resources beyond the couple dyad, and work from an assumption that love – not pathology – brought them to psychological treatment.

In forming therapeutic alliance and navigating treatment, the psychotherapist considers how societal and cultural constructs shape patient presentation. For example, cultural and societal norms dictate how people express pain – both psychic and physical – acceptable forms of coping and when to seek help. Similarly, as Nightingale et al. (2019) observe, societal assaults on Black womanhood and manhood may influence how Black American couples express themselves in therapy. For example, some may appear to be emotionally withdrawn not because they are not emotionally invested in their relationship or treatment but rather as an attempt to navigate a world that has rendered them largely invisible or threatening. Moreover, many Black Americans have learned that there can be a high price to pay for non-Blacks feeling uncomfortable by their expression of views and emotions and are acutely aware that they live in a society that places them under high levels of scrutiny and surveillance in which even benign verbal and physical expressions can lead severe reprisals, such as people calling the police for the slightest discomfort and attempt to exert their agency over them. In creating a framework specifically for Black men, Franklin and Boyd-Franklin (2000) discuss the concept of the invisibility syndrome whereby one develops a psychological sense of invisibility from repeated racial slights and devaluating messages from society about one's worth which includes a "conceptual model for understanding the intrapsychic processes and outcomes in managing the personal stress arising from racial slights and the subjective experience of invisibility among African Americans" (p. 33). Accordingly, therapists should be aware that African American behavior may be shaped by the contours of a broader society that seeks to project their pathology onto Black populations. Therapists who are highly reactive to emotionality among Black American couples or who seek to view them through a gaze of deficiency to confirm negative stereotypes will impede treatment and afflict harm. However, therapists who continually monitor and interrogate these factors and how they may loom in the shadows of treatment are better suited to provide a supportive and safe psychological environment. Moreover, the therapist is then better positioned to help the couple resolve conflicts in the presence of medical condition, identify and reinforce strengths that will serve to empower the couple, recenter and strengthen relational bonds, and help them regain a sense of control and adjust in the face of medical uncertainty. In sum, working with Black American couples facing medical illness offers mental health professionals a rich opportunity to facilitate adjustment to diagnosis, enhance patients' ability to manage illness and incorporate culturally sensitive relationship interventions to improve relational stability.

Discussion Questions

1. Why is it important to consider the role of both illness and disease when working with Black couples facing medical illnesses?
2. How do experiences of racist events impact illness and disease in Black couples?
3. How might a therapist educate clients about the impact of systemic racism on their health who are not consciously aware of the connection?
4. What are the benefits of using an ecological approach when working with Black couples experiencing chronic medical conditions?

REFERENCES

American Psychological Association. (2012). *Fact sheet: Health disparities and stress*. https://www.apa.org/topics/racism-bias-discrimination/health-disparities-stress
  (2017). *Mental health disparities: African Americans*. Psychiatry.org. https://www.psychiatry.org/File%20Library/Psychiatrists/Cultural-Competency/Mental-Health-Disparities/Mental-Health-Facts-for-African-Americans.pdf
Awosan, C. I. (2014). *Never married heterosexual Black male–female intimate romantic experiences: A phenomenological study* [Unpublished doctoral dissertation]. Drexel University.
Baucom, D., Porter, L., Kirby, J., & Hudepohl, J. (2012). Couple-based interventions for medical problems. *Behavior Therapy, 43*, 61–76.
Berg, C. A., & Upchurch, R. (2007). A developmental-contextual model of couples coping with chronic illness across the adult life span. *Psychological Bulletin Journal, 133*, 920–954.
Berry, E., Davies, M., & Dempster, M. (2017). Exploring the effectiveness of couples interventions for adults living with a chronic physical illness: A systematic review. *Patient Education and Counseling, 100*(7), 1287–1303.
Boyd-Franklin, N. (2003). *Black families in therapy: understanding the African American experience*. Guilford Press.
Bronfenbrenner, U. (1977). Toward an experimental ecology of human development. *American Psychologist, 32*(7), 513–531.
Bronfenbrenner, U., & Ceci, S. J. (1994). Nature–nuture reconceptualized in developmental perspective: A bioecological model. *Psychological Review, 101*(4), 568–586.

Centers for Disease Control and Prevention. (2017, July 3). *African American health*. https://www.cdc.gov/vitalsigns/aahealth/index.html

Chae, D. H., Wang, Y., Martz, C. D., Slopen, N., Yip, T., Adler, N. E., Fuller-Rowell, T. E., Lin J., Matthews, K. A., Brody, G. H., Spears, E. C., Puterman, E., & Epel, E. S. (2020). Racial discrimination and telomere shortening among African Americans: the coronary artery risk development in young adults (CARDIA) study. *Health Psychology, 39*(3), 209–219. https://doi.org/10.1037/hea0000832

Clark, R., Anderson, N. B., Clark, V. R., & Williams, D. R. (1999). Racism as a Stressor for African Americans: A Biopsychosocial Model. *American Psychologist, 54*, 805–816.

Cooper, R. S., Wolf-Maier, K., Luke, A., Adeyemo, A., Banegas, J. R., Forrester, T., Giampaoli, S., Joffres, M., Kastarinen, M., Primatesta, P., Stegmayr, B., & Thamm, M. (2005). An international comparative study of blood pressure in populations of European vs. African descent. *BMC Medicine, 3*, 2. https://doi.org/10.1186/1741-7015-3-2

El-Bassel, N., Caldeira, N. A., Ruglass, L. M., & Gilbert, L. (2009). Addressing the unique needs of African American women in HIV prevention. *American Journal of Public Health, 99*(6), 996–1001.

Engel, G. L. (1977). The need for a new medical model: A challenge for biomedicine. *Science, 196*(4286), 129–136.

Farrell, A. K., & Simpson, J. A. (2017). Effects of relationship functioning on the biological experience of stress and physical health. *Current Opinion in Psychology, 13*, 49–53. https://doi.org/10.1016/j.copsyc.2016.04.014

Franklin, A. J., & Boyd-Franklin, N. (2000). Invisibility syndrome: A clinical model of the effects of racism on African-American males. *American Journal of Orthopsychiatry, 70*(1), 33–41. https://doi.org/10.1037/h0087691

Gatchel, R. J., Peng, Y. B., Peters, M. L., Fuchs, P. N., & Turk, D. C. (2007). The biopsychosocial approach to chronic pain: Scientific advances and future directions. *Psychological Bulletin, 133*(4), 581–624.

Geronimus, A. T., Hicken, M., Keene, D., Bound, J. (2006). "Weathering" and age patterns of allostatic load scores among blacks and whites in the United States. *American Journal of Public Health, 96*, 826–833.

Greenberg, L. S., & Johnson, S. M. (1988). *Emotionally focused therapy for couples*. Guilford Press.

Hardy, K. V., & Awosan, C. I. (2019). Therapy with heterosexual Black couples through a racial lens. In M. McGoldrick & K. V. Hardy (Eds.), *Re-visioning family therapy* (pp. 419–432). Guilford Press.

Johnson, S. M., Bradley, B., Furrow, J., Lee, A., Palmer, G., Tilley, D., & Woolley, S. (2005). *Becoming an emotionally focused couples therapist: The workbook*. Brunner/Routledge.

Johnson, S. M., & Greenberg, L. S. (1985). Emotionally focused couples therapy: An outcome study. *Journal of Marital and Family Therapy, 11*(3), 313–317.

Johnson, S. M., & Greenman, P. S. (2006). The path to a secure bond: Emotionally focused couple therapy. *Journal of Clinical Psychology*, *62*(5), 597–609.

Kelly, S., & Boyd-Franklin, N. (2009). Joining, understanding, and supporting Black couples in treatment. In M. Rastogi & V. Thomas (Eds.), *Multicultural couple therapy* (pp. 235–254). Sage.

Kelly, S., & Floyd, F. J. (2006). Impact of racial perspectives and contextual variables on marital trust and adjustment for African American couples. *Journal of Family Psychology*, *20*, 79–87. https://doi.org/10.1037/0893-3200.20.1.79

Kiecolt-Glaser, J. K., & Newton, T. L. (2001). Marriage and health: His and hers. *Psychological Bulletin*, *127*, 472–503.

Kiecolt-Glaser, J. K., & Wilson, S. J. (2017). Lovesick: How couples' relationships influence health. *Annual Review of Clinical Psychology*, *13*, 421–443. https://doi.org/10.1146/annurev-clinpsy-032816-045111

Kochhar, R., & Cilluffo, A. (2017, November 1). *How wealth inequality has changed in the U.S. since the Great Recession, by race, ethnicity and income.* Pew Research Center. https://www.pewresearch.org/fact-tank/2017/11/01/how-wealth-inequality-has-changed-in-the-u-s-since-the-great-recession-by-race-ethnicity-and-income/

Martire, L. M., Schulz, R., Helgeson, V. S., Small, B. J., & Saghafi, E. M. (2010). Review and meta-analysis of couple-oriented interventions for chronic illness. *Annals of Behavioral Medicine*, *40*(3), 325–342. https://doi.org/10.1007/s12160-010-9216-2

McLean, L. M., & Nissim, R. (2007). Marital therapy for couples facing advanced cancer: Case review. *Palliative & Supportive Care*, *5*(3), 303–313.

Meghani, S. H., Byun, E., & Gallagher, R. M. (2012). Time to take stock: a meta-analysis and systematic review of analgesic treatment disparities for pain in the United States. *Pain Medicine (Malden, Mass.)*, *13*(2), 150–174. https://doi.org/10.1111/j.1526-4637.2011.01310.x

Nightingale, M., Ibilola Awosan, C., & Stavrianopoulos, K. (2019). Emotionally focused therapy: A culturally sensitive approach for African American heterosexual couples, *Journal of Family Psychotherapy*, *30*(3), 221–244. https://doi.org/10.1080/08975353.2019.1666497

Petersen, E. E., Davis, N. L., Goodman, D., Cox, S., Syverson, C., Seed, K., Shapiro-Mendoza, C., Callaghan, W. M., & Barfield, W. (2019). Racial/ethnic disparities in pregnancy-related deaths – United States, 2007–2016. *MMWR Morbidity and Mortality Weekly Report*, *68*, 762–765. DOI: http://dx.doi.org/10.15585/mmwr.mm6835a3

Pinderhughes, E. B. (2002). African American marriage in the 20th century. *Family process*, *41*(2), 269–282.

Robles, T. F., Slatcher, R. B., Trombello, J. M., & McGinn, M. M. (2014). Marital quality and health: A meta-analytic review. *Psychological Bulletin*, *140*, 140–187. https://doi.org/10.1037/a0031859

Rolland, J. S. (1994). In sickness and in health: The impact of illness on couples' relationships. *Journal of Marital and Family Therapy, 20*(4), 327–347.

Schwartz, R. C., & Feisthamel, K. P. (2009). Disproportionate diagnosis of mental disorders among African American versus European American clients: Implications for counselling theory, research, and practice. *Journal of Counseling & Development, 87*(3), 295–301.

Shaver, P., & Hazan, C. (1987). Being lonely, falling in love. *Journal of Social Behavior and Personality, 2*(2), 105–124.

Shields, C. G., Finley, M.A., Chawla, N., & Meadors, W. P. (2012). Couple and family interventions in health problems. *Journal of Marital and Family Therapy, 38*(1), 265–280. https://doi.org/10.1111/j.1752-0606.2011.00269.x

Shrout, M. R. (2021). The health consequences of stress in couples: A review and new integrated Dyadic Biobehavioral Stress Model. *Brain, Behavior, & Immunity – Health, 16*, 100328.

Singhal, A., Tien, Y. Y., & Hsia, R. Y. (2016). Racial-ethnic disparities in opioid prescriptions at emergency department visits for conditions commonly associated with prescription drug abuse. *PloS ONE, 11*(8), e0159224. https://doi.org/10.1371/journal.pone.0159224

Williams, D. R., & Collins, C. (2001). Racial residential segregation: A fundamental cause of racial disparities in health. *Public Health Reports, 116*(5), 404–416. https://doi.org/10.1093/phr/116.5.404

Williams, D. R., Lawrence, J. A., Davis, B. A., & Vu, C. (2019). Understanding how discrimination can affect health. *Health Services Research, 54*(S2), 1374–1388. https://doi.org/10.1111/1475-6773.13222

Index

363

Milton Keynes UK
Ingram Content Group UK Ltd.
UKHW021454060823
426405UK00008B/134